Clinical Cases in Obstetrics, Gynaecology and Women's Health

3e

T0357949

We wish to thank all our students who provided helpful feedback and criticism of the first and second editions of this text.

Clinical Cases in Obstetrics, Gynaecology and Women's Health

3e

CAROLINE DE COSTA

The Cairns Institute, James Cook University, Cairns

STEPHEN ROBSON

Department of Obstetrics and Gynaecology, Australian National University Medical School, Canberra

BOON LIM

Department of Obstetrics and Gynaecology, Canberra Health Services and Australian National University Medical School, Canberra

KIARNA BROWN

Department of Obstetrics and Gynaecology, Royal Darwin Hospital, Darwin

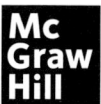

This third edition published 2022
First edition published 2007
Second edition published 2013

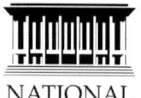

NATIONAL
LIBRARY OF AUSTRALIA

A catalogue record for this book is available from the National Library of Australia
Title: Clinical cases in obstetrics, gynaecology and women's health/ Caroline de Costa, Boon H Lim, Stephen Robson, Kiarna Brown
Edition: 3rd edition
ISBN: 9781743768174

Published in Australia by
McGraw Hill Education (Australia) Pty Ltd
Level 33, 680 George Street, Sydney NSW 2000
Publisher: Rochelle Deighton
Permissions Manager: Rachel Norton
Cover design: Christa Moffitt, christabella designs
Cover image: Pressmaster/Shutterstock
Typeset by MPS Limited
Printed in Singapore by Markono Print Media

Contents

Contents by subject matter

About the authors

Caroline de Costa was Professor of Obstetrics and Gynaecology at James Cook University, Cairns from 2004 to 2021. She is currently Adjunct Professor at The Cairns Institute, Cairns, Queensland.

Stephen Robson is Professor of Obstetrics and Gynaecology at the Australian National University Medical School, Canberra, ACT.

Boon Lim is Clinical Associate Professor at Australian National University Medical School, and Director and Senior Staff Specialist in Obstetrics and Gynaecology at Canberra Health Services, Canberra, ACT.

Kiarna Brown is a clinical Staff Specialist in Obstetrics and Gynaecology at Royal Darwin Hospital, Darwin, Northern Territory.

Introduction

The health of women is fundamental to the health of our communities, and so deserves a special place in medical school curricula. Despite this, there are moves in some postgraduate medical courses—in Australia and elsewhere—to reduce or even eliminate formal terms in obstetrics, gynaecology and women's health. We believe that all doctors should be confident and competent in providing high-quality healthcare and advice to the women they care for. For these reasons, we have developed the third edition of this book to address the core curriculum for medical courses in Australia, New Zealand and the United Kingdom. The book also has been tailored for doctors-in-training at the resident level as well as trainees in general practice and other women's-health-focused speciality streams. We have aimed to cover, in broad terms, the entire syllabus for medical students and the commonest and most important obstetric and gynaecological conditions likely to be encountered by busy junior hospital doctors, as well as those in general practice and primary care.

Since the last edition—published now over eight years ago—there have been a number of important advances in our knowledge of conditions, in management approaches and indeed in new technologies brought to bear in our care. As examples, next generation genetic sequencing has led to major advances not only in fetal screening and diagnosis, but also in pre-pregnancy carrier screening options for women and couples and cancer genetics. Indeed, new understanding of the genesis of ovarian cancer has led to a paradigm shift in risk reduction options for women at increased heritable risk. We have updated this edition to include all of these new medical options, and to put them into context for women in their own social situations. We are also delighted to welcome our new co-author, Dr Kiarna Brown, who brings a wealth of clinical experience from her home city of Darwin in northern Australia.

In this new edition we have striven to make the cases as inclusive as possible. We have actively worked to include issues relating to migrant and refugee women, and women who have English as a second language. We have included cases of Indigenous women to ensure there is an awareness of the extra complexities that can arise for certain population groups. We acknowledge the importance of doctors being culturally safe and we wish for healthcare workers to have some confidence in providing culturally respectful clinical care. We have sought to put women's healthcare in the context of the broad social determinants of health and to consider issues relating to transgender patients and to avoid heteronormative stereotypes where possible.

Our approach in this book is based on the problem-based learning (PBL) scenarios with which most recently graduated doctors will be familiar. PBLs introduce students to typical clinical situations and focus on the key elements of history-taking and on relevant examination approaches, then guide the reader through decision-making about the most useful investigations. Using these techniques, students are guided through treatment and management of common and important conditions and complications.

Our approach of questioning the reader as each of the cases progress will, hopefully, encourage exploration of management options based on the current evidence. In addition to the purely clinical aspects of each case, the emotional, social and psychological aspects of management of the individual woman— and her family—are examined. In each case, we list additional resources to further illuminate the principles and evidence underpinning management.

Each of the cases histories commences with a description of the clinical situation and follows the woman as the case progresses. Along the way important points in clinical examination and diagnosis, as well as complications, investigations and managements, are integrated into the text as a conversation with the reader. Essential points are highlighted in boxes, and 'clinical pearls' are attached in the hope that these points will stay with the reader in years to come.

In the chapters dealing with obstetrics and gynaecology we address the reader as a house or resident medical officer charged with direct care of the patient in a busy hospital setting. We also, at times, include tips for junior doctors facing women's health problems in the outer urban or rural setting, since facilities for care and the advice of senior practitioners may be more limited in those surroundings. Importantly, care pathways vary considerably across countries. In the section dealing with ambulant women's health issues, we address the reader as a general practitioner in an urban or non-urban setting, women's health clinic, or family planning service. Where conditions initially seen in general practice later are referred for care in more specialised services we continue to follow the patient through the journey.

In preparing this new edition we have had invaluable help and guidance from our colleagues including Professor Michael Peek of the Australian National University, and Dr Darren Russell, director of the Cairns Sexual Health Clinic, who kindly provided Case 25. We hope that you find the latest edition of this book a valuable and accessible resource in providing care to the women whose health underpins our communities.

Abbreviations

ACE	angiotensin-converting enzyme
AFI	amniotic fluid index
AMH	anti-Müllerian hormone
ANRQ	Antenatal Risk Questionnaire
APCR	activated protein C resistance
ARM	artificial rupture of membranes
β-hCG	beta human chorionic gonadotropin
bd	*bis die* (twice a day)
BMI	body mass index
BPD	biparietal diameter
bpm	beats per minute
BSL	blood sugar level
BV	bacterial vaginosis
CASA	cancer-associated serum antigen
CBAVD	congenital bilateral absence of the vas deferens
CDMR	caesarean delivery on maternal request
cfDNA	cell-free DNA
CGH	comparative genomic hybridisation
CGM	continuous glucose monitoring
CMV	cytomegalovirus
COCP	combined oral contraceptive pill
CRL	crown–rump length
CRP	C-reactive protein
CS	caesarean section
CST	cervical screening test
CT	computerised tomography
CTG	cardiotocograph
CVP	central venous pressure
D&C	dilatation and curettage
DASS	Depression Anxiety Stress Scale
DC	dichorionic
DCDA	dichorionic diamniotic
DM	diabetes mellitus

DMPA	depot medroxyprogesterone acetate
DNA	deoxyribonucleic acid
EC	emergency contraception
ECG	electrocardiogram
ECV	external cephalic version
ED	emergency department
EDC	expected date of confinement
EDD	expected date of delivery
EFT	estimated fetal weight
EMA	early medical abortion
eMR	electronic medical record
EPDS	Edinburgh Postnatal Depression Scale
ERCS	elective repeat caesarean section
EUA	examination under anaesthesia
FAST	focused assessment with sonography for trauma
FBC	full blood count
fFn	fetal fibronectin
FISH	fluorescence in-situ hybridisation
FNT	fetal nuchal translucency
FSH	follicle stimulating hormone
FTA-AbS	fluorescent treponemal antibodies
FVL	factor V (Leiden) gene mutation
FVS	fetal varicella syndrome
GA	general anaesthetic
GBS	group B streptococcus
GDM	gestational diabetes mellitus
GnRH	gonadotrophin releasing hormone
GP	general practitioner (family doctor)
GTD	gestational trophoblastic disease
GTT	glucose tolerance test
Hb	haemoglobin
HbA_{1c}	glycosylated haemoglobin
hCG	human chorionic gonadotropin
HCV	hepatitis C virus
HELLP	haemolysis, elevated liver enzymes, low platelets
HMB	heavy menstrual bleeding
HPV	human papillomavirus
HSG	hysterosalpingogram
HSIL	high-grade squamous intraepithelial lesion
HSV	herpes simplex virus
HT	hormone therapy

HZV	herpes zoster virus
IgA	immunoglobulin A
IgM	immunoglobulin M
IM	intramuscular
IMI	intramuscular injection
IQR	interquartile range
IU	international unit(s)
IUCD	intrauterine contraceptive device
IUGR	intrauterine growth restriction (or retardation)
IV	intravenous
IVF	in vitro fertilisation
LBC	liquid-based cytology
LDH	lactate dehydrogenase
LFT	liver function test
LH	luteinising hormone
LLETZ	large loop excision of the transformation zone
LMP	last menstrual period
LMWH	low-molecular-weight heparin
LNG	levonorgestrel
LNG-IUS	levonorgestrel-releasing intrauterine system
LSIL	low-grade squamous intraepithelial lesion
MCMA	monochorionic monoamniotic
MMR	measles, mumps and rubella
MRCS	maternal-request caesarean section
MRI	magnetic resonance image/imaging
MSU	midstream urine
MTHFR	methyltetrahydrofolate reductase
NAAT	nucleic acid amplification test
NCSP	National Cervical Screening Program
NHS	National Health Service
NIPT	non-invasive prenatal (diagnostic) test
NSAID	non-steroidal anti-inflammatory drug
OA	occipito-anterior
OGTT	oral glucose tolerance test
PAPP-A	pregnancy-associated plasma protein
PCOS	polycystic ovary syndrome
PCR	polymerase chain reaction
PCT	Primary Care Trust
PET/CT	positron emission tomography and computed tomography
pHSIL	possible high-grade squamous intraepithelial lesion

PI	pulsatility index
PID	pelvic inflammatory disease
pLSIL	possible low-grade squamous intraepithelial lesion
PMB	postmenopausal bleeding
po	*per orem* (by mouth)
POGTT	pregnancy oral glucose tolerance test
PPROM	preterm prelabour rupture of membranes
PrEP	pre-exposure prophylaxis
PTB	preterm birth
PUL	pregnancy of unknown location
PV	*per vaginam* (by vagina)
RBC	red blood count
RMI	risk of malignancy index
ROMA	risk of malignancy algorithm
RNA	ribonucleic acid
RPR	rapid plasma reagin
RUQ	right upper quadrant
SCBU	special care baby unit
SCC	squamous cell carcinoma
SFH	symphysial fundal height
SGA	small for gestational age
SHBG	sex hormone binding globulin
SSRI	selective serotonin reuptake inhibitor
STI	sexually transmissible infection
TOL	trial of labour
TOLAC	trial of labour after caesarean
TOP	termination of pregnancy
TPHA	*Treponema pallidum* haemagglutination antibody
TPL	threatened preterm labour
TSH	thyroid-stimulating hormone
TTTS	twin-to-twin transfusion syndrome
UEC	urea, electrolytes and creatinine
UFH	unfractionated heparin
UPA	ulipristal acetate
UPC	urine protein:creatinine ratio
USS	ultrasound scan
UTI	urinary tract infection
VDRL	venereal disease research laboratories
VIN	vulvar intraepithelial neoplasia
VSCC	vulvar squamous cell carcinoma

VTE	venous thromboembolism
VZIG	varicella zoster immune globulin
VZV	varicella zoster virus
WHO	World Health Organization

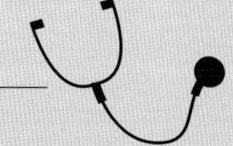

Part 1

Taking an obstetric or gynaecological history

The principles underlying history taking related to symptoms and signs suggesting obstetric or gynaecological conditions do not differ from those applied to history taking in every other field of medicine. However, we do emphasise several points.

1. People with female genitalia may not necessarily identify themselves as women. It is important to be aware of the gender identity of the person consulting you, to be sensitive with your history taking and appropriate with language especially with regard to the use of pronouns. However in order to facilitate the flow of the text in this book we have used the words 'woman' and 'women' throughout to refer to all people presenting for care in pregnancy, and for screening or complaints involving the female genital tract.

2. Be aware of the cultural background of the person presenting for care; their cultural beliefs may impact significantly on how your history taking and examination are conducted. Professional interpreters are available across Australia, although in regional areas and for some languages their services may be accessible only by telephone. For women from certain ethnic backgrounds female doctors may be requested and this request should be granted when it is feasible. It is also important to acknowledge the sensitivities and the needs of women of Indigenous background. The services of the appropriate liaison officers should be discussed and offered to provide extra support.

3. Although the presenting complaint may direct you immediately to the genital tract (e.g. major vaginal bleeding), do not neglect other body systems or the psychological and emotional aspects of the person's presentation.

Taking a gynaecological history

- Presenting complaint—what has brought the woman to see you (e.g. pain, bleeding, failure to conceive, urinary incontinence, sexual difficulties)?

- History of the presenting complaint—how long have the symptoms bothered the woman? How severe are they? Are there any related symptoms? This history may include questions about menstrual disturbance, bleeding problems, premenstrual symptoms, lower abdominal pain, dyspareunia, infertility, pelvic floor dysfunction, menopausal symptoms and so on.
- General gynaecological history—note the age of the woman, date of the last menstrual period, date of the last cervical screening test (CST) or Pap smear in New Zealand, any breast screening, contraception, parity, previous gynaecological surgery and previous gynaecological investigations and results. A reminder to the woman of the need for regular well-woman checks, CSTs and mammograms (in women over 40 years of age) is almost always useful.
- General medical and surgical history—obstetric history, family history, any current medications, allergies.
- Social history—family support, cigarette smoking, use of alcohol and recreational drugs, work situation.
- Sexual history—the details of this depend on the presenting complaint and other aspects of the individual woman's history. Establish whether or not the woman is currently sexually active (any form of sex, not just intercourse) and, if not (depending on her age), whether she has been in the past. History taking should include any previous sexually transmissible infections (STIs) and possible symptoms of current STIs. Sexual dysfunction or difficulty, current or previous, should not be overlooked. It is not uncommon, especially in general practice, for women to present initially with a physical symptom, such as heavy menstrual bleeding, when their main concern is of a sexual nature. This information needs to be elicited by sensitive and non-judgemental history taking.

Additionally, as already noted, you will need to establish whether the woman identifies as heterosexual, lesbian, bisexual, transgender or other. Don't forget that women who currently identify a certain way may have had different relationships in the past; for example, a woman now identifying as lesbian may have had previous heterosexual relationships, including some resulting in the birth of children.

We recommend that when concluding your history and before commencing your examination of the woman you ask a broad question such as 'Are there any other things about you or your health that you think I should know?' This may enable the woman to speak about personal matters that are worrying her. It also provides you with the assurance that from a medicolegal point of view you have endeavoured to obtain all relevant information.

Make sure that you document the history legibly and with sufficient detail, including the date and, if appropriate, the time.

Taking an obstetric history

In many cases, as a general practitioner or junior doctor consulted for the first time by a pregnant woman presenting with an apparent complication of pregnancy, you will have accessible copies of hospital booking notes, a shared care card or increasingly, access to electronic medical records (eMR), all containing much relevant information. However, with or without this preexisting information, we recommend you to note the following points:

- presenting complaint (e.g. pain, bleeding, rupture of membranes, absence of fetal movements), and the duration and severity of the symptoms
- age of woman; gravidity and parity; date on which her last menstrual period began; the length and regularity of her menstrual cycles; her expected date of confinement (EDC) by date of LMP; results of any ultrasound scans (USS) that may have been performed; previous contraception; last Pap smear
- past obstetric history, including all full-term pregnancies, vaginal births, caesarean sections, miscarriages, terminations of pregnancy, ectopic pregnancies, perinatal deaths, preterm labours, postnatal complications
- past gynaecological, surgical and medical history, including any sexually transmitted infections, any current medications, allergies
- cigarette smoking, alcohol and recreational drug use, social history (i.e. family support, work situation), family history, any history of intimate partner violence

Again, make sure that all documentation is complete and legible.

Conducting an examination

Examination of the adult gynaecological patient

1. Relevant general examination—assessment of vital signs appropriate to the case (pulse, blood pressure, temperature) and examination of other systems and organs (heart, lungs, thyroid and breasts, in particular) should be conducted as indicated.
2. Examination of the abdomen—inspection for scars of previous surgery, striae, palpation for tenderness, masses (whether arising from the pelvis or elsewhere), ascites. Do not omit to palpate for an enlarged liver or spleen and don't forget a renal examination.
3. Vaginal examination—note that this is not always necessary at the initial visit. If a vaginal examination is performed, you need to be clear in your mind why you are doing the examination and what you are looking for. The vast majority of women find vaginal examination invasive to some degree, uncomfortable at best. However, this should not serve as an excuse for not performing a vaginal examination if it is required. This excuse is too often used by junior doctors and general practitioners who perhaps feel uncomfortable or inexperienced in this situation. Serious pathology, in particular cervical cancer, can be missed because this examination has been avoided due to specious reasoning. It is essential that the woman herself understands why you are performing the examination and what you are looking for, has consented verbally to the procedure and is given the result so far as is possible when the examination is concluded. It is our practice and recommendation to have a female chaperone present for all breast and genital examinations, irrespective of the gender of the practitioner, but we appreciate that this is not possible in all practices. The woman should be able to undress and dress again in privacy and should have the results of your findings and other matters explained and

discussed only when she is fully dressed and sitting back in the consulting room. It is inappropriate for a fully dressed doctor (or other health professional) to be holding a discussion with a partly dressed woman lying on a gynaecological couch.

Vaginal examination is usually conducted with the woman in the dorsal position. Examination of the vulva (looking for erythema, atrophic changes, swellings, suspicious lesions) should be performed prior to the vaginal examination itself.

It is vital to explain the examination to the woman before you start. An explanation of why the examination is being performed is helpful for the woman. Always obtain consent prior to commencing the examination and ensure the woman is ready before you start touching her or inserting a speculum.

4. Speculum examination—it is generally recommended that this be performed before a bimanual vaginal examination if a CST is to be performed, to avoid displacing cells from the surface of the cervix. However, a gentle one-finger vaginal examination prior to passing the speculum is permissible; this enables you to know whether the cervix is lying posteriorly high in the vagina because the uterus is anteverted (the case in about 75% of women) or is more anterior because the uterus is retroverted (as it is in the remaining 25%). Where the cervix lies anteriorly, the speculum should be gently passed more in this direction. The procedure for conducting a speculum examination is as follows:
   - Warm the speculum. A gel-type lubricant may be used if a CST is not being performed, but warm water is usually a sufficient lubricant.
   - Sometimes, placing the patient's fists or a cushion underneath her buttocks will assist in making the examination more comfortable and the cervix more easily visible.
   - Note the appearance of the cervix—normal/abnormal?
   - Note the presence and characteristics of any vaginal discharge.
   - The left lateral position using a Sims speculum may give a more complete view when assessing uterovaginal prolapse.

5. Bimanual examination—this is normally performed with two fingers of the dominant hand intravaginally and the other hand palpating the lower abdomen, so that the fundus of an anteverted uterus can be balloted between the two hands, and any pelvic masses examined likewise. Using the two hands, the following features should be assessed:
   - uterus—size, position, shape, consistency, any tenderness, mobility

- adnexae—presence or absence of any masses or tenderness (normal ovaries are not usually palpable as discrete masses but may be tender if pressed between the examining hands)
- uterosacral nodularity/tenderness/tethering, which may suggest endometriosis

 CLINICAL PEARLS

If as a junior doctor (or a student) you are uncertain about what you are seeing or feeling on vaginal examination, do not be afraid to say this and consult a senior colleague. All of us have learnt vaginal examination by experiencing such situations.

In women of high BMI it may be difficult even for very experienced practitioners to establish the size and position of the internal genital organs.

Examination of the pregnant woman

As with gynaecological patients, a general physical examination should not be neglected in the pregnant patient. The woman should be made as comfortable as possible; in late pregnancy it may be appropriate either to ask the woman to turn slightly towards you or to place a pillow or wedge beneath her so that the weight of the fetus does not obstruct venous return, leading to syncope. You must also explain to the woman what you are doing and why.

Blood pressure should always be taken, preferably in a standard manner. In our clinics we take blood pressure in the right arm with the patient sitting up on the couch, her feet resting on a stool. If the circumference of the upper arm is greater than 27 cm, a large cuff should be used.

Abdominal examination

1. **Inspection**
   Is the abdomen distended? Are there any scars? Are there needle marks from the use of subcutaneous injections, such as for insulin or anticoagulants? Striae from the current or previous pregnancies may be apparent.
2. **Palpation**
   The uterus is palpable in the abdomen from 12 weeks of pregnancy (this may be difficult to determine if the woman is obese). Its

size, shape, consistency and any tenderness should be noted. Fetal parts are palpable from between 24 and 28 weeks dependent on the thickness of the abdominal wall. From 28 weeks onwards the lie of the fetus (relationship of the longitudinal axis of the fetus to the longitudinal axis of the uterus) can be determined. The nature of the presenting part (that part of the fetus lying in the lower uterine segment) may also be evident on palpation from 28 weeks onwards, although again this depends on the degree of thickness of the abdominal wall—it may be difficult on occasion to confidently distinguish breech presentation from cephalic even for experienced practitioners. With cephalic presentations the degree of descent of the fetal head in relation to the pelvic brim should be noted from 36 weeks' gestation onwards.

Note should also be made of any abdominal tenderness or enlargement of other abdominal organs.

3. **Measurement**

   Measure the pregnant uterus in centimetres from the symphysis pubis to the top of the uterus—this gives the fundal height. This examination is done from 20 weeks' gestation, when the fundus will be approximately level with the umbilicus. The height (in cm) should correspond approximately with the gestation in weeks.

4. **Auscultation**

   This is mainly of use in obstetrics for identifying the fetal heart sounds, which are most easily heard with an electronic Doppler device; a standard stethoscope is unable to detect fetal heart sounds easily.

The use of ultrasound in obstetrics and gynaecology

Ultrasound examination has become a fundamental part of care in all aspects of women's health. In many specialist clinical settings, including antenatal clinics, ultrasound is available at the bedside and is commonly seen as an extension of clinical examination. It is likely students will encounter ultrasound during their clinical attachments. When considering the use of ultrasound, it is important to be aware of its potential limitations as well as the benefits it can bring.

Ultrasound waves travel relatively freely through soft tissues and fluids in the body but are reflected by more solid structures (such as bones) and particularly by interfaces between structures of markedly differing density. These phenomena can give rise to 'artefacts', which can make

continued

continued

the interpretation of ultrasound images challenging in some cases. The addition of Doppler techniques—which measure the average speed of moving fluids, such as blood in vessels—allows for assessment of 'flows', such as the speed of flow in an umbilical vessel or in the vessels of the heart and brain in a fetus. Doppler can also aid in assessing blood flow to ovarian cysts or other pelvic masses.

The common uses of ultrasound in obstetrics are to accurately date the pregnancy and to image the anatomy of the fetus. Accurate dating of a pregnancy is usually performed between 7 and 13 weeks of gestation. Fetal anatomical assessment is best conducted from the middle trimester (approximately 12–28 weeks of pregnancy) and allows very accurate visualisation of structures such as the fetal brain. However, it is important to realise that, even in the best and most experienced hands, there are many fetal malformations that diagnostic ultrasound cannot detect. Large studies have revealed that more than one-third of fetal malformations are not visible on routine antenatal ultrasound.

References and further reading

Migrant & Refugee Health Partnership. Competency standards framework. https://culturaldiversityhealth.org.au/competency-standards-framework/

Stroumsa D, Wu J. Welcoming transgender and nonbinary patients: expanding the language of 'women's health'. *Am J Obstet Gynecol.* 2018; 219(6):585.e1–e5.

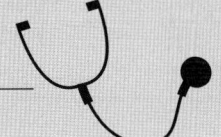

Part 2
Clinical cases in general practice

Case 1
Kate wants to talk about contraception. . .

Kate is a 19-year-old university student who has made an appointment to see you in general practice for a script for her pill. You have been Kate's family doctor since she was 10 years old. Apart from normal childhood illnesses, Kate has always been in good health.

At the age of 14, she presented with primary dysmenorrhoea for which you prescribed mefenamic acid, after normal findings at a general physical examination. This was effective for 2 years but at the age of 16, Kate developed more severe dysmenorrhoea. Examination at that time was again unremarkable, and Kate told you that she had never been sexually active. She was commenced on a combined oral contraceptive pill (COCP)—ethinyloestradiol 30 µg, levonorgestrel 150 µg—and this has completely controlled her period-related pain ever since. When Kate presented for her annual prescription last year, she told you that she had been sexually active for the past year. You reminded her about safe sex and she replied that she and her boyfriend were using condoms.

How do you commence your consultation with Kate?

Kate reports that she is well. She has continued on the COCP and has no concerns about this but she does wonder whether it is safe to continue indefinitely—she reminds you that she has now been taking it consistently for 3 years. She tells you that she has continued with the same boyfriend; confident that they are in a monogamous relationship, she has agreed to stop using condoms and rely on the COCP for contraception. She has been doing this for 6 months. Her last menstrual period (or more accurately withdrawal bleed) was 2 weeks previously.

What do you answer to Kate's questions about the 'pill'?

You explain to Kate that in the six decades that the pill has been available there have been major changes in formulation, with current preparations now containing much smaller doses of both oestrogen and progestogens. There are three main concerns about the safety of the COCP: thromboembolic disease, cardiovascular disease and breast cancer. Although statistically Kate's chances of developing any of these are slightly raised by long-term pill-taking, since she is a healthy young nonsmoker taking a second-generation pill, her absolute risk is extremely small for all conditions. You also briefly outline for Kate the advantages of the COCP. You point out that, as with any medication, there are always risks and benefits, and that ultimately it is her choice to make an informed decision about this medication.

 ## CLINICAL COMMENT

Numerous types of COCPs have been developed and used since the 1960s, and a number of different preparations are available for women:

- 'Second-generation' COCPs containing oestrogen (usually 20–30 µg) plus the progestogen levonorgestrel or norethisterone.
- 'Third generation' COCPs containing oestrogen plus desogestrel or gestodene.
- COCPs containing oestrogen, newer progestogens or anti-androgens, e.g. cyproterone acetate, drospirenone, dienogest or nomegestral acetate. These are used for women affected by acne, mild hirsutism or other androgenic signs of the polycystic ovarian syndrome, to provide both cycle control and contraception.
- The oestrogen in the COCP is usually ethinyloestradiol but may be oestradiol or oestradiol valerate.
- Pill formulations may be monophasic (same dose of oestrogen and progestogen in every active pill), biphasic (a two-step progestogen dose with constant oestrogen dose) or triphasic (three-step progestogen dose, two-step oestrogen dose). Triphasic pills offer few advantages over monophasic types, cannot be taken in continuous regimens and are associated with more breakthrough bleeding than monophasic pills.
- COCPs are extremely effective contraceptives with a Pearl Index of 0.1. The Pearl Index method failure rate (number of pregnancies per 100 woman-years) is derived from the formula: = (total accidental pregnancies × 1200)/total months of exposure. (Note that the Pearl Index refers to 'method failure'; in real life, 'failure' of a method may also be attributable to 'user failure'.)

The vaginal ring is an effective and acceptable alternative to the COCP for some women, providing oestrogen and progestogen for 3 weeks followed by a hormone-free week. It does not require daily compliance, and SMS services are available to remind the woman to insert a fresh ring each month. It may be useful in some women with gastrointestinal disorders interfering with COCP absorption and may possibly be associated with less breakthrough bleeding than the COCP.

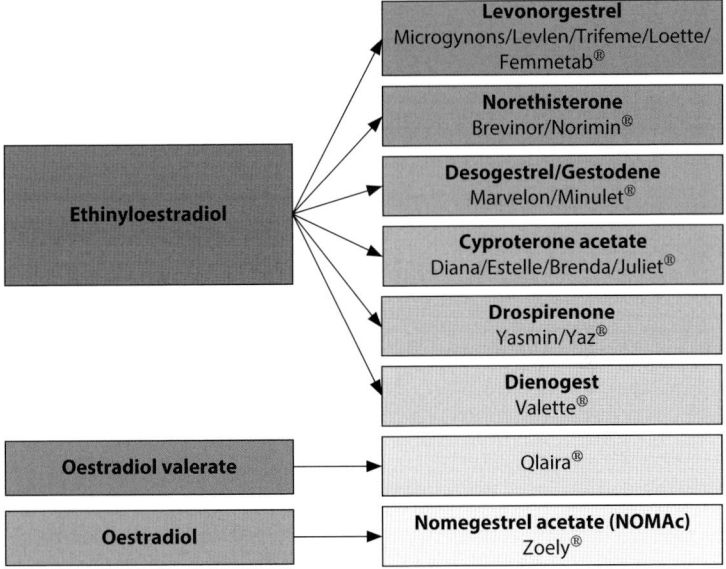

Figure 1.1 COCP types in Australia (not all generics are included)
Source: Reproduced with Permission from Stewart, M. Chaar, B. Bateson, D. Combined oral contraceptives. The Royal Australian and New Zealand College of Obstetricians and Gynaecologists (O&G Magazine). 2014

Safety of the combined oral contraceptive pill

- Thromboembolic disease. This is a rare but serious potential risk of COCP use. The rate of venous thromboembolism in pill users is about 10 per 100 000. This compares to a rate of about 5 per 100 000 reproductive-age women who do not take hormonal contraception. However, to put this in perspective, the rate of thrombosis in women during the puerperium is more than 300 per 100 000. Evidence suggests no difference in the risk between available COCP types, although studies are conflicting.

continued

continued

- Arterial thrombosis is more common in women with other risk factors, such as poorly controlled hypertension and/or diabetes, and in smokers and those with a family history. The COCP is not contraindicated in well-controlled hypertension or diabetes, although women with these conditions should be kept under regular observation. Migraine with aura is a contraindication to the pill because of increased stroke risk.
- Breast cancer. The best available evidence suggests that women using oral contraception are at a slightly increased risk of breast cancer, particularly younger women. However, this risk returns to normal 10 years after use of the pill is discontinued.
- There is a possible small increase in the risk of cervical cancer for users of the combined pill. The importance of regular cervical screening should be emphasised to all women. Hepatic adenoma is a rare risk of the combined pill.

Other uses of the COCP

As well as being an extremely reliable contraceptive method, the COCP is a very effective treatment for primary dysmenorrhoea. It reduces the amount of menstrual blood loss and therefore reduces the incidence of anaemia, and it allows for the manipulation of cycle length. It also reduces the incidence of ovarian cysts, ovarian cancer, endometrial cancer, benign breast disease and premenstrual syndrome. Important conditions such as endometriosis and fibroids can be treated effectively with oral contraception, and use may provide some protection against pelvic inflammatory disease.

Contraindications to the combined oral contraceptive pill

- High risk of thromboembolic disease, e.g. history of thromboembolism, known thrombogenic mutation or major surgery with prolonged immobilisation
- Breast cancer
- Liver disease: cirrhosis, active viral hepatitis or hepatocellular cancer

- High risk of cardiovascular disease, e.g. history of stroke or ischaemic heart disease, complicated valvular or congenital heart disease, uncontrolled severe hypertension, poorly controlled diabetes or diabetes complicated by vascular disease, migraine with aura, being over 35 years and smoking more than 15 cigarettes per day, Raynaud's disease with lupus anticoagulant and systemic lupus erythematosus with antiphospholipid antibodies
- Active gallbladder disease
- Being less than 6 weeks postpartum

What else should you discuss with Kate?

You explain to Kate that although the COCP will offer her protection against pregnancy, it does not protect her from sexually transmitted infections. Although Kate is in a long-term relationship, you offer her a chlamydia screening test as part of her well-woman check, explaining that the prevalence of *Chlamydia trachomatis* infection in young women is some areas is as high as 20% and that asymptomatic chlamydia can have serious consequences.

You conduct a general examination of Kate, including measuring her blood pressure and examining her abdomen. You also pass a vaginal speculum to inspect the cervix and take a swab for chlamydia PCR testing; chlamydia testing can also be done on a first-catch urine specimen (i.e. the first amount of urine to be passed), provided urine has not been passed for at least 2 hours. After the speculum examination, you perform a bimanual vaginal examination. All of your examination findings are within normal limits. You renew her prescription for the COCP. She feels happy with this and wishes to continue. You advise her that your practice will write to her with the results of her chlamydia test in 2–3 weeks' time.

 CLINICAL PEARLS

- Always take a holistic view of women's health—ask about concerns, take blood pressure, inquire about current contraception and plans for future pregnancy.
- Discussion of contraceptive options should prioritise the woman's choice and safety, and be evidence-based.
- Chlamydia can be screened for on a first-catch urine specimen if this is more appropriate or more acceptable to the woman concerned.

References and further reading

De Leo V, Musacchio MC, Cappelli V, et al. Hormonal contraceptives: pharmacology tailored to women's health. *Hum Reprod Update.* 2016;22(5):634–46.

Family Planning New South Wales, Family Planning Victoria, True Relationships and Reproductive Health. Contraception: an Australian clinical practice handbook. 4th ed. Sydney: FPNSW; 2016.

Powell A. Choosing the right oral contraceptive pill for teens. *Pediatr Clin North Am.* 2017;64(2):343–58.

Case 2
Hannah presents for a well-woman check. . .

Hannah is a 25-year-old teacher who has made an appointment to see you in general practice for a 'well-woman check'. Hannah tells you that she has never previously had any cervical screening and now that she is 25 years old, she is keen to ensure that she has no risk of getting cervical cancer.

What questions will you ask Hannah?

Hannah was first sexually active at the age of 19. She has had 3 sexual partners. She commenced the combined oral contraceptive pill (COCP) at age 18. She has been with her current partner for 3 years. She has never been pregnant and they are not considering starting a family any time soon. Hannah is keen to travel and work overseas before she gets married.

Hannah has regular periods on the pill. She does not get any intermenstrual bleeding. She never experiences any bleeding after intercourse.

You ask Hannah if she had the human papillomavirus (HPV) vaccine. She thinks she had it while she was at school. She would like more information about cervical screening generally and, in particular, wants to understand more about HPV infection and its consequences. Hannah does not smoke cigarettes. You explain to her the Australian guidelines for cervical screening.

1. Australian rates of cervical cancer fell by half after the introduction of the National Cervical Screening Program (NCSP) in 1991. In December 2017, this program saw some major changes. These included:
   - a 5-yearly cervical screening test (CST) replacing the 2-yearly Pap test.
   - age of commencement of screening changed to 25 years of age, continuing until 74 years.
   - cytology as the primary screening method replaced with testing for oncogenic HPV, and liquid-based cytology (LBC) used to determine the recommended clinical pathway if HPV is detected.
   - a new National Cervical Screening Register.

continued

continued

> **2.** Self collection of a vaginal sample for screening is available for patients aged 30 years or over who have declined to have a cervical sample collected by a clinician and are either:
> - overdue for screening by two years or more, or
> - have never been screened.
>
> **3.** In New Zealand, cervical cytology tests are taken in the conventional manner. Women between 25 and 70 years of age are encouraged to have regular cervical smears at 3-yearly intervals. It is planned to change to HPV testing, but at the time of writing (2021) a date has not been set for this.

Cervical cancer is one of the most preventable of all cancers. It is the second commonest cancer in women worldwide, but the commonest in developing countries, comprising 12% of cancer in women. Up to 90% of squamous cell carcinoma can be prevented if cell changes can be detected and treated early.

Should Hannah have a cervical screening test?

Yes. First, you explain to Hannah that HPV infection is a common although usually transient condition in women her age around the time they become sexually active. HPV is so common that exposure to the virus may be seen as a normal consequence of becoming sexually active. There are almost 200 types of HPV. Some of these (e.g. types 2, 6, 11) may cause visible papillomata or warts on the vulva, in the vagina, on the cervix or around the anus, but many can be present without causing visible warts. Some types (especially types 16 and 18, but also others) present a high risk for the development of premalignant change in the cervical epithelium or, less commonly, the vaginal or vulval epithelium. While HPV is necessary for premalignant change, other factors are commonly involved—cigarette smoking has been implicated as an associated factor. You note with approval that Hannah does not smoke.

In the majority of cases, infection with HPV in young women is transient—their own immune systems deal with the virus and in most cases it is eradicated without further consequences. In about 3% of women infected with types 16, 18 and more rarely other types, dysplastic changes occur and, if undetected and untreated, these may progress to a high-grade squamous intraepithelial lesion (HSIL) and eventually to invasive cancer of the cervix. The time required for high-risk HPV infection to lead to HSIL is usually prolonged, a minimum of 6 years. If invasive cancer arises, this generally occurs over many years—often decades.

You explain to Hannah that it is recommended that she participate in a cervical screening program. A CST refers to testing for the presence of oncogenic HPV in the cervix. If HPV is detected, a subsequent LBC test is performed on the sample to assess for any dysplastic cellular change. The chances of detecting premalignant change are high. Cervical screening is really about *preventing* the development of cervical cancer.

> *Are cervical screening tests 100% effective at preventing cancer?'* Hannah wants to know.

You explain that in countries where cervical screening programs have been introduced, rates of invasive cervical cancer have fallen by half and survival has improved. The development of vaccines against high-risk types of HPV is likely to further reduce the incidence of cervical cancers in the coming years.

You also offer Hannah a chlamydia screening test as part of her well-woman check, explaining that the prevalence of *Chlamydia trachomatis* infection in young women in some areas is as high as 20% and that asymptomatic chlamydia can have serious adverse consequences.

> A CST is a screening test, not a diagnostic test.

CLINICAL COMMENT

Characteristics of a screening test

- The purpose of a screening test is to give a reasonable probability that the disease or condition being screened for is or is not present. All screening tests will have a certain proportion of false positive results (i.e. the test is positive but the condition is not present) and false negative results (i.e. the test is negative although the condition is, in fact, present) and the percentages of these should be known to those performing the tests. An ideal screening test should have high sensitivity (i.e. a high chance of detecting the condition if it is present) and a low false positive rate. A negative CST result in a woman with worrying symptoms such as postcoital bleeding, intermenstrual bleeding or abnormal vaginal discharge should not be regarded as an exclusion of cancer.
- If a screening test is positive, further tests may be offered to reach a definite diagnosis (specific tests).

continued

21

continued

- A screening test should be minimally invasive, not harmful and relatively inexpensive since it is being offered to large numbers of people.
- Effective treatment should exist for the condition being screened for.

💬 *'Should my boyfriend be tested?'* Hannah asks.

You explain that HPV infection in men is very common as well, but cancer of the penis is rare. Even if Hannah returns a positive result there is no reason for her partner to be examined unless visible warts (papillomata) are present. If this is the case, these can be treated, although it is worth noting that visible warts are usually caused by low-risk HPV types.

What examination does Hannah require?

You conduct a general examination of Hannah, including measuring her blood pressure and examining her abdomen, then pass a vaginal speculum to inspect the cervix and take a CST (Fig. 2.1). After the speculum examination, you perform a bimanual vaginal examination. All of your examination findings are within normal limits.

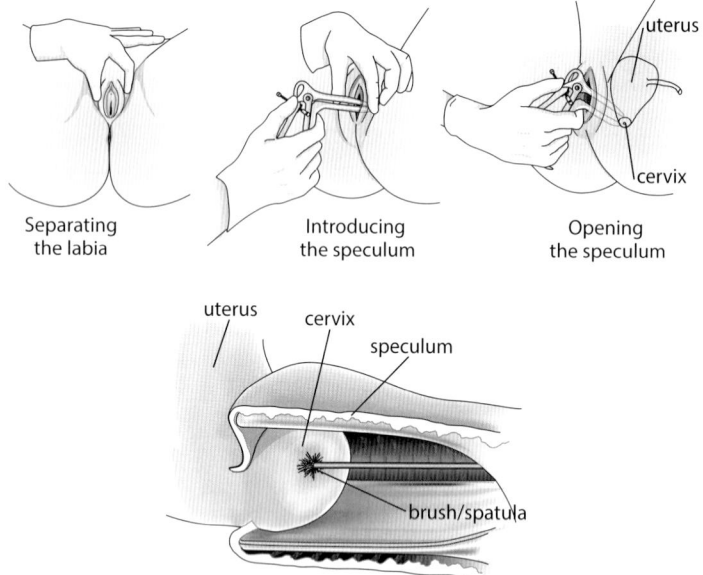

Figure 2.1 Collecting a cervical screening test sample

1. After the patient is prepared and comfortable, begin the speculum examination by examining the external genitalia for any abnormalities, then:
   - warm the speculum and apply a small amount of water-based lubricant.
   - gently part the labia and encourage the patient to breathe out while you slowly insert the closed speculum into the vagina using slight downward pressure, keeping the lower blade against the posterior wall of the vagina.
   - ask the patient if she is in any discomfort and encourage feedback throughout.
   - open the blades just slightly, then tilt the speculum forward a little to allow maximum visualisation of the external orifice of the cervix uteri (external os).
2. Once the cervix is visualised, inspect for the following features:
   - colour, size, shape, position
   - abnormal areas, discharge
   - the transformation zone, which may or may not be visible
3. The objective is to sample cells from the transformation zone, where HPV is present and cell abnormalities are usually found. Collect a sample using a brush or broom sampling device. Swirl the collection vigorously in the vial. It is optimal for the sample to contain both ectocervical and endocervical cells.

> *'When will I get my results?'* Hannah asks. 💬

You advise Hannah that your practice will write to her with the results of her CST in 2–3 weeks' time and that her name will be placed on the cervical screening register. Furthermore, your own practice will send her a reminder letter for her next CST, depending on the result. You renew her prescription for the COCP at her request.

Table 2.1 Cervical screening test results for clinician-collected sample

Risk of significant cervical abnormalities	HPV test result	Reflex LBC result	Recommended management
Low-risk result	HPV not detected		Return to screening in 5 years

continued

continued

Risk of significant cervical abnormalities	HPV test result	Reflex LBC result	Recommended management
Intermediate-risk result	HPV not 16/18 detected	Negative, possible LSIL or LSIL	Repeat HPV test in 12 months
Higher-risk result	HPV not 16/18 detected	Possible HSIL or HSIL	Refer to specialist (Colposcopy)
	HPV 16/18 detected	Any LBC results	
Unsatisfactory for evaluation	Unsatisfactory HPV test	–	Collect new sample for HPV in 6–12 weeks
Unsatisfactory for evaluation	HPV not 16/18 detected	Unsatisfactory	Collect new sample for HPV in 6–12 weeks

CLINICAL COMMENT

The Australian National Cancer Screening Register supports the NCSP by providing a safety net to patients and healthcare providers to support usual care. All information is confidential and protected by the latest state-of-the-art data security measures, in accordance with strict security requirements and legislation.

Women presenting for CST automatically have their names included on the Register unless they specifically ask not to be included ('opt out' registration). The Register sends reminders to women who are overdue for routine screening and attempts to follow up women with abnormal cytology reports for whom no record of investigation and/or treatment is known. They also provide nationwide data collection.

The Register will support you to manage your patient's personal information and participation in the NCSP and may also send you notifications to indicate that your patient has not attended important clinical follow-up tests or examinations.

In the United Kingdom, the national office of the National Health Service (NHS) Cancer Screening Programmes is responsible for improving the overall performance of the programs. Every Primary Care Trust (PCT) has a nominated person responsible for its cervical screening program and implementing the national guidelines. Regional directors of public health are responsible for the quality-assurance network in their region.

CLINICAL PEARLS

- Always take a holistic view of patients' health—ask about concerns, take blood pressure, inquire about current contraception and plans for future pregnancy.
- Visually inspect the cervix as well as taking a cervical screening sample.
- Make sure that the patient knows how her CST results will be communicated to her.

References and further reading

Australian Government Department of Health and Ageing. National cervical screening program. Canberra: DHA; 2020. www.health.gov.au/initiatives-and-programs

Cancer Research UK. About cervical screening. London: Cancer Research UK; 2020. www.cancerresearchuk.org/about/cancer/cervical-cancer/getting-diagnosed/screening/about

National Screening Unit, Ministry of Health. Clinical practice guidelines for cervical screening in New Zealand. Wellington: Ministry of Health; 2020. www.nsu.govt.nz/system/files/resources/final_ncsp-guidelines-for-cervical-screening-new-zealand-5_june_2020.pdf

Case 3
Felicity is recalled after an abnormal cervical screening test report. . .

Felicity is a 31-year-old woman you are seeing to discuss the result of her cervical screening test (CST) that you performed 2 weeks previously. You first met Felicity last year when she was due for her routine cervical screening. Felicity commenced screening at 25 years of age. Her first CST was low risk. She presented last year for her routine 5-yearly test. Last year her result was:

> RESULT: Intermediate risk for significant cervical abnormality
> HPV 16: Not detected
> HPV 18: Not detected
> HPV other: Detected
> LIQUID-BASED CYTOLOGY: Low-grade squamous intraepithelial lesion (LSIL), Endocervical component present

You advised Felicity to come back for a repeat test in 1 year, which she did. She sees you today for the results. Felicity also tells you that although she is taking the oral contraceptive pill, she wants to stop this soon to try to become pregnant.

Felicity's CST report now reads:

> RESULT: Higher risk for significant cervical abnormality
> HPV 16: Not detected
> HPV 18: Not detected
> HPV other: Detected
> LIQUID-BASED CYTOLOGY: Possible high-grade squamous intraepithelial lesion (HSIL), Endocervical component present

When Felicity arrives in your consulting room she is obviously very nervous.

How do you manage Felicity's understandable anxiety?

You explain clearly to Felicity that she is very unlikely to have cancer, but that there are changes reported in her cervical screening result that will require investigation and probably some minor surgery and follow-up. You emphasise this test is a screening test and it does not supply a final diagnosis, merely an indication for further investigation. She will be wise to continue with the contraceptive pill until the investigation and any treatment is complete, but thereafter she will be able to try for a pregnancy. She may need to be carefully watched in a pregnancy following treatment to her cervix as there is a slightly increased risk of miscarriage or preterm labour following these cervical procedures. You take the opportunity to mention to Felicity that prior to trying to conceive, it is important she should commence regular folic acid supplements and be screened for rubella immunity, so that she can be immunised if her immunity is low.

You then explain that HSIL is a premalignant condition that may progress to cervical cancer if left untreated.

> '*What kind of treatment will I have?*' asks Felicity.

The next step is to undergo a colposcopy (Fig. 3.1). The gynaecologist will carefully inspect the cervix using the magnification of the colposcope for close examination and identification of any abnormal areas and the extent of these. A biopsy may be taken from areas suspicious for dysplasia. If histological examination of the biopsy confirms a high-grade lesion, then either laser treatment or a loop excision procedure using diathermy (large loop excision of the transformation zone, LLETZ) may be recommended. Less commonly, a cone biopsy may be performed, using a scalpel to excise a portion of affected tissue. The laser is used with local anaesthesia; LLETZ may be done with local or general anaesthesia. In both types of treatment, the doctor will first inspect the cervix again with a colposcope to identify the abnormal area or areas in order to try to remove all abnormal tissue. Following the procedure there will be some vaginal discharge for 7–10 days.

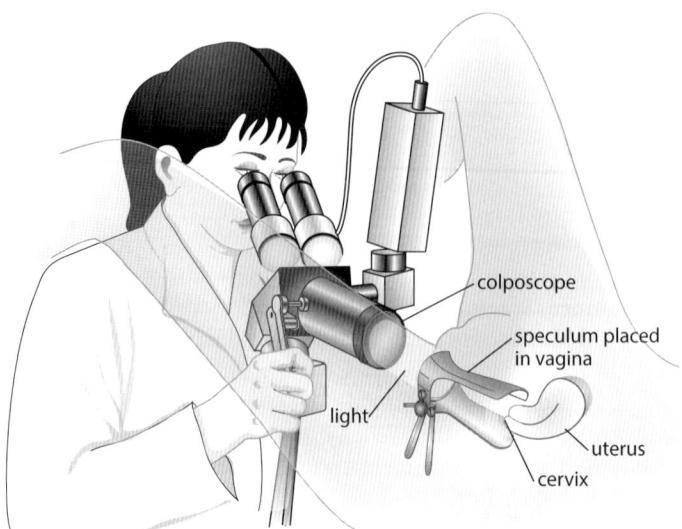

colposcope

speculum placed
in vagina

light

uterus

cervix

Figure 3.1 Colposcopy procedure. Through the colposcope a magnified view of the cervix is obtained. Abnormal areas are inspected and directed biopsies can be taken

'Are there any risks to these procedures?' Felicity wants to know.

Rarely, there may be moderate to severe bleeding requiring a return to hospital and possible diathermy or suturing of bleeding points. However, subsequent bleeding is usually mild and due to secondary infection. Such bleeding is usually treated with broad-spectrum antibiotics. Complications following cone biopsy are more frequent than those following the LLETZ procedure. Cervical stenosis causing dysmenorrhoea (painful periods) or reduced or absent periods (amenorrhoea) can occur; cervical stenosis can also interfere with the ability to become pregnant.

'When can I try to become pregnant after all this?' Felicity asks.

It is recommended that patients who have received treatment for a high-grade abnormality should complete test of cure surveillance to confirm their treatment has been successful. Test of cure surveillance is a co-test (HPV and LBC test) performed 12 months after treatment, and annually thereafter, until the patient receives a negative co-test on two consecutive occasions.

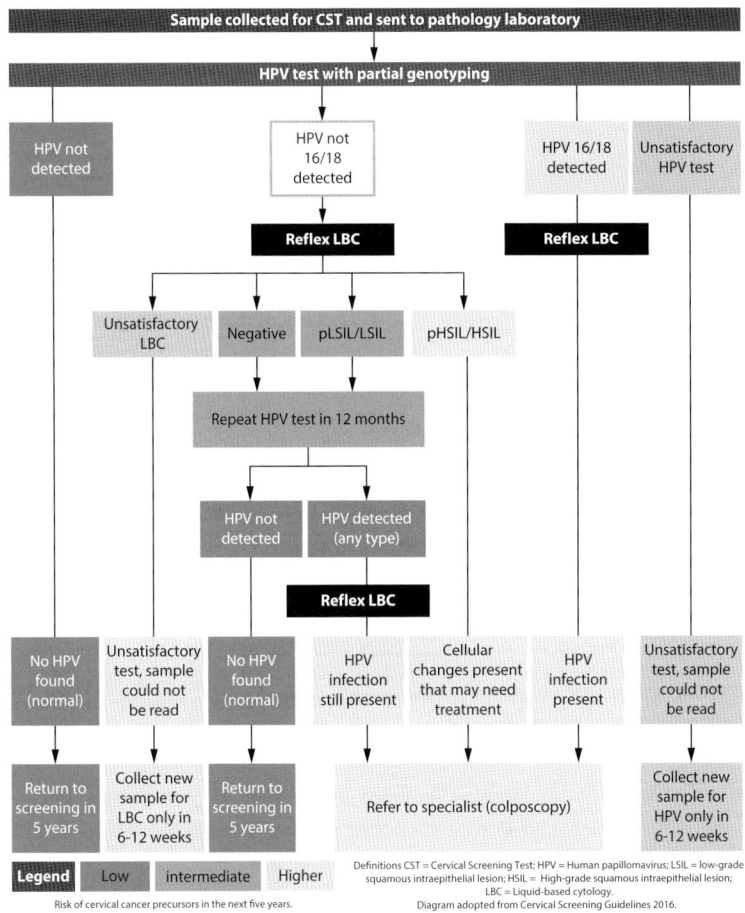

Figure 3.2 Cervical screening pathway for the clinician-collected sample
(Adapted from Australian Institute of Health and Welfare: National Cervical
Screening Program monitoring report. Canberra: NHMRC; 2019).

It is advisable that Felicity wait for normal results from the 12-month check before trying for a pregnancy. However, testing can be carried out safely during pregnancy provided the correct equipment is used.

> *'How much will the treatment affect my chances of becoming pregnant or continuing with the pregnancy?'* Felicity specifically wants to know the answers to these questions.

After the surgery the cervix heals, with the formation of a new squamo-columnar junction. In most cases the cervix functions normally and does not interfere with subsequent conception. Very occasionally as already mentioned, cervical stenosis may follow a LLETZ procedure or a cone biopsy, and dilatation of the cervix or other treatment may be needed. Following a LLETZ procedure there is also a slightly increased incidence of miscarriage or preterm labour due to cervical incompetence. Repeated LLETZ procedures or cone biopsy of the cervix are more likely to result in shortened cervical length and therefore predispose to cervical incompetence. In such cases careful specialist assessment is needed and insertion of a cervical suture during pregnancy may be advised.

> Felicity has one final question: *'Does the new vaccine prevent these changes happening?'*

The National HPV Vaccination Program commenced for girls in 2007 and for boys in 2013, using a quadrivalent vaccine against HPV types 6, 11, 16 and 18 (Gardasil). This vaccine is effective in preventing infection with the oncogenic HPV types (16 and 18) that cause 70–80% of cervical cancer in Australia. It is also effective against lesions (warts) related to HPV 6 and 11 infections.

In 2018, Australia commenced using the nonavalent HPV vaccine Gardasil9, replacing the quadrivalent vaccine Gardasil, protecting against an additional 5 strains of HPV (types 6, 11, 16, 18, 31, 33, 45, 52 and 58). The Gardasil9 program reduces the number of doses from 3 to 2 (spaced 6–12 months apart).

Vaccine-induced protection appears to last for many years, although further follow-up is in place. Generally, the vaccines are well tolerated but they may produce local discomfort or pain, redness, fatigue, headache and muscle pains in the day or so after administration.

So your answer to Felicity is—yes, we hope that in future this will be the case for women who have undergone a full course of vaccination, now widely available.

CLINICAL PEARLS

Each year in Australia approximately 900 new cases of cervical cancer are diagnosed and over 200 women die from the disease. It is the 14th most common cancer in Australian women. Australian rates of cervical cancer incidence and death are among the lowest in the world. This is largely attributed to the successful introduction in 1991 of the National Cervical Screening Program (NCSP). From 2012 to 2016, 74% of women survived their cervical cancer for 5 years or more.

With regular cervical screening and appropriate treatment when abnormalities are detected, most cervical cancer could be prevented. The introduction of vaccines that are protective against the two common high-risk types of HPV (types 16 and 18) will hopefully contribute even more significantly to the prevention of the majority of cervical cancers in the near future.

References and further reading

Australian Government Department of Health. National Cervical Screening Program. www.cancerscreening.gov.au/internet/screening/publishing.nsf /Content/health-care providers and www.health.gov.au/initiatives-and -program/national-cervical-screening-program

Australian Institute of Health and Welfare. Cancer data in Australia. Canberra: AIHW; 2020. www.aihw.gov.au/reports/cancer/cancer-data-in-australia /contents/summary

Cancer Council Australia, Cervical Cancer Screening Guidelines Working Party. National cervical screening program: guidelines for the management of screen-detected abnormalities, screening in specific populations and investigation of abnormal vaginal bleeding. Sydney: Cancer Council Australia; 2020. https://wiki.cancer.org.au/australia/Guidelines:Cervical _cancer/Screening

Case 4
Mai Ling is missing school because of heavy periods. . .

Mai Ling is a 14-year-old schoolgirl who is brought to see you by her mother. Mai Ling has had very heavy periods for the past 12 months. She is feeling tired and listless, and is missing several days of school each month at the time of her period.

What are the important points to note in your first consultation with Mai Ling?

It is important to understand the sensitivities of dealing with a young teenager with menstrual problems. She may be embarrassed by the visit and need her mother's help in answering questions. Alternatively, she may be quite confident and may actually prefer not to have her mother present. Note: It is appropriate to suggest that you spend part of the consultation with Mai Ling alone. You can explain to both Mai Ling and her mother that this is your normal practice with patients of Mai Ling's age. If she and her mother agree, this will give her the opportunity to raise issues of concern to her. If she indicates that she has become sexually active, you can take the opportunity to talk about effective contraception and the importance of safe sex.

You need to be sensitive and circumspect when inquiring about sexual activity in a minor. There is no perfect way to handle this question, but it is important to ask. If she is sexually active and her mother is unaware of this, you should encourage her to tell her mother, but you should preserve patient–doctor confidentiality. This is a complex social and medicolegal situation, and advice should be sought if you think she is in any danger from her activity.

What history do you take from Mai Ling?

Mai Ling's menarche was at age 11, and for the first 12 months her periods were irregular, light and painless. About 12 months ago, they became more regular, occurring once a month (indicating the onset of regular ovulation), but they have become increasingly heavy. She bleeds heavily for 7 days, regularly every 28 days, and is experiencing moderate cramping menstrual pain on day 1. She uses large pads, changes every 2 hours, on days 1–2 of bleeding. She has never used tampons. She has been vaccinated against human papillomavirus (HPV). Otherwise there is no relevant medical or surgical history; Mai Ling has always been in good health.

Is there a family history of bleeding abnormalities?

Mai Ling's mother tells you there is no known history of bleeding abnormalities in the family.

What examination of Mai Ling is indicated?

You conduct a general examination of Mai Ling and specifically look for signs of anaemia. You find that she does have pale conjunctivae and is mildly tachycardic—pulse rate 90 beats per minute (bpm) at rest. Abdominal examination reveals no masses. Mai Ling then tells you that she has never been sexually active. You explain to her that there is no reason for you to perform a vaginal examination for her.

> You should never perform a vaginal examination on a young woman who has never had sexual intercourse. An abdominal examination is all that is required. Rectal examination to detect any uterine masses is not warranted either in a young and potentially vulnerable girl. In the rare event of abdominal palpation detecting a mass arising from the pelvis or if there is a suspicion of a pelvic pathology, an ultrasound scan may be performed prior to specialist referral.

What investigations do you order for Mai Ling?

Mai Ling should have a full blood count (FBC) performed. You also order a coagulation screen for her and testing for von Willebrand factor. A week later, she returns to see you for the results of these tests:

- FBC: haemoglobin—90 g/L, with evidence of a hypochromic, microcytic picture.
- Coagulation screen, including testing for the absence or deficiency of von Willebrand factor—normal.

Bleeding diatheses must be excluded in this group of patients: von Willebrand disease is the most common. Consider referral to a haematologist if there are blood coagulation abnormalities or a family history.

How do you now manage Mai Ling's problem?

You recommend oral iron-folate supplementation for Mai Ling, as she has iron-deficiency anaemia secondary to her excessive menstrual blood loss. You also recommend that she take a 50 µg ethinyloestradiol COCP in order to control her heavy periods, and discuss the use of this with Mai Ling and her mother. You explain that the pill has roles other than contraception. You advise her about the common initial side effects of nausea and headache, explaining that these will generally resolve quickly with continued use of the medication. You also explain that the pills may be taken continuously—up to 3 months at a time is common practice, reducing periods to 4 times a year, and that this has no harmful short-term or long-term effects while also decreasing the amount of blood loss.

CLINICAL COMMENT

Treating heavy menstrual bleeding in teenagers

- Oral iron supplementation is usually required for only 2–3 months.
- In general, triphasic oral contraceptive pills are not useful for symptom control, as 30% of women still ovulate on these pills, which may not control symptoms such as menorrhagia or dysmenorrhoea. Even a 30 µg monophasic pill may not sufficiently inhibit the menstrual cycle of a teenager, so a 50 µg pill may be more appropriate.
- You must remember to tell the patient to take the pill every day. Missed pills will result in breakthrough bleeding or, if used for contraception, possible unplanned pregnancy.
- The COCP is also helpful in controlling menstrual pain. Other possible alternative treatments include NSAIDs and tranexamic acid, but the COCP is the easiest and most effective treatment in this age group.
- The LNG-IUD may be considered if medical treatment is not successful and the teenager is sexually active.

When do you arrange to see Mai Ling again?

You see Mai Ling 3 months later. Her haemoglobin level is now normal and she is no longer experiencing symptoms of anaemia. Her periods now last for 3 days, and are light and pain-free. They are no longer interfering with her school and sporting life. She wants to know how long she should remain on the pill. You advise her that she may continue safely on the pill until such time as she wants to have a baby but that she should return for annual checkups with your practice. You further explain that if and when she becomes sexually active she should return to see you to make sure she completely understands the contraceptive effects of the pill and what other precautions should be taken.

 CLINICAL PEARLS

When assessing the effect of the COCP on menstrual symptoms, it is important to wait for 2–3 cycles to judge the outcome, as symptom control may not occur immediately. It is important not to assume therapeutic failure and change the COCP to a different variety each month, trying to control the symptoms. This will not be effective and can result in severe bleeding due to inappropriate hormonal manipulation.

References and further reading

Australian Commission on Safety and Quality in Health Care. Heavy menstrual bleeding clinical care standard. Sydney: The Commission; 2017. www.safetyandquality.gov.au

Fareeda H, Sass A, Dietrich J. Heavy menstrual bleeding in adolescents. *J Pediatr Adolesc Gynecol.* 2017;30(3):335–40.

Moon L, Perez-Milicua G, Dietrich J. Evaluation and management of heavy menstrual bleeding in adolescents. *Curr Opin Obstet Gynecol.* 2017; 29(5):328–6.

National Institute for Health and Care Excellence. Heavy menstrual bleeding: assessment and management. London: NICE; 2020. www.nice.org.uk/guidance/NG88

Case 5
Carrie's periods are becoming heavier. . .

Carrie is a 41-year-old nurse who attends your practice intermittently. Carrie's menstrual periods have become increasingly heavy over the past few years.

What history do you take from Carrie?

Carrie tells you that when she last saw you for a cervical screening test (CST) 6 years ago, her periods were normal. She consulted you at that time for a referral for sterilisation as she had completed her family and wanted to stop taking the COCP. A laparoscopic clip sterilisation was performed 6 months later at the local hospital. Since then, her periods have become heavier. During the first 4–5 days of her period, she passes large clots, and also has flooding, which is enough to overwhelm both a tampon and a large menstrual pad. She has had some 'accidents' with blood on her clothes, which she finds mortifying. Her periods still occur regularly every 28 days but have lengthened to 7–8 days' duration, although the heavy bleeding is limited to the first 4–5 days. Carrie has some crampy pain related to passing the larger clots, but otherwise experiences only mild discomfort during menstruation. She feels tired and worn out most of the time, which she attributes to her long working hours and the pressures of having to bring up a young family. Carrie is wondering if she should have a dilatation and curettage (D&C), in the hope that her periods will return to normal.

> Menstrual loss is usually significantly reduced with COCP use—it is possible that the COCP had effectively prevented Carrie's heavy menstrual loss, which was revealed after she ceased taking the pill after the sterilisation. When counselling women taking the COCP about sterilisation procedures, it is important to explain that stopping the pill will result in natural cycles returning—if these were previously heavy, this may be the case again.

CLINICAL COMMENT

- Heavy menstrual bleeding (HMB) (formerly called menorrhagia or dysfunctional uterine bleeding) is a common problem affecting up to 25% of women of reproductive age.
- Heavy menstrual bleeding has been defined by the National Institute for Health and Care Excellence as 'excessive menstrual blood loss which interferes with a woman's physical, social, emotional and/or material quality of life. It can occur alone or in combination with other symptoms.'
- Around 50% of women referred to secondary care for heavy menstrual bleeding experience severe or very severe pain, even when they do not have any uterine pathology, and many women who seek medical help do so because of disabling pain.
- Remember to perform a cervical screening test if your patient is due (or overdue) for the next screen.
- Obtaining effective menstrual hygiene can be expensive if a woman has very heavy periods.
- Dilatation and curettage is a diagnostic procedure and does not have any therapeutic effect.

What are the important points to note in your consultation with Carrie?

Important points to note when taking a history include the following:

- the woman's sexual and reproductive health, her desire for future fertility and cervical screening status
- the duration, timing, heaviness and chronicity of the bleeding and its impact on her daily activities and quality of life (postcoital and intermenstrual bleeding are different from heavy menstrual bleeding and require investigation)
- symptoms including pelvic pain or pressure, and fatigue
- symptoms suggesting a bleeding disorder
- symptoms associated with polycystic ovarian syndrome (PCOS) including acne, hirsutism and irregular bleeding

You should also ask if she has been experiencing any symptoms of menopause, such as missed periods or hot flushes.

Carrie reports that she does not have any of these symptoms.

What examination do you conduct for Carrie?

First, you explain that you would like to examine her, including a pelvic examination and a CST, as she is overdue for this test. You examine Carrie's conjunctivae and nail beds to assess clinical signs of anaemia and note that she does appear quite pale. Next, you examine her abdomen, looking for any masses, in particular to assess whether there is an enlarged uterus arising from the pelvis. Then, you perform a speculum examination and CST, noting that Carrie's cervix appears normal. Finally, you perform a bimanual pelvic examination to assess the size, consistency and position of her uterus, and palpate both adnexae to exclude any masses, also noting whether any part of the examination elicits pain or tenderness (Fig. 5.1). You find that Carrie has a normally sized anteverted uterus with no adnexal masses or tenderness.

(a)   (b)

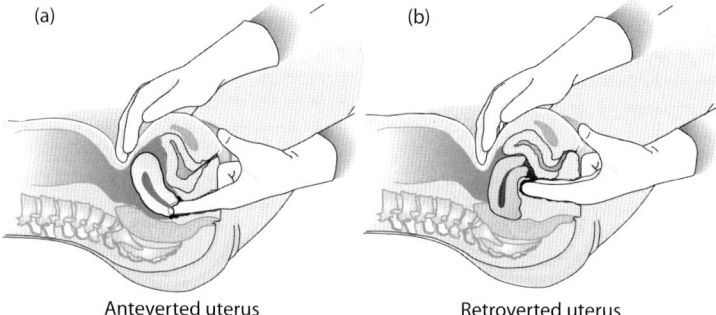

Anteverted uterus   Retroverted uterus

Figure 5.1 Performing a bimanual vaginal examination. The uterus is palpated for size, shape and position, and the adnexae are palpated for enlargement or tenderness. (**a**) Anteverted uterus (**b**) Retroverted uterus

Heavy menstrual bleeding—important clinical points

- Heavy menstrual periods can result in anaemia.
- Always examine the woman fully, including blood pressure and abdominal and bimanual pelvic examination.
- The uterus may not necessarily be enlarged.
- If the uterus is enlarged, the diagnosis may be uterine fibromyomata (fibroids) or adenomyosis. However, a normal-sized uterus may still be the site of pathology including polyps

and endometrial hyperplasia. Pelvic ultrasound may be useful in this circumstance.
- Malignancy (endometrial carcinoma) is rare in the premenopausal age group. You should always inquire about intermenstrual bleeding, postcoital bleeding and abnormal vaginal discharge. Referral to a gynaecologist is mandatory with these symptoms. Women over the age of 45 or obese women (who are at greater risk of endometrial cancer) may also need to be referred early for specialist opinion.

What investigations are indicated for Carrie?

You arrange a full blood count (FBC), to assess the possibility of anaemia, and an ultrasound scan (USS), and discuss the likely causes of the heavy bleeding with Carrie. At this stage, you feel that there is no need to refer her to a gynaecologist as the periods, although heavy, are not alarming, there are no symptoms to suggest malignancy and there are no abnormal findings on examination to suggest uterine fibroids, endometriosis or pelvic inflammatory disease. You explain to her that a D&C does not have a therapeutic effect and will be unlikely to return her periods to normal. There are several possible treatment options for Carrie, both medical and surgical. She is keen to avoid surgery as she cannot afford the time off work. You explain that common medical treatments include nonsteroidal anti-inflammatory drugs (NSAIDs), tranexamic acid, the COCP and the levonorgestrel-releasing intrauterine device (LNG-IUD, e.g. Mirena© or Kyleena©). For completeness, you also explain to her that the surgical options include endometrial ablation and hysterectomy.

 CLINICAL COMMENT

Medical options for the treatment of heavy menstrual bleeding
- NSAIDs (e.g. mefenamic acid, naproxen) can bring about up to a 25% reduction in menstrual loss. Ideally, they should be commenced 5–7 days prior to menstruation. They are also helpful for reducing menstrual pain. The main side effect is gastric irritation.
- Tranexamic acid, an antifibrinolytic, can produce up to a 40% reduction in menstrual loss. It is usually taken on the first three days of bleeding, when it is most commonly heavy. The

continued

continued

most common side effects are nausea and abdominal bloating. Tranexamic acid can be taken in conjunction with NSAIDs.

- Periods are lighter and less painful on the monophasic COCP. Various types of COCP can be tried if an earlier choice is unsuccessful, but they need to be continued for three cycles before the effect can be gauged. They are useful if contraception is required and allow timing of commencement of NSAIDs in women with otherwise irregular cycles.
- The levonorgestrel-releasing intrauterine device (LNG-IUD) is the most effective medical therapy for HMB, with an 80% reduction in menstrual loss, and it can remain in situ for 5 years. The most common complaint is daily spotting and cramps for the first 3–5 months; women should be warned in advance that this may happen. The IUD also provides contraception for women requiring this.

Surgical options for the treatment of heavy menstrual bleeding

- Endometrial ablation—50% of patients become amenorrhoeic, 40% have reduced periods and 10% are unchanged. There are a variety of different methods available, but meta-analysis suggests that radiofrequency ablation techniques are the most effective. The procedure is best reserved for women whose families are definitely complete, for example, if either the woman or her partner has been sterilised. It is not a contraceptive and, if sterilisation has not been performed or is not performed concurrently, contraception must be provided.
- Hysteroscopic resection—this method is effective if the HMB is caused by endometrial polyps or fibroid polyps.
- Hysterectomy—this may be abdominal, vaginal or laparoscopic. There is a 100% guarantee of success, but it remains major surgery with all of the associated risks. In general, it should be considered only when other options have been unsuccessful.
- Uterine artery embolisation—this is performed by interventional radiology for multiple large fibroids as a uterine sparing procedure in order to preserve the reproductive function of the uterus. This is performed in specialised units.

How do you follow up Carrie?

Two weeks later, Carrie returns to you for the results of her tests and her decision regarding treatment. Her CST report is normal, and you remind her when the next one is due, following national screening program recommendations (see Case 2). You provide her with a reminder card. Her USS has been reported as showing a normal pelvis with, in particular, no endometrial abnormality. Her FBC shows a haemoglobin (Hb) value of 95 g/L and you place her on oral iron supplements until the treatment for reducing the degree of menstrual blood loss is successful. She has decided to try tranexamic acid because she feels this will suit her circumstances best. You arrange for her to see you again in 3 months' time, with a menstrual calendar recording her loss so you can both review the success of this approach.

CLINICAL PEARLS

- A woman with heavy but regular periods and with normal findings on general clinical examination and investigation in general practice does not require immediate gynaecological referral—medical treatment can be tried.
- Remember to ask about intermenstrual or postcoital bleeding—these symptoms, or any history of irregular bleeding, mean that the woman should be further investigated before any treatment is commenced.
- Do not overlook general health concerns and remember to take a CST.

References and further reading

Australian Commission on Safety and Quality in Health Care. Heavy menstrual bleeding clinical care standard. Sydney: The Commission; 2017. http://www.safetyandquality.gov.au/

National Institute for Health and Care Excellence. Heavy menstrual bleeding: assessment and management. London: NICE; 2020. www.nice.org.uk/guidance/NG88

Case 6
Chloe has severe period pains. . .

Chloe is a 13-year-old schoolgirl brought along by her mother to see you because of increasingly severe period pain. Each month for the past 3 months Chloe has needed 2 days away from school because of period-associated pain. This is interfering with her ability to play competition netball, which she loves. Chloe has tried paracetamol, aspirin and hot-water bottles for the pain, with only partial success. Her last period, the most painful yet, has just finished.

What is the likely diagnosis here?

The most likely diagnosis is primary dysmenorrhoea due to prostaglandins produced by the disintegrating endometrium, causing painful uterine contractions. However, it is important not to overlook occasional rare causes of lower abdominal pain in young teenagers. Chloe should also be reassured so that she does not start to see her normal bodily functions in a negative light.

How do you manage this consultation?

You take a history from Chloe, with her mother present. Her first period occurred when she was 11, and for several months cycles were irregular and periods pain-free. Over the past year, her cycles have gradually become regular, with bleeding every 30 days lasting 4–5 days. Pain is cramping in nature and begins at the same time as the bleeding, on day 1, not resolving completely until day 3. Bleeding is not particularly heavy, by both Chloe's and her mother's estimates.

Chloe's health is otherwise good. She has occasional mild asthma but no history of allergy to any medication, including NSAIDs. She had her appendix removed at the age of 8, and her tonsils when she was 10. She is in Year 8 at school and is fitting well into school life.

Characteristically, primary dysmenorrhoea does not occur in the first cycles after the menarche, which are anovulatory, but only begins following ovulation, when the cycle usually becomes more regular. This happens 1–2 years after menarche.

What examination do you make?

You conduct a brief general physical examination of Chloe. She looks well, with no signs of anaemia, and is neither overweight nor underweight. Her heart sounds are normal. Abdominal palpation reveals no tenderness or masses.

Is it necessary to perform a vaginal examination?

No. If the abdominal examination is unremarkable and the girl has a characteristic history of primary dysmenorrhoea, it can be assumed that the pelvic organs are normal. In the rare event of a lower abdominal mass being found or if you suspect some pelvic pathology, an ultrasound scan should be performed. You should not perform a vaginal examination in a teenager who has not had penile-vaginal sex.

What treatment do you suggest for Chloe?

You explain to Chloe and her mother that period pain like hers is common among girls of her age but that she appears to be experiencing more pain than most. You also explain the principle of using NSAIDs in a prophylactic manner to try to prevent the dysmenorrhoea.

Prostaglandin synthetase inhibitors, by preventing the formation of prostaglandins in the endometrium, reduce future pain but are ineffective against prostaglandins already formed.

You recommend Chloe take one of the common over-the-counter NSAIDs, such as naproxen or mefenamic acid. You suggest that she keep a menstrual calendar so that she can take the NSAIDs a day before her period starts. She can continue this treatment regularly over the first 2 days of bleeding, which is when she experiences the most pain. You warn her about gastrointestinal symptoms and recommend taking it with food or milk.

> Chloe's mother then tells you that she herself suffered painful periods for years and eventually had a hysterectomy. She is worried that Chloe may be on the same course. How do you respond?

You explain that Chloe's symptoms are quite normal and not necessarily an indication of future problems. You reinforce your approval of Chloe's already healthy lifestyle and arrange to see her in 3 months' time to assess the benefits of your therapy. You stress that surgery such as laparoscopy or dilatation and curettage (D&C) would not be appropriate.

CLINICAL PEARLS

- It is important when dealing with situations such as this that the girl does not come to see her normal physiology from a negative point of view.
- Surgery has no place in the management of primary dysmenorrhoea.

References and further reading

Burnett M, Lemyre M. Primary dysmenorrhea. *J Obstet Gyneccol Can.* 2017;39(7):585–95.

Ryan S. The treatment of dysmenorrhea. *Pediatr Clin North Am.* 2017;64(2):331–42.

Society of Obstetricians and Gynecologists of Canada. Primary dysmenorrhea consensus guidelines. Ottawa: SOGC; 2017. www.sogc.org

Case 7
April is bothered by facial hair. . .

April is a 19-year-old Aboriginal woman who comes seeking your help with facial hair. She tells you that over the last few years she's been growing more and more hair over her jaw and chin. She has tried various removal techniques such as plucking and waxing but with limited success. She says to you, 'My mum thinks I might need some medicine for it, but I don't know how that will help.'

What is your response to April?

You explain that you first need to know more about April and take a full history. She tells you that the hair is most marked on her face but is also present on her chest and back. She is very embarrassed by it. It is dark and coarse. She is also bothered by acne on her face and back.

What history do you take from April?

You take a full menstrual history from April. Her periods began when she was 14. They have always been irregular and unpredictable. Her cycles vary from 1 to 3 months in length, and the periods themselves are sometimes light but sometimes heavy with the passage of clots and dysmenorrhoea. On questioning, April also says that she has had a tendency to put on weight for the past 3 years, although she states she's always been a 'big girl'. She played football when she was at high school, but doesn't exercise much anymore.

In the past, April has had no serious illness or surgical operations and the only relevant family history is her mother's type 2 diabetes. She does not have a boyfriend and has never been sexually active.

What examination do you perform for April?

You then conduct a physical examination for April. General examination shows a young woman of height 165 cm and weight 80 kg, yielding a body mass index (BMI) of 29.4 kg/m². She has a moderate degree of hirsutism around her jaw and below her chin, and a mild degree of acne. The hair is also visible on her back and chest. Her BP is 130/70 mmHg. You inspect and palpate her abdomen; nothing abnormal is detected.

Should you perform a vaginal examination?

No. April has indicated that she is not sexually active, and no useful information is likely to be gained from the examination anyway.

What is your clinical impression and what is your next step?

April's history and examination provide a diagnosis of polycystic ovarian syndrome (PCOS)—she has signs of androgen excess (hirsutism and acne), irregular menstrual cycles suggestive of unopposed oestrogen and a tendency to obesity.

PCOS is a significant public health issue with reproductive, metabolic and psychological features. PCOS is one of the most common conditions in reproductive-aged women, affecting 8–13% of reproductive-aged women, with up to 70% of affected women remaining undiagnosed. Presentation varies by ethnicity and in high-risk populations such as indigenous women, prevalence and complications are higher. Women with PCOS present with diverse features including psychological (anxiety, depression, body image), reproductive (irregular menstrual cycles, hirsutism, infertility and pregnancy complications) and metabolic features (insulin resistance, metabolic syndrome, prediabetes, type 2 diabetes (DM2) and cardiovascular risk factors.

 CLINICAL COMMENT

Polycystic ovarian syndrome

- Diagnosis and treatment of PCOS remain controversial and challenging due to significant clinical heterogeneity, ethnic differences and variation in clinical features across a woman's life course.
- This leads to delayed diagnosis, poor diagnosis experience and dissatisfaction with care reported by women all over the world.
- Consider PCOS if women present with menstrual irregularity, overweight, hirsutism, acne, fertility issues, prediabetes, gestational diabetes or early-onset type 2 diabetes.

What investigations should you arrange for April?

A diagnosis of PCOS can be made on the grounds of irregular cycles plus clinical hyperandrogenism so long as other causes have been excluded such as a thyroid disorder or hyperprolactinaemia (Table 7.1).

A pelvic ultrasound is not indicated as April is <8 years after menarche.

Table 7.1 Diagnosis of PCOS

Step 1: Irregular cycles + clinical hyperandrogenism = diagnosis	**Irregular cycles** In women >3 years post menarche to perimenopause: • <21-day or >35-day cycles In adolescents: • No period by age 15 • >1 year post-menarche cycles >90 days • >1 to <3 years post-menarche cycles <21 or >45 days **Clinical hyperandrogenism** • hirsutism • acne • alopecia
Step 2: If no clinical hyperandrogenism Test for biochemical hyperandrogenism = diagnosis	**Biochemical androgens** • Measure after 3-month cessation of COCP • Measure sex hormone binding globulin (SHBG), total testosterone and free androgen index
Step 3: If ONLY irregular cycles OR hyperandrogenism: ultrasound	**Adolescents** • Ultrasound should not be used for the diagnosis in those <8 years after menarche, due to the high incidence of multi-follicular ovaries in this life stage • Should be considered 'at risk' and receive follow-up assessment **Adults** • In patients with irregular menstrual cycles and hyperandrogenism, an ovarian ultrasound is not necessary for PCOS diagnosis

How do you manage this situation?

You tell April that she has PCOS. You explain that PCOS is the most common endocrine problem in women of reproductive age. You carefully explain to April that PCOS may cause difficulties in reproductive health, including an irregular menstrual cycle, but also later in life may cause fertility difficulties.

You reassure her that it is very common to feel depressed or anxious about this and that a psychologist can help her with this; you can offer her a referral.

You also mention that young women with PCOS have a higher incidence of diabetes, hypertension and cardiovascular disease in later life—April's family history of diabetes is significant in this regard. The most important thing for April is to achieve and maintain a healthy weight. You point out that attention to diet and undertaking regular exercise can have a positive impact on April's health generally and reduce the undesirable effects of PCOS. You offer her a referral to see a dietitian.

You then recommend April start the COCP, to regulate her menstrual cycles as well as help improve her facial hair issues. You warn her, however, that it may take several months for her to observe this improvement. She is agreeable to this. You tell her to commence it at the time of her next period and you arrange to review her in 3 months' time.

 CLINICAL PEARLS

> The high prevalence of PCOS found in high-risk populations such as Indigenous women means that healthcare providers need to be aware of both diagnosis and best-practice management of PCOS. A lower threshold for screening Indigenous women for PCOS may be necessary.

References and further reading

Boyle JA, Cunningham J, Norman RJ, et al. Polycystic ovary syndrome and metabolic syndrome in Indigenous Australian women. *Intern Med J.* 2015;45(12):1247–54.

Jean Hailes for Women's Health. PCOS health professional tool. www.jeanhailes.org.au/resources/pcos-health-professional-tool

Teede H, Misso M, Costello M, et al. International evidence-based guideline for the assessment and management of polycystic ovary syndrome 2018. Melbourne: Monash University on behalf of the NHMRC, Centre for Research Excellence in PCOS and the Australian PCOS Alliance; 2018. www.monash.edu/__data/assets/pdf_file/0004/1412644/PCOS_Evidence-Based-Guidelines_20181009.pdf

Case 8
Michelle still hasn't started her periods. . .

Michelle comes to see you with her mother. You have been caring for the family for a number of years and have known Michelle since she was a young girl. She is now aged 17, in the final year of high school, and has not had her first period. This didn't trouble Michelle initially—she is a sporty girl who is a keen runner and swimmer and plays basketball. She knows that women who are slim and train regularly can have sparse periods.

Her mother doesn't see it that way, as Michelle's breast development began 4 years earlier and she read in a family medical guide that the periods should have started within 2 years of that event. Her mother wants you to confirm that there are no underlying problems.

Puberty

Michelle is the middle child in a sibship of three. Her older brother is 19 and has joined the navy, where he is studying to be an officer. He is a healthy man and had no medical problems or developmental delays. Michelle's younger sister is only 12 and she too is fit and well; she has not yet had any periods. Both of Michelle's parents are healthy and well, and your review of the family history reveals no evidence of any developmental problems.

Michelle developed normally as a girl, always meeting her milestones. She is a strong performer at school and seems to have a healthy diet and normal appetite. Discussion with her teachers has revealed no abnormal stresses at school, and Michelle enjoys her studies. You know from your contact with her family over the years that her home environment is loving and supportive. Her immunisations are up to date. Apart from a febrile convulsion as a toddler, she has never had any major health problems and there are no allergies.

Her mother tells you that breast development began when Michelle was 10 years old, and she developed body hair from about 13 years of age. She reached her current height, 170 cm, last year and in all respects seems to have normal adult development (Table 8.1, Fig. 8.1).

Table 8.1 Normal sequence of puberty changes in females

Thelarche	Initial development of the breasts	Usually between 10 and 12 years
Pubarche	Growth of pubic hair	Up to 6 months after breast thelarche
Menarche	The first period	About 2 years after thelarche

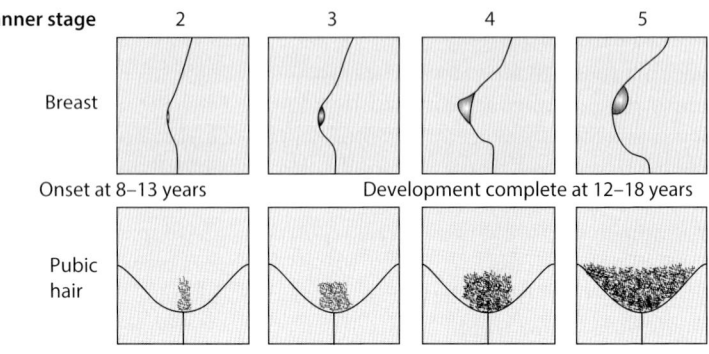

Tanner stage	2	3	4	5
Breast				

Onset at 8–13 years   Development complete at 12–18 years

Pubic hair

Menarche occurs at 10–16 years, correlating most closely with T4 development. Growth spurt at 5–8 cm/year and 3–8 kg/year, peaking at T3–4.

Figure 8.1 Tanner stages of breast and hair development

You see Michelle in private

You take the opportunity to speak with Michelle without her mother present, explaining that this is your normal practice, and find out that although she is attracted to boys, she does not have a boyfriend and has not yet been sexually active. She is very interested in sports, particularly amateur horseriding, and is motivated to become a vet, so she has been studying hard to achieve good marks. On examination, her weight is 62 kg, yielding a BMI of 21.4 kg/m², which is in the normal range—she is not noticeably underweight. Her distribution of body hair is normal for her age. Blood pressure and heart sounds are normal, and her thyroid appears normal. You find no specific abnormality on general examination. Michelle's abdomen is soft with no masses. Since she is not sexually active, you do not perform an internal examination. However, her external genitalia appear normal and mature.

Since Michelle's mother seems particularly concerned to rule out a problem, you sit down and speak with both of them. You explain that there is a wide variation in normal, but that you will undertake some preliminary tests to exclude major pathologies (Table 8.2). You arrange a check of Michelle's FSH, LH, prolactin level and TSH and a pelvic ultrasound scan (USS), and arrange to see them in 2 weeks with the results.

Table 8.2 Causes of primary amenorrhoea and relevant investigations

Condition	Diagnostic investigation
Pregnancy	Positive β-hCG test
Hypothyroidism	Elevated serum TSH level
Hyperprolactinaemia	Elevated serum prolactin, possible pituitary adenoma on imaging
Hypogonadism	Low level of FSH—may be associated with constitutional delay, over-training, underweight, eating disorders, stress, hypopituitarism
PCOS	Elevated LH, typical ovarian appearances on USS
Premature ovarian failure	Elevated FSH, very low AMH—may be associated with chromosomal abnormality such as Turner syndrome (45 X karyotype) or fragile X syndrome
Anatomical abnormality	Vaginal obstruction with 'cryptomenorrhoea'—imperforate hymen; absent uterus
Feminised male	Androgen insensitivity, 46 XY karyotype

A distressing discovery

When you see Michelle and her mother again for their follow-up visit, they are both distressed by the news you have for them. Although the hormone levels—FSH, LH, TSH and prolactin—are all normal, the pelvic USS has revealed a major abnormality. The ovaries are present, although high on the pelvic side wall, but the uterus and cervix are absent. It appears that the upper part of the vagina is also absent, with only the lower portion visible on the ultrasound. This is uterine agenesis, or Mayer–Rokitansky–Küster–Hauser syndrome.

You refer Michelle to the adolescent gynaecology unit of the local tertiary hospital. About 3 months later, both Michelle and her mother return to see you. Michelle had an MRI that confirmed the ultrasound findings and also excluded any associated abnormality of the urinary tract. This information is important, since as many as one-third of women with anatomical abnormalities of the reproductive tract have additional abnormalities of the urinary tract. Michelle's karyotype was checked and she has been found to have a normal set of female chromosomes: 46 XX. The specialist team spent a lot of time with her and put her in touch with an online support group and an experienced local counsellor. The awkward issue of intercourse was discussed, and Michelle is aware that the use of graded dilators is likely to allow her to have satisfactory intercourse when she does wish to begin an intimate relationship. Because the embryological origin of the reproductive tract is quite separate from that of the ovaries, she will have a normal hormonal cycle with release of eggs, although pregnancy will not be possible. However, in the future she would be able to consider the use of a surrogate, so that, with IVF, her own eggs could be collected and embryos created that are transferred to the uterus of another woman.

You sense that Michelle will have a difficult time over the years ahead and explain that you are keen to maintain a good relationship and will always be happy to see her for consultation.

 CLINICAL PEARLS

- Any young woman who has not had her first period either 3 years after the first stages of breast development, or by the age of 16, should have an examination and some preliminary tests.
- Teenagers of both sexes are naturally anxious to be assured that they are 'normal', and major disorders of the reproductive system require great tact and empathy in management.

References and further reading

Klein D, Paradise S, Reeder R. Amenorrhoea: a systematic approach to diagnosis and management. *Am Fam Physician*. 2019;100(1):39–48.

Nisenblat V. Primary amenorrhoea. *O&G Magazine*. 2017;19(3 Spring). www.ogmagazine.org.au/19/3-19/primary-amenorrhoea

Case 9
Tracey and Ian are trying for a pregnancy. . .

Tracey is a 38-year-old woman married for the first time 10 months ago. Her husband Ian is aged 52. Ian was married previously and has two sons from that marriage, but Tracey has never been pregnant and the couple have been trying to conceive since their marriage. Both partners come to consult you about the matter.

What are the important facts you wish to establish at the beginning of your history taking with this couple?

Tracey is now quite late in her reproductive years and if a problem with fertility exists, she needs to be given help with this as soon as possible, in contrast to the situation with younger women where it is usual to wait for a full 12 months before commencing fertility investigations. It is important to establish that the couple are regularly achieving full sexual intercourse. Ian is at an age at which erectile dysfunction is becoming increasingly common. Since his sons were conceived, he may have experienced some health problem interfering with fertility or he may have undergone vasectomy and attempted reversal of this.

Initially you see both partners together. You then arrange to see and examine each partner individually. They are agreed that there is no problem achieving full intercourse and that this has occurred at least three or four times per week over the past 10 months. They are also agreed that they would wish to have some investigations if this seems appropriate but are not sure at this stage whether they would go as far as having in vitro fertilisation (IVF). You explain to them that, statistically, after the age of 40, Tracey will quite rapidly become less likely to conceive and that even at age 38 she is less likely to do so spontaneously than when she was under 35. However, the chances of successful spontaneous pregnancy are still quite high for the couple and IVF is certainly an increasingly successful possibility. You recommend that Tracey commence taking folic acid 0.5 mg daily.

At puberty, there are about 250 000 potential ova in a woman's ovaries. In each cycle about 30 ova commence development but normally only one matures fully and is released in the process of ovulation; the remainder are spontaneously inhibited and absorbed. In the course of a woman's reproductive years, she ovulates about 400 times, and by the time she reaches her 40s most of these events of ovulation have been completed. Taking the oral contraceptive pill does not delay this process: degeneration of ova continues while a woman is on the pill.

What history do you take from Tracey?

You find that Tracey is in good general health. Her periods began at the age of 13 and for many years have been regular, 4–5 days in a 29-day cycle. She reports no dysmenorrhoea or dyspareunia. Her last period was 3 weeks previously. In her 20s, she began taking the COCP and continued this with no problems until the age of 36; she has not been taking it recently. You confirm that Tracey has never been pregnant. She has no regular medications, no allergies and no serious illnesses or operations apart from a laparoscopic cholecystectomy at the age of 35; she does not smoke cigarettes; and she drinks alcohol socially. She has never had a sexually transmitted infection. There is no relevant family history; in particular, no history of breast or ovarian cancer or of endometriosis or of genetic disorders. She last had a cervical screening test, reported as normal, in your practice 5 years ago.

In taking a history from a woman presenting for investigation of fertility, it is important to be sure that there have been no previous pregnancies, including ectopic pregnancies, pregnancies ending in miscarriage or termination of pregnancy or full-term pregnancies after which the baby was surrendered for adoption. All of these have implications for current management. On occasion, a woman may not wish to reveal previous pregnancy to her current partner; this desire must be respected and the information kept confidential.

What examination do you perform for Tracey?

On examination, Tracey appears healthy with a BMI in the healthy normal range; BP is 120/80 mmHg. There is no hirsutism, which might suggest PCOS, or galactorrhoea, which might suggest a raised prolactin level. You find nothing remarkable in the cardiovascular or respiratory systems. You examine her abdomen—apart from the small scars of the cholecystectomy, there is nothing of note to find.

Should you perform a vaginal examination for Tracey at this stage?

Yes—apart from giving useful information about the genital organs that may be relevant to her presenting problem, you will also be able to take the CST, which is due.

You carry out a speculum examination looking at the vagina, which appears normal. The cervix also looks normal, with the central circular os characteristic of the nulligravida. You perform the CST. You then carry out a bimanual pelvic examination. You find that the uterus feels somewhat enlarged with irregularities suggestive of fibroids, but there is no tenderness, either on palpating the uterus or on feeling in the lateral fornices, and no masses palpable in the fornices.

What history and examination do you undertake for Ian?

Initially, you will take a general medical history. You find that Ian is also in reasonable health. He has been found to be hypertensive and to have elevated lipid levels; he currently takes a calcium channel blocker for hypertension and a statin to lower lipid levels. He has attended one of your partners recently for a check and both blood pressure and serum lipid levels have been found to be within the normal range. He admits to being overweight but a glucose tolerance test (GTT) returned a normal result. He has two sons aged 24 and 20 with his first wife. Apart from an appendicectomy and an arthroscopy, there is nothing else remarkable in his medical history. In particular, he has had no sexually transmitted infections and no testicular disease or surgery and has not had mumps; there is also no family history of genetic disorders.

> Type 2 diabetes is common in men in this age group, especially when obesity is present, and may be related to erectile dysfunction. It is important to screen for diabetes in a presentation of this type if this has not recently been done.

Should you examine Ian?

Yes—infertility/subfertility involves two people. You should perform a general physical examination and a genital examination. However, it must be said that in practice it is quite common to arrange a semen analysis for the male partner and only proceed to examination if the results are abnormal.

On examination, Ian is normotensive and moderately overweight. There is no evidence of gynaecomastia. Secondary sex characteristics (e.g. facial hair, male pattern body hair distribution) are normal. Genital examination reveals normal-sized testes and penis. A vas deferens can be palpated bilaterally. There is a small, left-sided vericocoele.

What investigations would you perform for Tracey and Ian?

You organise some basic tests for Tracey and Ian. Tracey needs a FBC and measurement of rubella and varicella antibody levels as part of pre-pregnancy screening, and a day-21 serum progesterone level test to see if this is in the ovulatory range. This result returns at 59 nmol/L, which is in the ovulatory range, so no further tests are required. If Tracey had not been ovulating, further tests would have been performed to ascertain a cause. Note that these tests are often ordered routinely but are superfluous if ovulation has been proven. However, a pelvic USS will give useful information about the size and shape of the uterus and ovaries.

Investigations of female infertility/subfertility in general practice

1. **Follicle stimulating hormone (FSH), luteinising hormone (LH)**
   - If these are elevated, this may indicate menopause or resistant ovary syndrome.
   - If these are low, this may indicate pituitary hypogonadism (e.g. anorexia nervosa).

2. **Prolactin**
   - Elevated serum prolactin interferes with pituitary function and may be due to a pituitary adenoma.

3. **Serum androgens, sex hormone binding globulin**
   - Rarely, testosterone-secreting tumours of the ovary or adrenal gland can present as infertility; they more commonly present as virilism.
   - Polycystic ovarian syndrome (PCOS) is the most common cause of anovulatory infertility in women.

4. **Thyroid function tests**
   - Both hyperthyroidism and hypothyroidism can cause anovulation.

Ian requires a semen analysis. You explain to Ian that this is best performed at a specialist andrology laboratory, which will provide a room for the collection. Alternatively, the specimen can be produced at home but it must be delivered to the testing laboratory for examination promptly, as motility of the sperm falls rapidly. The specimen is usually produced by masturbation. You explain to Ian that he must not have sexual intercourse or masturbate for at least 2 days prior to the test. As spermatogenesis takes approximately 3 months, an abnormal semen analysis may be a consequence of a febrile illness during this time. Consequently, all abnormal semen analyses should be repeated after 3 months.

 CLINICAL COMMENT

Semen analysis

Different laboratories may differ in their criteria but the following provides a guide:

- volume—should be greater than 2.5 mL
- sperm concentration—should be greater than 20 million per mL
- motility—more than 50% spermatozoa should show forward motility
- morphology—at least 20% spermatozoa should have a normal shape

Finally, you explain to the couple that you may need to refer them to an infertility specialist gynaecologist for further assessment and possible infertility treatment. You explain that the specialist may want to assess whether Tracey's fallopian tubes are patent, and that this can be done in one of two ways. A hysterosalpingogram (HSG) is an X-ray performed while radio-opaque dye is injected into the uterine cavity via the cervix. If the fallopian tubes are patent, dye can clearly be seen outlining the tubal lumen and spilling from the tubes. Hysterosalpingogram using ultrasound is another method of assessing tubal patency. Alternatively, a laparoscopy can be performed to assess tubal patency, but this requires a general anaesthetic and is usually performed only if there is a suspicion of other pathology, such as endometriosis.

However, considering Tracey's age the specialist may wish to perform more tests, such as the serum level of anti-Müllerian hormone (AMH), if one has not already been done, or an antral follicle count by ultrasound, both of which provide a guide to the reserves of the ovaries.

 CLINICAL PEARLS

- Natural conception requires regular sexual intercourse with ejaculation, the presence of healthy motile spermatozoa, patent fallopian tubes and otherwise normal anatomy, and regular ovulation in the female. Intercurrent health problems in either partner can interfere with conception. A good history and physical examination in general practice can identify many possible barriers to successful conception.
- It is important to emphasise to couples presenting with problems in conceiving that no procedure or treatment exists that can guarantee 100% success in achieving a pregnancy that leads to the birth of a live and healthy baby. Patients should be well-informed about the details, risks and success rates of all investigations and procedures and given time to decide whether or not they wish to be referred for more invasive procedures. It is also worth noting that many infertility treatments may be expensive.

References and further reading

Chambers GM, Harrison C, Raymer J, et al. Infertility management in women and men attending primary care—patient characteristics, management actions and referrals. *Hum Reprod.* 2019;34(1):2173–83.

Katz DJ, Teloken P, Shoshany O. Male infertility—the other side of the equation. *Aust Fam Physician.* 2017;46(9):1641–6.

Case 10
Sara would like to be pregnant. . .

Sara is a 28-year-old woman who comes to see you for a well-woman check but also has a number of other issues to discuss.

Sara is already well-known to you, having been a patient of your practice for at least 10 years. From the age of 18 she took the COCP, both for contraception and for the control of heavy painful periods. At 24, having been married a year, she stopped the pill with the intention of trying to become pregnant. However, within 9 months, her periods were again very heavy and irregular, and she had not conceived and was, in fact, experiencing some deep dyspareunia that was making her attempts to conceive difficult. You referred her to a gynaecologist, Dr Yu, who performed a laparoscopy and found a moderate degree of endometriosis. Areas of endometriosis, particularly on the uterosacral ligaments, were then resected. Tubal patency was confirmed by dye hydrotubation. Following explanation of the presence of residual endometriosis and her symptoms, Sara elected to have a 6-month course of medroxyprogesterone. 'I was fed up with bleeding all the time,' she said. 'I wanted some time to think over the whole thing.' Two years ago, at the time of her last well-woman check, she decided to go back on the COCP for at least a year before trying again to conceive. You renewed her prescription last year when she was well and have not seen her since.

> Endometriosis may be asymptomatic but when symptoms occur they are characteristically pelvic pain, dysmenorrhoea, deep dyspareunia, menorrhagia and infertility. Small areas of endometriosis may cause severe symptoms (e.g. nodules of endometriosis on the uterosacral ligaments may be the cause of severe dyspareunia); conversely, large areas of endometriosis with extensive pelvic adhesions may be asymptomatic. A definite diagnosis of endometriosis can only be made at laparoscopy or laparotomy, although the condition may be suspected from the history. There is also a familial tendency to endometriosis. Pelvic USS may help with the diagnosis of endometriosis affecting the ovaries, i.e. endometrioma, but will not detect pelvic deposits.

At this consultation, Sara tells you that she stopped the COCP 4 months ago. 'My periods are back,' she says, 'regular but not heavy and quite manageable. However, I'm still not pregnant although we're trying, and I'm afraid I've got this discharge. . .'

What history do you take from Sara?

She tells you that the discharge is watery and occasionally pink, not offensive and not burning, stinging or itching. It is most profuse after sex, and she finds this embarrassing and uncomfortable. She is absolutely certain there is no possibility of an STI and denies that either she or her partner has ever had an STI. She has been well since her last consultation with you; apart from her endometriosis and its associated symptoms, Sara has always enjoyed good health. She is on no medications, has had no surgery apart from the laparoscopy, does not smoke and has no allergies. Since she has been trying to conceive, she has abstained from alcohol and takes folic acid daily. Her partner, who is a patient of your practice, is also in good health, although he has never had a semen analysis performed.

What examination do you make for Sara?

You perform a short general examination, including checking the blood pressure and auscultating the heart. You inspect and palpate the abdomen, finding nothing remarkable and, in particular, no lower abdominal tenderness or masses. You then perform a vaginal examination.

What are your expected findings on vaginal examination?

Given that a discharge related to an STI is unlikely, there is the possibility of a candida infection or a cervical ectropion associated with COCP use.

On passing a speculum, however, what you observe is a large cervical polyp protruding on a stalk through the cervical os. This is very mobile but it is not possible to see the top of the stalk. On moving the polyp aside to take the Pap smear, you also note a moderate degree of cervical ectropion as expected in a woman who has been taking the COCP. The polyp appears benign.

Causes of vaginal discharge

- Physiological discharge—may be more marked when a degree of cervical ectropion (ectopy) is present
- Infections—cervical (chlamydia, gonococcal) or vaginal (candida, trichomoniasis, bacterial vaginosis, group B streptococcus, anaerobic bowel organisms)
- Cervical lesions—polyps, cancer, HSV, warts
- Foreign bodies (tampon, condom)
- Trauma to the vagina or cervix

In many women, especially those on the COCP or during or after pregnancy, the squamocolumnar junction is located well onto the vaginal surface of the cervix. The exposed endocervical tissue (ectropion) is mucus-producing and may be responsible for symptomatic discharge.

You also perform a bimanual examination for Sara. The polyp is easily palpable but otherwise the uterus is normal in size, anteverted and mobile. There is no tenderness in the fornices or over the uterosacral ligaments, and no palpable masses in the adnexae.

What is your next step?

You explain your findings to Sara when she is dressed and back in your consulting room. You explain that cervical polyps with the attachment of the stalk clearly visible can be removed easily with polyp forceps in your surgery but as you cannot see the top you will refer her back to Dr Yu for its removal at hysteroscopy (Fig. 10.1). Dr Yu will probably also inspect the remainder of the cervical canal and uterine cavity for further polyps.

> 'Could the polyp be stopping me getting pregnant?' Sara asks. 'And has it grown since my last cervical screening test?'

'Yes and yes,' you answer. 'The polyp is certainly physically blocking access to the cervical canal, as well as being the undoubted cause of the discharge. The polyp consists of the same tissue that lines the canal of your cervix, tissue that produces plenty of mucus, which is what the discharge is. The polyp needs to be removed anyway, to confirm that it is benign.'

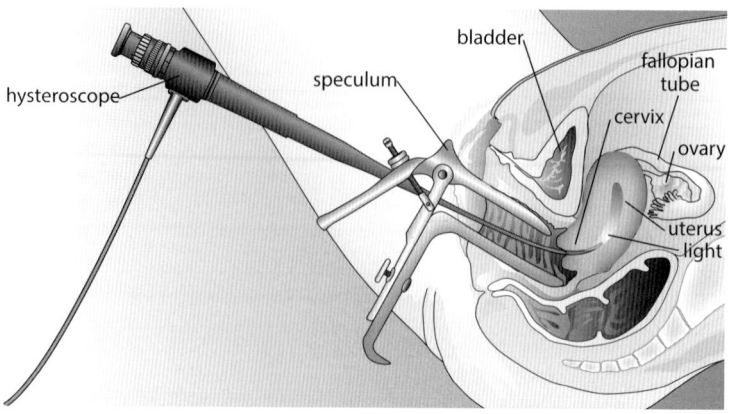

Figure 10.1 Hysteroscopy. The entire cavity of the uterus as well as the cervical canal is directly inspected during a diagnostic hysteroscopy. Using an operative hysteroscope, polyps and subserous fibroids may be resected, specimens taken directly from suspicious areas and the endometrium ablated or excised

An appointment is made for Sara with Dr Yu and you receive a letter saying that the polyp has been successfully removed. The histopathology report shows a benign endocervical polyp. No further abnormality was detected on hysteroscopy and an endometrial biopsy taken at the time shows normal secretory endometrium. Her Pap smear has also been reported as normal.

> Three months later, Sara comes to see you again. *'The discharge has gone,'* she says. *'Sex isn't a problem anymore and what's more, my period is a week overdue.'*

You perform a urinary β-hCG for Sara, which is positive. She is delighted with this news. You make a further appointment for her and her partner in 2 weeks' time to discuss arrangements for antenatal care.

Causes of dyspareunia

Superficial (at introitus)
- Vaginal infections (e.g. candidiasis)
- Vulval infections (e.g. herpes simplex virus, human papillomavirus)
- Atrophic vaginitis—lactational or postmenopausal

Deep (within pelvis)

- Endometriosis
- Pelvic infection (acute or chronic)
- Ovarian cysts or other ovarian lesions
- Adenomyosis

Dyspareunia may be psychosexual in origin or may be exacerbated by psychological and emotional factors.

CLINICAL PEARLS

New symptoms in a patient whose medical history is well-known should not be automatically attributed to the original condition; history, examination and investigation of the presentation is always warranted.

References and further reading

European Society of Human Reproduction and Embryology. Guideline on the management of women with endometriosis. Grimbergen, Belgium: ESHRE; 2013. www.eshre.eu/guidelines-and-legal/guidelines/endometriosis-guideline.aspx

Rolla E. Endometriosis: advances and controversies in classification, pathogenesis, diagnosis and treatment. *F1000Res*. 2019;8:F1000 Faculty Rev-529. https://f1000research.com/articles/8-529

Royal College of Obstetricians and Gynaecologists. Chronic pelvic pain, initial management. Green-top Guideline no. 41; 2012 (reviewed 2017). www.rcog.org.uk/en/guidelines-research-services/guidelines/gtg41

Case 11
Lara is followed through a normal pregnancy. . .

Lara, a 26-year-old woman, makes an appointment to see you. She reports happily that it is 7 weeks since her last menstrual period and a home pregnancy test is positive. She wants to know about options for antenatal care and delivery as this is her first pregnancy.

What do you tell Lara?

You congratulate Lara and ask her if she is well. She responds that she has had some slight nausea in the mornings but has no other problems. You tell her that where she chooses to book for the birth will be somewhat determined by her general health and the progress of the pregnancy, and that her options include obstetrician-led care through a hospital and midwife-led care.

Models of care in pregnancy and childbirth

- All care from a private obstetrician or general practitioner obstetrician and delivery by that doctor either in a private hospital or as a private patient in a public hospital.
- All care in the maternity unit of a public hospital and delivery in the birth suite of that hospital. Care may be shared with midwives if the woman is considered low-risk; care in clinics and intrapartum may be from doctors at junior, registrar or specialist level depending on the complexity of the case.
- Care by public hospital midwives and delivery in a birth centre within the hospital, in a freestanding birth centre adjacent to the main hospital or a planned homebirth, with the possibility of transfer to the conventional birth suite if problems arise.
- Shared care between public hospital and general practitioners—usually for women who are low or medium risk.
- Care from an independent midwife with planned homebirth is a recognised option in the United Kingdom and New Zealand but is available to only a very limited extent in Australia.

What history do you take from Lara?

You take a full history from Lara, commencing with the date of her last menstrual period (LMP) and cycle details. Her LMP is, in fact, a withdrawal bleed following discontinuing the COCP, which she has been taking for the previous 6 years. You calculate a tentative expected date of delivery (EDD) based on the menstrual information.

> Naegele's rule: Add nine months and seven days to the LMP of a woman who is certain of her menstrual dates and has regular 28-day cycles. It is not accurate in longer or shorter cycles, or as in Lara's case, the LMP with a withdrawal bleed; ethnicity may also influence the length of pregnancy. Dating with a first-trimester ultrasound scan is generally more reliable.

Apart from an appendicectomy at age 15, Lara has no relevant medical, surgical or gynaecological history. She has never been pregnant before and has never had a sexually transmitted infection. She takes folic acid 0.5 mg daily but no other medications and has no allergies. Her last cervical screening test 8 months previously was reported as negative.

What other history is relevant to Lara's pregnancy?

A family and a social history should be taken from all women. Lara tells you that her mother is a nonidentical twin and that her father has diabetes, a condition he developed at age 46. Her two younger sisters are non-identical twins. There is no history of other familial conditions or congenital anomalies that she is aware of. Lara is in a stable relationship and her partner Russell is thrilled about the pregnancy. Both partners work in banking. She discloses that she is in a safe environment at home and that Russell is supportive. Lara plans to stop working at 34 weeks of pregnancy, all being well, and take maternity leave to care for her new child.

You assess her risk of depression and anxiety in pregnancy. The commonly used and validated tool for screening for depression is the Edinburgh Postnatal Depression Scale (EPDS, see Case 16). A score of 13 or more on the EPDS has moderate sensitivity and high specificity for detecting possible depression in pregnant women and a score of 10 or more has moderate sensitivity and specificity. Be aware that anxiety disorder is very common in the perinatal period and should be considered in the broader clinical assessment. Anxiety disorders during pregnancy may have a negative influence on obstetric, fetal and perinatal outcomes, including more pregnancy symptoms (nausea and vomiting); more medical visits; increased alcohol or tobacco consumption or unhealthy eating habits; preeclampsia and preterm birth; and postnatal depression and mood disorders. High levels of maternal anxiety during pregnancy are associated with increased exposure of the fetus to maternal cortisol and risk of adverse neurodevelopmental outcomes. In the absence of a freely available practical screening tool for anxiety disorders with adequate evidence in the antenatal period, clinical judgement must be used. This may include consideration of items 3, 4 and 5 of the EPDS and relevant items from the Depression Anxiety Stress Scale (DASS), the K-10 and the Antenatal Risk Questionnaire (ANRQ). In carrying out the appropriate screening, it is important to be aware of the cultural sensitivities for the Indigenous population and also those of migrant and refugee women.

What examination do you conduct for Lara?

You carry out a full general examination for her, including checking her blood pressure, examining the cardiovascular and respiratory systems, inspecting the breasts to note any inversion of the nipples or other condition that may interfere with breastfeeding and examining the thyroid gland, abdomen and lower limbs. Her height and weight are recorded and body mass index (BMI) calculated.

Does Lara need a vaginal examination?

Lara had a well-woman check 8 months previously and has a negative cervical screening test report. She does not need a repeat vaginal examination performed; however, you arrange an ultrasound scan (USS) in the first few weeks of pregnancy because of her close family history of multiple pregnancy and uncertainty about her dates. A scan performed at this gestation will give a very accurate estimation of the EDD. This is performed 3 days later and confirms that Lara is pregnant—the crown–rump length (CRL) of the fetus is the mean for 7 weeks and 5 days and only one fetus is present.

> There is no reason to offer routine ultrasound simply to confirm an ongoing early pregnancy in the absence of any clinical concerns, pathological symptoms or specific indications. It is advisable to offer the first ultrasound scan when gestational age is thought to be between 11 and 13^{+6} weeks' gestation, as this provides an opportunity to confirm viability, establish gestational age accurately, determine the number of viable fetuses and, if requested, evaluate fetal gross anatomy and risk

of aneuploidy. In multiple pregnancy, the chorionicity is best assessed at this stage.

Up to 10 weeks' gestation, the USS measurement (CRL of the fetus) is accurate to ± 5 days.

At 10–14 weeks, the accuracy of the CRL is ± 7 days.

At 14–20 weeks, the accuracy of the head circumference is ± 10 days and at more than 20 weeks it is ± 14 days. CRL is no longer an accurate measurement.

What other tests should be ordered or offered to Lara in the first trimester?

Lara should have the full panel of routine antenatal blood and urine tests performed. These should be outlined to her by you before they are ordered. You should also inform Lara about screening tests for Down syndrome and other conditions in the first trimester (see Case 27).

When should Lara be booked in for hospital delivery?

Most hospitals with shared care arrangements would wish to see Lara as early in the pregnancy as possible (by 12 weeks' gestation) in order to confirm the most appropriate model of care and to inform her about antenatal classes and other services provided in preparation for childbirth. The hospital will then keep records of all tests performed for Lara and offer a shared care card (or 'patient hand-held record') to record all information derived as the pregnancy continues. Lara will be given this card to carry with her and take to all medical consultations during her pregnancy.

Increasingly, as electronic medical records systems are adopted, this information is likely to be provided electronically for pregnant women and their carers.

Antenatal panel of tests

- Full blood count (FBC)
- Blood group and antibody screen
- Rubella antibody screen
- Hepatitis B and C screening, human immunodeficiency virus (HIV) screening—not universally practised

continued

continued

- Rapid plasma reagin (RPR), venereal disease research laboratories (VDRL) or other syphilis screening
- Midstream urine (MSU)
- First-catch urine for polymerase chain reaction (PCR) (chlamydia and gonorrhoea)—not universal
- Endocervical swabs—not universal
- Ferritin level, screening for haemoglobinopathies and vitamin D measurement (in women with low exposure to sunlight)—may be appropriate in certain populations
- Early glucose tolerance testing (GTT) for women at high risk of gestational diabetes mellitus (GDM) (see Case 34)

You arrange all routine tests and refer Lara for booking to the local hospital. You also offer Lara noninvasive screening for Down syndrome (see Case 27).

Lara returns to see you at 13 weeks' gestation. She has booked into the hospital and is scheduled to commence antenatal classes with her partner at 20 weeks of pregnancy. Her morning sickness has settled down and she is having no difficulty coping with work.

What examination do you carry out for Lara at this and subsequent antenatal visits?

At each visit, after inquiring about Lara's general well-being and any specific concerns, you should check her blood pressure, examine the abdomen, auscultate the fetal heart and check for oedema of the lower limbs. Urine should be tested for protein only if the blood pressure is elevated. From 18 weeks onwards, the presence of fetal movements should be noted.

The abdomen should be visually inspected for the size and overall shape of the pregnant uterus in the latter part of pregnancy. From 24 weeks, it is important to measure the symphysial fundal height (SFH) and document it. Plotting the SFH on a validated chart will help to indicate if the fetus is at risk of growth restriction or macrosomia. Any deviation from the expected growth velocity would be an indication for ultrasound for fetal biometry. From approximately 28 weeks onwards, it is possible to feel fetal parts and usually to determine the lie and presentation of the baby (Fig. 11.1). From 36 weeks onwards, the descent of the head into the pelvis (measured in fifths above the pelvic brim) becomes increasingly relevant (Fig. 11.2).

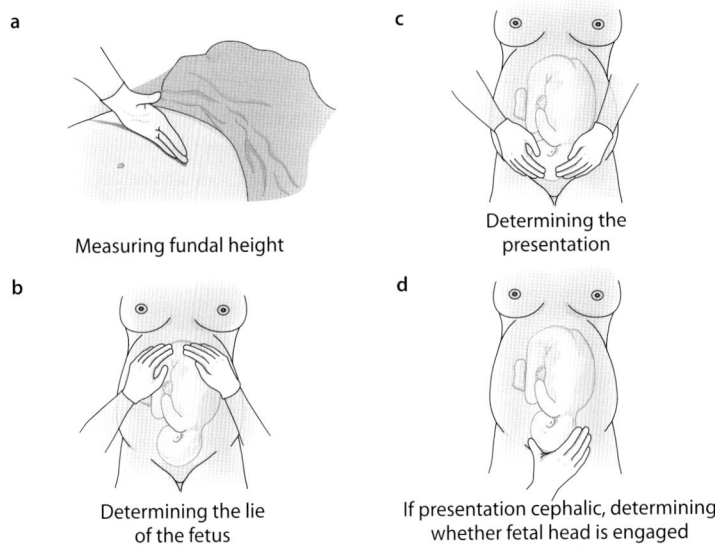

a

Measuring fundal height

b

Determining the lie
of the fetus

c

Determining the
presentation

d

If presentation cephalic, determining
whether fetal head is engaged

Figure 11.1 Palpation of the pregnant abdomen: (**a**) measuring symphysial fundal height; (**b**) determining the lie of the fetus; (**c**) determining the presentation; (**d**) when the presentation is cephalic, determining whether the fetal head is engaged

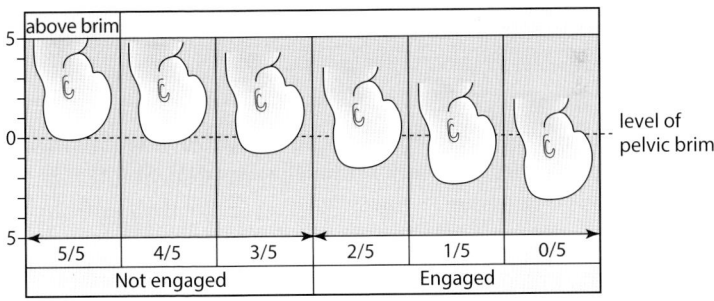

Figure 11.2 Determination of the descent of the fetal head in a cephalic presentation. The measurement of the head in 'fifths' is demonstrated. Once three-fifths of the fetal head has passed into the pelvis, the head is termed 'engaged'

Abdominal palpation in pregnancy

- Symphysial fundal height (SFH)—measured from the top of the pubic symphysis to the top of the uterine fundus; after 24 weeks' gestation, this measurement (in cm) corresponds approximately to the number of weeks' gestation
- Lie—the relationship of the long axis of the baby to the long axis of the uterus; may be longitudinal, transverse or oblique
- Presentation—the part of the baby occupying the lower part of the uterus; usually the head (cephalic presentation), less commonly the buttocks and/or feet (breech presentation) and rarely the shoulder or an arm (in cases of transverse lie)

Visits are, by convention, 4–6 weekly to 32 weeks, 2–3 weekly to 36 weeks and weekly until delivery, although this may be modified to suit the circumstances. Some hospitals wish to see shared care patients for a further visit in the third trimester and most will require a hospital visit if a woman has passed 41 weeks' gestation, although local protocols vary.

What further tests will you perform for Lara?

Lara should also be offered a fetal morphology ultrasound scan at 18–20 weeks of pregnancy. GTT is arranged at 24–28 weeks. Many centres offer routine glucose tolerance screening to all pregnant women regardless of risk category.

The Australian Diabetes in Pregnancy Society (ADIPS) recommends routine screening for all women with no history of GDM with a 75 g oral GTT at 24–28 weeks.

Women not known to have preexisting glucose abnormalities, but with risk factors for GDM, should be tested early in pregnancy. A tiered approach to early glucose testing is recommended.

Women of Asian, Indian subcontinent, Aboriginal, Torres Strait Islander, Pacific Islander, Maori, Middle Eastern or non-white African ethnicity, or with a BMI of 25–35 kg/m^2 as their only risk factors, should be considered as 'moderate risk' and should initially be screened with either a random or a fasting glucose test in early pregnancy, followed by a pregnancy OGTT (POGTT) if clinically indicated. The thresholds for further action are not clear at present and clinical judgement should be exercised.

High risk factors for GDM

- Previous GDM
- Previously elevated blood glucose level
- Maternal age ≥40 years
- Family history DM (first-degree relative with diabetes or a sister with GDM)
- BMI >35 kg/m²
- Previous macrosomic baby (with birth weight >4500 g or >90th percentile)
- Polycystic ovarian syndrome
- Medications: corticosteroids, antipsychotics

Women at 'high risk' of GDM (one high-risk factor or two moderate-risk factors) should undergo a 75 g POGTT at the first opportunity after conception, with venous plasma samples taken fasting, one hour and two hours after the administration of glucose. Women considered as moderate or high risk but with normal early pregnancy glucose testing should have a repeat POGTT at the usual time of 24–28 weeks' gestation. However, a POGTT should be performed at any earlier time during pregnancy, if clinically indicated.

In the United Kingdom, the NICE guidelines suggest GTT for at-risk women at booking (16–18 weeks) and, if normal, again at 24–28 weeks; they have not yet recommended universal GTT.

Lara's blood group is A Rhesus (D) positive and her antibody screen is negative. This screen should be repeated at 26–28 weeks. If Lara were Rhesus (D) negative, she would have antibody screening at 28 weeks and be offered anti-D prophylaxis at 28 and 34 weeks (in Australia) (Table 11.1). At 36 weeks, she will have an FBC performed; in areas where syphilis is prevalent RPR may be repeated at this time. Routine screening for group B streptococcus (by means of urine testing, vaginal or rectal swabs) varies from one centre to another. No other tests are indicated if Lara's pregnancy progresses otherwise uneventfully to term.

Table 11.1 Anti-D prophylaxis for Rhesus-negative women in pregnancy

	Timing	Anti-D dose (IU)
For each sensitising event[a]	1–12 weeks' gestation	No strong evidence to support administration
	Singleton pregnancy	250
	Multiple pregnancy	625
	>12 weeks' gestation	625
	Postpartum	625
Routine prophylaxis[b]	28 weeks' gestation	625
	34 weeks' gestation	625

(a) Sensitising events include genital tract bleed, normal delivery, ectopic pregnancy, miscarriage and termination of pregnancy, amniocentesis and chorionic villus sampling, external cephalic version and antepartum haemorrhage.

(b) The doses at 28 and 34 weeks are given in addition to any doses given for sensitising events.

Lara's pregnancy progresses uneventfully to 41 weeks. At this visit, all observations are within normal limits. Lara, however, is anxious that she has not yet had any signs of impending labour. Her fetal movements continue to be normal.

'How long must we wait?' she asks.

You explain that there is great natural variation in the timing of the onset of labour. Past 42 weeks' gestation (calculated from the first day of the LMP), there is an increase in perinatal mortality and morbidity. It is usual to offer induction at 41–42 weeks. She is referred to the day pregnancy unit for further assessment.

In the day pregnancy unit of the hospital, Lara has a cardiotocograph (CTG) trace performed, which shows a normal baseline, good reactivity and variability and no decelerations. She also has ultrasonic measurement of the amniotic fluid index (AFI) to assess the amount of liquor surrounding the baby; this is within the normal range. She is asked to return in 2 days' time for a further CTG with a view to planning induction of labour at 40 weeks + 12 days' gestation; however, that evening she commences labour spontaneously and proceeds to the uncomplicated birth of a healthy girl.

In cases of prolonged pregnancy, it is usual to provide some assessment of fetal well-being in the 41st week, usually CTGs plus AFI at 2-day to 3-day intervals, in addition to the usual antenatal visits.

 ## CLINICAL PEARLS

Maternal satisfaction with antenatal and intrapartum care is greatest when women themselves feel that they have been well-informed about their options and have been active participants in decisions about their care. Continuity of caregivers is also a strong predictor of women's satisfaction with their birth experience.

References and further reading

Australian Government Department of Health. Clinical practice guidelines: pregnancy care. Canberra: DoH; 2019. www.health.gov.au/resources/pregnancy-care-guidelines

Nankervis A, McIntyre HD, Moses R, et al. for the Australasian Diabetes in Pregnancy Society. ADIPS consensus guidelines for the testing and diagnosis of hyperglycaemia in pregnancy in Australia and New Zealand. Sydney: ADIPS; 2014. www.adips.org/downloads/2014ADIPSGDMGuidelin esV18.11.2014_000.pdf

National Institute for Health and Care Excellence. Antenatal care. Clinical guideline CG62. London: NICE; 2019. www.nice.org.uk/cg62

National Institute for Health and Care Excellence. Antenatal and postnatal mental health: clinical management and service guidance. Clinical guideline CG192. London: NICE; 2014. www.nice.org.uk/guidance/cg192

Qureshi H, Massey E, Kirwan D, et al. BCSH guideline for the use of anti-D immunoglobulin for the prevention of haemolytic disease of the fetus and newborn. *Transfus Med.* 2014; 24(1):8–20.

Royal Australian and New Zealand College of Obstetricians and Gynaecologists. Standards of maternity care in Australia and New Zealand. Melbourne: RANZCOG; 2018. www.ranzcog.edu.au

Case 12
Stacey is unsure about having vaccinations in pregnancy…

Stacey is a 25-year-old primigravida having midwife-led antenatal care at her local hospital. She has been advised by her midwife to consult you about vaccinations in pregnancy. It is now coming to the winter months and she is at 11 weeks gestation. She works as a primary school teacher.

What would you like to know about Stacey?

You review her history and note that she has a history of mild asthma, which is controlled with only occasional use of an inhaler. She is a nonsmoker and has no history of diabetes. There is no significant family history and she is not on any other medication. She has no known allergies. She lives with her husband, Tom, who is in good health. Her pregnancy has been progressing well and she has been advised to have hospital care in view of her weight.

On examination, she appears well and her BMI is 40. Her blood pressure is 120/80 mmHg and urinalysis is negative. General and abdominal examination revealed no abnormality.

What discussions will you have with her?

Stacey is worried about conflicting advice about flu vaccine on the internet. She understands that she could easily pick up the virus from the children at work.

How do you explain the risks and benefits of the flu injection?

You explain that flu vaccination is safe and is recommended for all gestations of pregnancy. It is an inactivated vaccine.

Most influenza infections cause a mild illness and mothers make a rapid and full recovery. However, the A2009/H1N1 virus has been shown to have potentially serious side effects on the mother and her developing fetus.

Effects of influenza

Effects of influenza on the mother

- A2009/H1N1 influenza is associated with an increased risk of hospital admission for pregnant mothers with severe illness.
- Pneumonia is the most common serious illness, and other serious complications include acute respiratory syndrome, secondary bacterial infection, septic shock, multiorgan failure and death.
- Risk factors include obesity, smoking, asthma, diabetes, heart disease and being Indigenous or from an ethnic minority.

Effects of influenza on the pregnancy

- There is no strong evidence linking the virus to an increased incidence of congenital abnormalities.
- In women with severe A2009/H1N1 infection, an increased incidence of preterm birth, stillbirth, neonatal death and low birth weight babies has been reported.

Stacey thanks you for your thorough explanation and says she has decided to have the vaccine.

Vaccination for influenza in pregnancy

- Routine vaccination for pregnant women is endorsed by the departments of health of Australia, New Zealand and the United Kingdom and the Centers for Disease Control and Prevention, USA.
- Flu injections are available from March in the southern hemisphere and from October in the northern hemisphere.
- Current vaccines incorporate the A2009/H1N1 vaccine.
- It is highly effective and it is estimated that vaccination of just five people will prevent one case of serious maternal or infant respiratory illness.
- The vaccine will confer protection to the infant for 6 months as a result of the transplacental transfer of maternal antibodies.

continued

continued

- The vaccine may cause flu-like symptoms for 48 hours and most side effects are local in nature, e.g. soreness at the injection site.
- No congenital abnormalities as a result of the vaccine have been reported.
- No increased risk of Guillain-Barré syndrome from the adjuvants or preservative thiomersal has been reported.
- The influenza vaccine is contraindicated for people with a history of allergy to eggs.

Stacey asks about other vaccinations in pregnancy.

You start by explaining that vaccination against whooping cough (pertussis) is routinely offered after 20 weeks' gestation.

Whooping cough (pertussis)

Pertussis, commonly known as whooping cough, is a disease of the respiratory tract caused by the bacterium *Bordetella pertussis*. It is highly infectious in unvaccinated people. In Australia, pertussis epidemics usually occur every 3–4 years.

Acellular pertussis-containing vaccine is recommended for:
- routine vaccination in infants, children and adolescents
- routine booster vaccination in adults, including those in special-risk groups or in contact with a special-risk group, such as
  - women who are pregnant or breastfeeding
  - healthcare workers
  - early childhood educators and carers
  - people in close contact with infants

Pertussis-containing vaccines are only available in Australia as combination vaccines that include other antigens such as diphtheria and tetanus.

Vaccination of pregnant women is recommended during each pregnancy, preferably between 20 and 32 weeks' gestation.

Chickenpox

- Chickenpox is caused by the varicella zoster virus (VZV), a DNA virus of the herpes family.
- Chickenpox is highly contagious and transmitted by respiratory droplets, by direct personal contact with vesicle fluid and indirectly via fomites. Most people in developed countries get chickenpox in childhood, when it is a mild infection causing a rash, or have been vaccinated.
- Over 90% of the antenatal population (these figures are from the United Kingdom and Ireland) are seropositive for VZV immunoglobulin (IgG) antibody, i.e. they have immunity.
- Women from tropical and subtropical countries are more likely to be seronegative and more susceptible to the development of chickenpox.

The incubation period is 1–3 weeks and the disease is infectious from 48 hours before the rash appears until the vesicles crust over, which usually happens within 5 days. The first signs are fever and feeling unwell. These signs are followed by the formation of watery blisters, which can appear anywhere on the body. The blisters itch. After a few days the blisters burst, crust over and then heal. This may take up to 2 weeks.

Following the primary infection, the virus remains dormant in the sensory root ganglia. If it is activated again, it causes a vesicular eruption in a dermatomal distribution and is called herpes zoster or shingles. The risk of contracting the zoster virus from nonexposed sites is very low.

Vaccination

Varicella vaccine is a live, attenuated vaccine and is contraindicated in pregnancy.

When given before pregnancy, it is very effective in reducing the incidence of and the morbidity related to chickenpox.

Pregnancy should be avoided for 3 months following vaccination.

Contact with chickenpox

- A woman who has previously had chickenpox is immune. A history of chickenpox infection is 97–99% predictive of the presence of serum varicella antibodies.
- If a woman has no history or an uncertain history of previous infection, or was born and raised overseas, it may be appropriate to undertake serum testing.

continued

continued

- If a woman is not immune to chickenpox and comes into contact
  with it during pregnancy, she may be given an injection of
  varicella zoster immune globulin (VZIG). This is a human blood
  product and can be given for up to 10 days after contact. VZIG
  does not work once blisters have developed.
- Once VZIG is given, the pregnant woman should be considered
  potentially infectious for 8–28 days.
- A second dose of VZIG may be required if a further exposure is
  reported and 3 weeks have elapsed since the last dose.

Effects on the pregnancy
Up to 28 weeks of pregnancy
- The risk of spontaneous miscarriage does not appear to be
  increased if chickenpox occurs in the first trimester.
- There is a small risk of fetal varicella syndrome (FVS) if the
  woman develops varicella in the first 28 weeks.
- FVS is characterised by one or more of the following:
  skin scarring in a dermatomal distribution, eye defects
  (microphthalmia, chorioretinitis, cataracts), hypoplasia of the
  limbs and neurological abnormalities (microcephaly, cortical
  atrophy, developmental delay and dysfunction of the bowel and
  bladder sphincters).
- FVS does not occur at the time of initial fetal infection but results
  from a subsequent VZV reactivation in utero and occurs only in a
  minority of infected fetuses.
- The risk of FVS appears to be lower in the first trimester (0.55%).

Between 28 and 36 weeks of pregnancy
- No case of FVS has been reported when maternal infection
  occurred after 28 weeks.
- The virus may become active again, causing shingles in the first
  few years of the child's life.

After 36 weeks and to birth
- The baby may become infected and could be born with
  chickenpox.

Around the time of birth
- If the baby is born within 7 days of the appearance of the rash in
  the mother, the baby may get severe chickenpox.

- Elective delivery should normally be avoided until 5–7 days after the onset of the maternal rash to allow for the passive transfer of antibodies from mother to child.

Up to 7 days after birth
- The baby may get severe chickenpox and will be treated.
- It is safe to breastfeed even if the mother has or had chickenpox during pregnancy.

Effects on the mother

Chickenpox in pregnancy is associated with greater morbidity, namely pneumonia, hepatitis and encephalitis. Chickenpox results in the death of 25 people per year in England and Wales, and 75% of these deaths occur in adults.

Oral aciclovir should be prescribed for pregnant women with chickenpox if they present within 24 hours of the onset of the rash and if they are more than 20 weeks' gestation. Aciclovir should be used cautiously before 20 weeks of gestation. VZIG has no therapeutic benefit once chickenpox has developed.

Women hospitalised with varicella should be nursed in isolation from babies, potentially susceptible pregnant women and nonimmune staff.

You explain about TORCH infections, an acronym that stands for toxoplasma, rubella, cytomegalovirus and herpes.

TORCH infections

Toxoplasmosis

Toxoplasmosis is a parasitic disease caused by the protozoan *Toxoplasma gondii*.

The main host in Australia is the domestic cat. Many other intermediate hosts—including sheep, goats, rodents, cattle, swine, chicken and birds—can carry an infective stage of *T. gondii* encysted in their tissues, especially the brain and muscles.

Clinical features
Toxoplasmosis infection is asymptomatic in 80% of people. The most common sign in symptomatic patients is enlarged lymph

continued

continued

nodes, especially around the neck. The illness may mimic glandular fever with other symptoms of muscle pain, intermittent fever and malaise.

Primary infection in pregnancy is rare, although up to one-third of these infections result in transplacental spread to the developing fetus. Primary infection in pregnancy can cause serious fetal disease. Infection in the first trimester results in a low fetal infection rate (15%) but a higher risk of serious disease. Infection later in pregnancy results in a higher infection rate but generally less severe disease. Diagnosis and treatment during pregnancy appears to reduce the effects on the baby.

In early pregnancy, brain damage as well as liver, spleen and eye disorders may occur. Infection in late pregnancy may result in persistent eye infection throughout life. Toxoplasmosis acquired after birth usually results in no symptoms or only a mild illness.

Method of diagnosis
Serological results require careful interpretation and should preferably be performed and discussed with a reference laboratory. In general, toxoplasma-specific IgG antibody appears 2–3 weeks after acute infection, peaks in 6–8 weeks and often persists lifelong. Testing paired sera taken 2 weeks apart is often helpful, as is IgG-antibody avidity testing. The presence of IgA antibodies is said to correlate with acute infection.

A specific PCR performed on amniotic fluid taken via amniocentesis may determine if a fetus has become infected.

Mode of transmission
Adults most commonly acquire toxoplasmosis by eating raw or under-cooked meat infected with tissue cysts. Consumption of contaminated, unpasteurised milk has also been implicated.

Preventive measures
No immunisation is available. Pregnant women and immunosuppressed people should be advised to:

- cook meat thoroughly (until it is no longer pink) and avoid uncooked cured meat products.
- not consume unpasteurised milk or its products.
- wash all raw fruit and vegetables carefully before eating.
- wash hands thoroughly before meals and after handling raw meat.

- delegate the cleaning of cat litter trays to others wherever possible and, if this is not possible, wear gloves during cleaning and wash hands well afterwards.
- empty cat litter trays daily and regularly disinfect them with boiling water to dispose of the oocysts before they become infective.

Treatment

Specific antiprotozoal treatment may be indicated in infections during pregnancy or where there is eye or other organ involvement. Specialist advice should be sought. Spiramycin is the most commonly used antimicrobial in pregnancy for the treatment of acute toxoplasmosis.

Isolation of the patient is not required.

Rubella

Rubella (German measles) is usually a mild infectious disease in children and adults that is clinically difficult to diagnose because the clinical features are transient and are common to a number of other virus infections.

It is asymptomatic in 25–50% of cases and is spread by respiratory airborne droplet transmission. The transient erythematous rash characteristically begins on the face and spreads to the trunk and extremities. It will usually resolve within 3 days in the same order in which it appeared (face first, then body).

The incubation period is 14–23 days and the period of infectivity is from 1 week before until 4 days after the onset of the rash. Rubella is a notifiable disease.

Effects on the pregnancy

Maternal rubella infection in the first 8–10 weeks of pregnancy results in fetal damage in up to 90% of affected pregnancies, usually with multiple defects.

Abnormalities associated with congenital rubella syndrome include:
- developmental delay
- eye abnormalities (cataracts and retinopathy)
- sensorineural deafness
- cardiac abnormalities
- microcephaly
- intrauterine growth restriction, short stature
- inflammatory lesions of the brain, liver, lungs and bone marrow.

continued

continued

The risk of fetal damage declines to 10–20% by 16 weeks' gestation and there are rare reports of abnormalities resulting from maternal infections up to 20 weeks. The prominent abnormality in the second trimester is sensorineural deafness. Maternal reinfection in immune women carries a risk of fetal damage of less than 5%.

Following birth, these infants have persistent infection, shedding virus for 6–12 months.

Termination of pregnancy should be discussed if maternal infection is confirmed in the first trimester and fetal testing should be considered following maternal infection in the second trimester.

Diagnosis
Routine antenatal screening for rubella IgG is recommended for all pregnant women at their first visit. All pregnant women who have contact with rubella or clinical features consistent with rubella-like illness should be screened for the presence of rising antibody titre and/or rubella-specific IgM. Serological confirmation is required before rubella can be diagnosed.

Maternal management
Obtain a maternal history of infection and immunisation. The vaccine is usually given in the form of the measles, mumps and rubella (MMR) vaccine.

When immunisation is given as part of pre-pregnancy planning, the woman should be advised to avoid pregnancy for 28 days after vaccination.

If the mother is seronegative on her antenatal screen, she should be advised of this and immunised in the postnatal period.

Cytomegalovirus
Cytomegalovirus (CMV) is a beta-herpesvirus with a worldwide distribution. The incidence of primary CMV infection in pregnancy in Australia is estimated to be 6 per 1000 pregnancies. Most primary CMV infections are asymptomatic but carry a 50% risk of transmission to the fetus.

In Australia, CMV causes abnormalities in 200–600 babies each year, such as:
- deafness
- mental disability
- hepatitis

- pneumonitis
- blindness

Awareness of CMV infection in pregnancy is low in Australia among pregnant women and health professionals. Only one in six women who are pregnant or planning a pregnancy know about CMV, and only one in ten health professionals routinely discuss CMV prevention with pregnant women.

Prevention through hygiene and behavioural interventions reduces maternal infection during pregnancy. Provision of information regarding congenital cytomegalovirus prevention strategies to pregnant women improves their knowledge, is acceptable to them and results in no significant increased anxiety.

Women need to be given advice about prevention strategies regardless of their serological status. Women who are aware of their CMV-negative status are more likely to adhere to prevention strategies.

Hygiene precautions and behavioural interventions to prevent cytomegalovirus infection in pregnant women

- Do not share food, drinks, or utensils used by young children.
- Do not put a child's dummy/soother/pacifier in your mouth.
- Avoid contact with saliva when kissing a child.
- Thoroughly wash hands with soap and water for 15–20 seconds, especially after changing nappies, feeding a young child or wiping a young child's nose or saliva.
- Other precautions that can be considered, but are likely to less frequently prevent infection, include cleaning toys, countertops and other surfaces that come into contact with children's urine or saliva, and not sharing a toothbrush with a young child.

Route of transmission

CMV is shed in saliva, urine and breastmilk. Intermittent shedding is common, particularly in infected infants, children and pregnant women. Infection with CMV can also occur via respiratory airborne droplets, sexual contact, blood transfusions and vertical transmission from mother to fetus.

Diagnosis

A good history may help. Obtain maternal serology for CMV: an IgG-positive, IgM-negative result indicates past exposure, while

continued

continued

seroconversion (IgG negative to positive) or a significant rise in IgG indicates a recent primary CMV infection.

Serologic testing for CMV is recommended for women in pregnancy who:
- have a history suggestive of CMV illness.
- have been exposed to a known CMV-infected individual or blood product.
- are immunocompromised.
- have abnormalities on routine antenatal ultrasound (usually at 18 weeks).

Features associated with symptomatic congenital infection include:
- microcephaly
- ascites
- hydrops fetalis
- oligohydramnios or polyhydramnios
- hepatomegaly
- pseudomeconium ileus
- hydrocephalus (ventricular dilation)
- intrauterine growth restriction (IUGR)
- pleural or pericardial effusions
- intracranial calcification
- abdominal calcification

Diagnosis may be confirmed by detecting viral RNA by PCR in amniotic fluid by amniocentesis.

There is no specific treatment or vaccine for CMV.

Genital herpes simplex

Genital herpes is caused by the herpes simplex virus type 1 or 2 (HSV-1 or HSV-2). After infection, the virus travels along the nerves connected to the affected skin and lies dormant within nerve ganglia. The virus can reactivate later and travel along the nerve to the skin surface on or near the genitals, causing a recurrence of tender fluid-filled vesicles containing the virus. The vesicles are highly contagious.

Most genital HSV infections (primary, non-primary and recurrent) are asymptomatic, i.e. most mothers of infants with neonatal HSV disease were previously unaware of their own infection.

Effects on the pregnancy
- Primary infection in the first trimester is associated with an increased risk of early miscarriage. Continuation of the pregnancy does not lead to congenital abnormalities.
- In early primary infection (before 30 weeks), the risk of shedding HSV during a normal birth is 7%, with an overall risk of ≤ 3% for neonatal HSV disease.
- In late primary infection (after 30 weeks), a vaginal birth may lead to severe neonatal disease due to ascending infection after rupture of membranes; however, intrauterine infection accounts for less than 5% of reported cases.
- In women with multiple recurrent lesions, suppressive aciclovir reduces the risk of neonatal transmission at birth.
- In a woman with active genital herpes who has spontaneous rupture of the membranes, caesarean section should be performed as soon as possible, ideally within 6 hours, as it reduces the risk of HSV transmission.
- If there is a history of early primary infection (in the first and second trimesters) and there is evidence of seroconversion (usually by 30–34 weeks), vaginal birth is suitable.
- Consider suppressive therapy with antiviral therapy (aciclovir) from 36 weeks until delivery.
- Neonatal herpes is a viral infection with a high morbidity and mortality that is most commonly acquired at or near the time of delivery.
- Neonatal herpes is classified into three subgroups: disease localised to the skin, eye and mouth; local central nervous system disease (encephalitis) alone; and disseminated infection with multiple organ involvement.

Aciclovir is the mainstay of treatment of primary and recurrent infections.

Parvovirus

- Slapped face syndrome (previously called 'slapped cheek syndrome') is caused by parvovirus B19.
- The virus blocks the development of RBCs and induces inflammation, forming the characteristic facial rash. The rash can also be seen on the hands, wrists and knees.

continued

continued

- Transmission of the virus is by respiratory droplets, e.g. via sneezing and coughing.
- The incubation period ranges from 4 to 14 days after exposure but may be as long as 3 weeks.
- Up to 50% of pregnant women are susceptible to the virus; however, only a small percentage of them will be infected with it. Women are more vulnerable if they are immunocompromised or have a preexisting haematological condition.
- If a pregnant woman develops the infection, there is a 30% chance of fetal transmission, with a 5–10% rate of fetal loss, though most neonates are born healthy.
- Infected fetuses, where there is tissue inflammation and RBC destruction, are particularly at risk.
- The maternal symptoms of the virus are usually short-lived but fetal complications can occur, including hepatitis, severe anaemia, myocarditis, cardiac failure and fetal death.
- The risk of fetal death is linked to gestational age at infection. Maternal infection in the first trimester is associated with a risk of fetal death of 19%. Infection between 13 and 20 weeks is associated with a 15% chance of fetal death and this falls to 6% after 20 weeks.
- In the third trimester, fewer fetal complications occur because there is a decreased need for a high number of RBCs, and RBC life span increases.
- There is no specific antiviral therapy or vaccine available for parvovirus B19 infection. If a fetus is infected, regular ultrasound scans should be done to detect fetal anaemia and cardiac failure.
- Management can include cordocentesis and fetal transfusion to correct fetal anaemia.

Novel coronavirus (SARS-CoV-2) (COVID-19)

Novel coronavirus (SARS-CoV-2) is a new strain of coronavirus causing COVID-19, first identified in Wuhan City, China, towards the end of 2019. A pneumonia of unknown cause was first reported to the World Health Organization (WHO) Country Office in China on 31 December 2019. The outbreak was declared a Public Health Emergency of International Concern on 30 January 2020. On 11 February 2020,

WHO announced a name for the new coronavirus disease: COVID-19. On 11 March 2020, WHO declared the COVID-19 outbreak a global pandemic as the novel coronavirus continued to rapidly spread worldwide.

The picture of this pandemic is rapidly evolving and at the time of going to press (April 2021), the number of confirmed positive cases in the world is approaching 100 million and numbers of deaths from the disease are approaching two million.

Much is still to be learnt about the effects of COVID-19 on pregnancy and the newborn.

It is known that, although pregnant women are not necessarily more susceptible to viral illness, physiological pregnancy-related changes to their immune system in pregnancy can be associated with more severe symptoms. This is particularly true in the third trimester.

Most pregnant women will experience only mild or moderate cold/flu-like symptoms. Cough, fever, shortness of breath, headache, anosmia and loss of taste are other relevant symptoms. More severe symptoms which suggest pneumonia and marked hypoxia are widely described with COVID-19 in older people, the immunosuppressed and those with chronic conditions such as diabetes, cancer or chronic lung disease. The symptoms of severe infection are no different in pregnant women, and early identification and assessment for prompt supportive treatment are key.

At the time of writing this book there is good evidence that vaccination against COVID-19 is safe for pregnant and breastfeeding women.

Risk factors that appear to be associated with hospital admission with COVID-19 illness include:

1. Black, Asian or minority ethnicity
2. overweight or obesity
3. preexisting comorbidity
4. maternal age >35 years

Effects of COVID-19 on the fetus

There are currently no data suggesting an increased risk of miscarriage in relation to COVID-19. In the UK Obstetric Surveillance System cohort, the median gestational age at birth was 38 weeks (IQR 36–39 weeks). Of women who gave birth, 27% had preterm births: 47% of these were iatrogenic for maternal compromise and 15% were iatrogenic for fetal compromise, with 10% of term babies requiring admission to the neonatal unit. Six (2.5%) babies had a positive test for SARS-CoV-2 during the

continued

continued

first 12 hours after birth; three of these were in babies born by caesarean section before labour commenced. One of these babies required admission to the neonatal unit. It was unclear from the report whether two perinatal deaths were related to coexisting maternal COVID-19. A review of 71 neonates delivered to women with COVID-19 in the third trimester reported that neonatal infection was diagnosed in 4 cases (5.6%) within 48 hours of delivery by PCR tests of cord and neonatal blood samples.

CLINICAL PEARLS

- Pregnant women should be encouraged to have the influenza vaccine. It is safe at all gestations.
- Common viral illnesses can present in a nonspecific manner in pregnancy, so a good history and high index of suspicion will lead to appropriate testing to confirm the diagnosis.
- Once fetal abnormalities develop secondary to a viral infection, it is important to seek the input of the fetal medicine specialist.
- Severe viral infections need to be managed by a multidisciplinary team.
- COVID-19, a novel coronavirus infection, is a new disease that is still being understood. The effects on pregnancy are still being studied; vaccines are just becoming available at the time of writing.

References and further reading

Australian and New Zealand Intensive Care Influenza Investigators, Australasian Maternity Outcomes Surveillance System. Critical illness due to 2009 A/H1N1 influenza in pregnant and postpartum women: population based cohort study. *BMJ.* 2010;340:c1279.

Australian Government Department of Health. Clinical practice guidelines: pregnancy care. Canberra: DoH; 2019.

Australian Technical Advisory Group on Immunisation (ATAGI). Australian immunisation handbook. Canberra: Australian Government Department of Health; 2018. www.immunisationhandbook.health.gov.au

Bouthry E, Picone O, Hamdi G, et al. Rubella and pregnancy: diagnosis, management and outcomes. *Prenat Diagn.* 2014;34(13):1246–53.

Knight M, Bunch K, Vousden N, et al. Characteristics and outcomes of pregnant women admitted to hospital with confirmed SARS-CoV-2 infection in UK: national population based cohort study. *BMJ.* 2020;369:m2107.

Knight M, Lim B. Immunisation against influenza during pregnancy. *BMJ.* 2012;344:e3091.

Lim BH, Mahmood TA. H1N1 in pregnancy. *Obstet Gynaecol Reprod Med.* 2010;20(4):101–6.

Meijer WJ, van Noortwijk AGA, Bruinse HW, Wensing AMJ. Influenza virus infection in pregnancy: a review. *Acta Obstet Gynecol Scand.* 2015;94(8): 797–819.

Practice bulletin no.151: cytomegalovirus, parvovirus B19, varicella zoster, and toxoplasmosis in pregnancy. *Obstet Gynecol.* 2015;125(6):1510–25.

Royal College of Obstetricians & Gynaecologists. Educational and support resources for coronavirus (COVID-19). London: RCOG; 2020. www.rcog. org.uk/en/guidelines-research-services/coronavirus-covid-19-pregnancy-and-womens-health/educational-and-support-resources-for-coronavirus-covid-19

Shrim A, Koren G, Yudin MH, Farine D. No. 274-Management of varicella infection (chickenpox) in pregnancy. *J Obstet Gynaecol Can.* 2018;40(8):e652–e657.

Vogel JP, Tendal B, Giles M, et al. Clinical care of pregnant and postpartum women with COVID-19: living recommendations from the National COVID-19 Clinical Evidence Taskforce. *Aust N Z J Obstet Gynaecol.* 2020;60(6):840–51.

Case 13
Diane has diabetes and wants to have a baby...

Diane is a 27-year-old woman who was diagnosed with type 1 diabetes at the age of 11. She has been a patient of your general practice for her entire life. You can see from the voluminous case notes that although she had some episodes of poor sugar control in the first years of diagnosis, and was a little rebellious about her need for insulin in her teenage years, she has been well-controlled for the past 9 years. Diane married 2 years ago and she is currently taking the COCP. She comes to see you today to ask about planning a pregnancy. She is aware that her diabetes poses particular problems for women like herself.

What are the initial points to be established in your discussion with Diane?

You have a short chat with Diane to confirm that her diabetes is well-controlled. You find that she is assiduous with regular checks using her home glucometer. She measures her blood sugar levels up to four times daily and adjusts her insulin regimen when necessary over the telephone with the local diabetes centre. Her control is generally good and her glycosylated haemoglobin (HbA_{1c}) is within the normal range. She has regular ophthalmology checkups, and her endocrinologist reports that she has no evidence of renal disease or hypertension.

> Diane asks you, 'What are the risks of pregnancy for me and my baby?'

As she herself has no evidence of significant diabetic vasculopathy, pregnancy will not have an adverse effect on her health. If blood glucose levels are not well-controlled in early pregnancy, fetal abnormalities can occur—the risk is approximately double that of the background risk of 2–3%. Poor control later in pregnancy can lead to the fetus developing macrosomia, and there is an increased risk of stillbirth. Macrosomia does not simply mean the baby is large. These babies have an abnormal distribution of fat over the upper body, and the fetal hyperinsulinaemia causing the syndrome may result in metabolic dysfunction leading to stillbirth.

> Pregnancy in a woman with diabetes can have an adverse effect on her health if there is preexisting renal impairment, hypertension secondary to renal disease or severe retinopathy. Blindness or renal failure requiring dialysis may result from continuing the pregnancy. Termination of pregnancy must be discussed in such cases.

> Diane then asks, *'Is there any way to reduce the risks to my baby?'*

You emphasise the need for good sugar control both before and after conception, and suggest that Diane also visit her endocrinologist prior to attempting to conceive as there may be a need to alter her insulin regimen. Continuous glucose monitoring (CGM) and flash glucose monitoring are now fully subsidised in Australia through the National Diabetes Services Scheme for women with type 1 diabetes who are planning a pregnancy, are pregnant or are immediately postpartum. You arrange for her to have a FBC and rubella and varicella antibody screening. You recommend that Diane take folic acid 5 mg daily from now until at least the end of the first trimester to reduce the risk of fetal neural tube defect. You also explain the need to report back early once she thinks she may be pregnant so that the pregnancy can be confirmed.

A first-trimester ultrasound scan for very accurate dates is important in diabetic pregnancies. Noninvasive screening for Down syndrome and related chromosomal abnormalities can be offered from 11 weeks (see Case 11). A further ultrasound scan at 19 weeks, preferably by an experienced obstetric ultrasound specialist, is required to maximise the chance of detecting fetal anomalies. A second tertiary scan at 22–24 weeks is often advised to assess fetal cardiac anatomy, since preexisting diabetes is an important risk factor for fetal cardiac anomalies. Cardiac anomalies represent about 50% of all abnormalities in pregnancies in women with diabetes and these are more easily demonstrated at this gestation, as the fetal heart is larger and more easily assessed. You explain that in the event of a severe fetal abnormality being detected, termination of the pregnancy can be readily offered.

Fetal abnormalities associated with diabetes

- neural tube defects
- cardiac abnormalities
- bowel abnormalities
- urinary tract abnormalities
- sacral agenesis

What do you need to explain to Diane about her care in later pregnancy?

As well as careful control of blood sugar levels, Diane will need regular assessment of fetal growth by ultrasound from 24 weeks, looking for evidence of macrosomia and also for a disproportionate abdominal circumference growth rate and polyhydramnios.

Fetal macrosomia is associated with shoulder dystocia during vaginal delivery and an increased incidence of caesarean section for obstructed labour due to fetal size and 'macrosomic' morphology. Fetal death in utero (and subsequent stillbirth) is associated with poor control of blood glucose levels and fluctuating fetal insulin levels in the final weeks of pregnancy.

The infants of mothers with diabetes are more prone to hypoglycaemia, respiratory distress syndrome, hypocalcaemia, hypomagnesaemia, polycythaemia and neonatal jaundice. However, you emphasise to Diane that with good sugar control, and careful obstetric and neonatal care, she can expect to have a live and healthy baby.

 CLINICAL PEARLS

> The key to a successful outcome to pregnancy in a woman with diabetes lies in tight control of blood sugar levels before and throughout the pregnancy. Care should always involve a multidisciplinary team, with close co-operation between obstetricians, endocrinologists, diabetes educators and paediatricians.

References and further reading

National Institute for Health and Care Excellence. Diabetes in pregnancy: management from preconception to the postnatal period. NICE guideline NG3. London: NICE; 2015. www.nice.org.uk/guidance/ng3

Rudland V, Price S, Callaway L, et al. ADIPS 2020 position paper on pre-existing diabetes in pregnancy. *Aust N Z J Obstet Gynaecol.* 2020; 60(6):831–9.

Rudland V, Price S, Hughes R, et al. ADIPS 2020 guideline for pre-existing diabetes and pregnancy. *Aust N Z J Obstet Gynaecol.* 2020; 60(6):e18–52.

Case 14
Maria has a twin pregnancy. . .

Maria is a 38-year-old woman who comes to consult you in general practice. Maria is pregnant for the fifth time. She has had four uncomplicated pregnancies resulting in the spontaneous vaginal births of four healthy sons now aged 16, 14, 12 and 9. Maria and her husband have used the ovulation method of natural family planning for the past 9 years with no problems. She keeps accurate menstrual records and tells you that she has had no bleeding since her last period 8 weeks previously and is quite sure that she is pregnant. This pregnancy was unplanned, but the couple are now happy with the idea of a fifth child. Maria, however, tells you that she is experiencing much more marked symptoms of early pregnancy than she remembers from her other pregnancies. She feels nauseated and exhausted for much of the day. She is suffering from heartburn, urinary frequency and nocturia, and thinks she is putting on weight very rapidly.

What further history do you need from Maria?

You need to be aware of any intercurrent medical problems Maria may have. In fact, she has been a patient of your practice for 20 years and from her notes you see that her past medical history is unremarkable. Her cervical screening tests are up to date.

What examination do you make for Maria?

You organise a urine beta-human chorionic gonadotrophin (β-hCG) test to confirm the pregnancy and then conduct a general examination. Maria's BP is 120/70 mmHg, and general examination reveals no unexpected abnormality. Palpation of her lower abdomen, however, reveals a central mass arising from the pelvis and reaching to 4 cm above the pubic symphysis. After informing Maria that you think her uterus is larger than expected you use your small portable ultrasound machine to perform a transabdominal scan and have no difficulty demonstrating to Maria two distinct pregnancy sacs with two viable fetuses, each with a CRL corresponding to 8 weeks' gestation, and two fetal hearts. Maria has a twin pregnancy.

The causes of the finding of a 'large-for-dates' uterus on examination include wrong dates, multiple pregnancy, molar pregnancy and the coexistence of uterine pathology such as fibroids with normal singleton pregnancy.

While understandably Maria is somewhat overwhelmed by this news, she tells you that she is quite happy about it and feels her family will be too. There is no family history of twins that she is aware of.

Are they identical?' she asks.

You explain that the presence of two separate sacs may suggest the twins are nonidentical—statistically and because of Maria's age this is also more likely. However, there is also a chance they may be identical.

Types of twin pregnancies

Dizygotic twins (conception occurring with two ova released in the same cycle, and two sperm) will each have a chorion and an amnion surrounding the developing embryo, and this pattern is known as dichorionic diamniotic (DCDA). Monozygotic twins occur when a single fertilised egg separates into two embryos: if this occurs between days 1 and 3 after conception each embryo develops a separate amnion and chorion (DCDA); between 4 and 7 days there will be a single chorion but separate amnions (monochorionic diamniotic, MCDA); and after day 7 the twins will be monochorionic and monoamniotic (MCMA). Conjoined twins occur if the egg splits at around 13 days. Monochorionic twins have poorer outcomes than dizygotic twins, with greater rates of early pregnancy loss, preterm delivery and perinatal mortality and morbidity.

Epidemiology

The incidence of monozygotic twins is constant worldwide, approximately 4 per 1000 births. Approximately two-thirds of twins are dizygotic. Birthrates of dizygotic twins vary by race (10–40 per 1000 births in Black women, 7–10 per 1000 births in White women and approximately 3 per 1000 births in Asian women) and maternal age (i.e. the frequency rises with increasing

continued

continued

> maternal age ≤ 40 years). Dizygotic twin birthrates are also influenced by
> other factors, such as parity and mode of fertilisation (e.g. most artificially
> conceived twins are dizygotic, but 6–10% are monozygotic).

PLACENTATION OF TWINS

MONOCHORIONIC DIAMNIOTIC
SINGLE PLACENTA, 1 CHORION, 2 AMNIONS

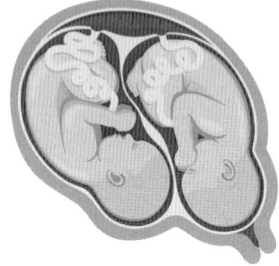

MONOCHORIONIC MONOAMNIOTIC
SINGLE PLACENTA, 1 CHORION, 1 AMNION

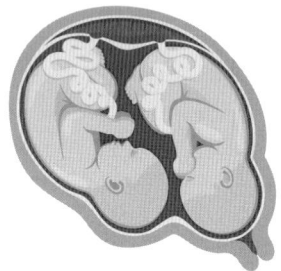

DICHORIONIC DIAMNIOTIC
FUSED PLACENTAE, 2 CHORIONS, 2 AMNIONS

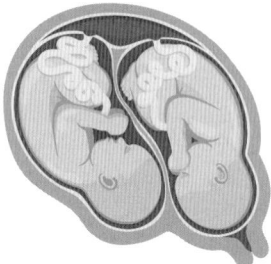

DICHORIONIC DIAMNIOTIC
SEPARATE PLACENTAE, 2 CHORIONS, 2 AMNIONS

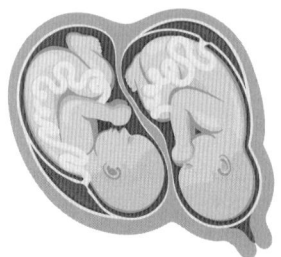

Figure 14.1 Types of twin pregnancies
Source: logika600/Shutterstock.

> 'How will this pregnancy be different from the others?' Maria asks,
> 'and how will the babies be delivered?'
> 'It's quite a while since I had a baby', she points out. 'After four boys,
> we'd love a girl but our main concern would be that the babies are
> healthy.'

Given her age, her parity and the fact of the twin pregnancy, you recommend that Maria have all her care in the hospital antenatal clinic. You also explain that at the age of 38 she faces an increasing risk of a fetus with Down syndrome. There are screening tests and diagnostic tests for Down syndrome (see Case 27), but with a twin pregnancy, the interpretation of such tests has to be made in conjunction with the type of twins. Measurement of fetal nuchal translucency (FNT) in the window between 11 and 13 weeks ± 6 days can be undertaken for each twin, with a sensitivity of more than 80%. Combining the nuchal translucency result with biochemical markers (the free subunit of β-hCG and pregnancy-associated plasma protein [PAPP-A]) improves the sensitivity to more than 85%, especially in the context of a dichorionic twin pregnancy. Noninvasive prenatal diagnostic test (NIPT) is a useful alternative to measure the cell-free DNA; (cf)DNA screening in twin pregnancies presents unique challenges. Although the total fetal fraction in twins is approximately 1.6 times that reported in singletons, the average fetal fraction per twin is lower. Placental volume and chorionicity affect the fetal fraction. Monochorionic (MC) and dichorionic (DC) placentas have comparable total volumes and weights. Theoretically, the sensitivity for trisomy screening in MC twins should be as good as or better than screening in singletons. This is because MC twins are almost certainly genetically identical and the combined fetal fraction (1.6 × singletons) is representative of both twins. In contrast, the sensitivity for DC (usually genetically nonidentical) twins may be lower because the average fetal fraction per twin is 0.8 × that of singletons. When a trisomy is present in DC twins, usually only one twin is affected. It is important to remember that while the NIPT is a very sensitive test for the major chromosomal abnormalities, it is still a screening test, and that any abnormality noted should be confirmed by invasive testing such as amniocentesis or chorionic villus sampling, depending on the gestation of the pregnancy.

You further explain that if Down syndrome were diagnosed, termination of one or both pregnancies would be an option, but that making such a decision can be extremely stressful for parents. Maria should also have a morphology scan at 18–20 weeks to screen for fetal abnormalities.

Maria tells you that she will discuss this with her husband. While their religion is opposed to abortion, and she herself has always felt negative about the procedure, she is certain she would not be able to cope with twins with Down syndrome. She thinks she will probably decide to have fetal nuchal translucency (FNT) screening performed as it is noninvasive and a negative result would give her a measure of reassurance.

USS carried out before 14 weeks' gestation is invaluable for determining chorionicity of the twin pregnancy and this is important because it determines the outlook for the pregnancy and the schedule of monitoring.

Chorionicity and amnionicity are determined at the time of detecting a twin pregnancy by ultrasound using:

- the number of placental masses.
- the presence of amniotic membrane(s) and membrane thickness.
- the lambda (dichorionic) or T-sign (monochorionic).

Monochorionic twin pregnancies have an overall poorer outlook than dichorionic twins. The most important complication in monochorionic twins is twin-to-twin transfusion syndrome (TTTS), where the donor twin can become severely anaemic and the recipient twin develops heart failure due to polycythaemia. This is due to anastomoses between the fetal vessels as a result of the shared placenta. It does not happen in dichorionic twins. It is recommended that monochorionic twins undergo ultrasound scans fortnightly from 18 weeks to try to pick up early signs of TTTS. Scans on a 4-weekly basis are recommended for dichorionic twins to monitor growth.

What other information do you give Maria about the earlier part of her pregnancy?

You tell Maria that generally everything that can occur in a singleton pregnancy is more pronounced with twins. 'Great!' she answers. She had been about to change from a part-time to a full-time teaching job. Now you suggest that she stay with part-time work and consider stopping altogether at about 28–30 weeks' gestation. The good news, you tell her, is that since she is already 8 weeks pregnant and both fetal hearts are visible it is likely that the pregnancy will continue; miscarriage or loss of one twin is uncommon at this stage. You reassure her that vaginal birth is a possibility, although there is a greater chance of needing caesarean delivery under certain circumstances. Her morning sickness should improve after 12 weeks' gestation. Meanwhile, she should eat small, regular meals and take an iron-folate preparation.

 CLINICAL COMMENT

The 'minor discomforts' of pregnancy are all more marked in multiple pregnancy.

Table 14.1 The minor discomforts of pregnancy and their management

Problem	Solutions
Nausea and vomiting— more pronounced due to higher levels of β-hCG	Small frequent meals Ginger preparations, pyridoxine, doxylamine Oral antiemetics (e.g. metoclopromide, antihistamines, ondansetron)
Reflux oesophagitis	Avoid caffeine Elevate the bedhead Oral antacids (e.g. Mylanta, Gaviscon) H_2 histamine receptor antagonists (e.g. ranitidine)
Abdominal pressure and distension, discomfort	Rest (routine bed rest for multiple pregnancies is not beneficial)
Striae gravidarum	A vitamin E cream may help alleviate itch
Back pain	Rest, physiotherapy, water immersion
Leg oedema and varicose veins	Compression stockings Elevation of the lower limbs whenever possible

You supply Maria with information about the local multiple-birth support group, which she is interested in contacting. Before she leaves your surgery, with a letter of referral to the hospital antenatal clinic, you also suggest to Maria that she and her husband might like to consider their options for family planning once this pregnancy is over. Natural family planning depends on a woman having regular cycles and being able to interpret the signs of ovulation. As Maria enters her 40s, her periods may become less regular as progesterone levels decline. She may experience anovulatory cycles interspersed with normal cycles. Although she may wish to continue with the method, she should be aware of differences in how her body is functioning. Maria promises to discuss all this with her husband.

CP CLINICAL PEARLS

- Almost every minor and major side effect and complication of singleton pregnancy occurs with greater frequency in pregnancies with twins and higher multiples.
- Many women gain great psychological support and emotional benefit from contact with groups of other mothers who have experienced multiple births.

References and further reading

Lowe SA, Armstrong G, Beech A, et al. SOMANZ position paper on the management of nausea and vomiting in pregnancy and hyperemesis gravidarum. *Aust N Z J Obstet Gynaecol.* 2020;60(1):34–43.

National Institute for Health and Care Excellence. Twin and triplet pregnancy. NICE guideline 137. London: NICE; 2019. www.nice.org.uk/guidance/ng137

Royal Australian and New Zealand College of Obstetricians and Gynaecologists. Management of monochorionic twin pregnancy. C-Obs 42. Melbourne: RANZCOG; 2017. www.ranzcog.statements-guidelines/obstetrics/monochorionic-twin-pregnancy/Management-of-Monochorionic-Twins-(C-Obs-42)-review-July-2017.pdf

Case 15
Anula is depressed after the birth of her baby. . .

Anula is a 36-year-old patient of your practice who gave birth to her first baby six weeks ago at the local hospital where you provide shared care. She has been a patient of your practice for many years and you know her well. Anula and her partner Ranjit had faced a long and distressing period of infertility and this pregnancy was the result of several IVF attempts. Anula was delighted to be pregnant, but was very anxious during the pregnancy. You provided most of her antenatal care, sharing this with the hospital. You have received a discharge summary from the hospital stating that Anula gave birth to a healthy baby girl by emergency caesarean section, with a birthweight of 3570 g. Anula is seeing you today for her 6-week routine postnatal check. You have been somewhat surprised that she had not come by to show you and your staff her new baby, as she promised to do so before the birth. On checking her medical records, you see that she is due for her routine CST.

The first consultation

Anula enters the room without her baby, looking very tired and flat. She doesn't give you the normal bright greeting you've come to expect from her over the years. You ask her how she is, and whether has she brought her baby, as you had been looking forward to seeing her.

'I'm OK, doctor. I've left Kamala at home because she is having another one of her crying fits, and I didn't want to bring her today.' Anula moves quite slowly and looks very tired. You ask her if she is getting enough rest. 'Not really. I was exhausted after the birth and she cries a lot. I haven't really been getting much sleep.' Her husband has been trying to help but because she has been off work, he is working extra shifts at the factory to help their finances. Her mother has come from interstate for the birth, but Anula's relationship with her mother has always been difficult and she feels her mother's presence is not of much benefit. 'She's critical of everything, and everything is always my fault—the baby crying, the breastfeeding problems, the caesarean—she makes me feel like a total failure.' At this point, Anula starts crying and is difficult to console.

What are your concerns in this situation and how do you proceed?

You offer Anula time to speak, some tissues and a comforting hand. When she stops crying you ask further about her problems. You make it clear that this will be a prolonged consultation and you have plenty of time to listen. Anula tells you that her husband hasn't really been at home much, and she finds it hard to confide in him, particularly with her mother being present. She had to have an emergency caesarean section for obstructed labour, and she feels as if she has somehow 'failed as a woman'. Breastfeeding is proving more difficult than she had imagined, and she does not know where to turn for help.

You decide that you will defer the CST until a later visit, as Anula's other concerns are more pressing. However, you do examine her abdomen and confirm the caesarean section incision is well-healed, with no evidence of infection. You perform a breast examination—Anula's nipples are both cracked and inflamed. You ask her to complete the Edinburgh Postnatal Depression Scale (EPDS) questionnaire, and when you score her responses, the calculation is 15—well above the triage cut-off score of 13.

What immediate practical help can you offer to Anula?

You explain to Anula that she would benefit from additional help and support, and arrange a referral to the local day centre for new mothers where a lactation consultant visits to provide assistance with breastfeeding. You advise her that she should probably thank her mother for her help, but suggest that she is no longer required and should return home. You explain to Anula that both she and the baby are healthy, and that she should not feel as if she has failed by requiring a caesarean section. It is most important that she not blame herself for this outcome. You go over the indications for the caesarean with her—the operation was performed for a good medical reason, as she was not progressing in labour. You explain that this is a common scenario with a first labour and not an indicator of any failure.

To exclude possible biological contributors to Anula's first presentation you arrange a blood test of her thyroid function and iron studies, along with a check of her vitamin D, vitamin B_{12} and folate. You then arrange to see Anula the following week to see how she is getting along, and ask her to bring Kamala too so you can perform her 6-week baby check. If the blood test results are normal and there is no improvement in her mental state, you intend to discuss the potential benefits and risks of antidepressant medication and a referral to a perinatal mental health service.

Breastfeeding problems are common. Most hospitals have lactation consultants, midwives who specialise in breastfeeding and its difficulties and are freely available to help and encourage new mothers. As well, many cities have mother-and-baby day centres to help postnatal women with these common difficulties.

The second consultation

The following week Anula returns to see you. Again, she has not brought Kamala. Your receptionist tells you that the baby has been left at home with Anula's husband because 'she was crying too much'. You have heard from the day centre that despite their best efforts Anula has stopped trying to breastfeed. During this visit, Anula appears remote and withdrawn, and answers your questions in a monosyllabic fashion. She is somewhat unkempt with unwashed hair and crumpled clothing, which concerns you as she is usually fastidious about her appearance. As she is not volunteering anything spontaneously, you start asking her specific questions:

'How is Kamala?'—*no reply.*
'Has your mother gone home?'—*'Yes, thank goodness.'*
'How is your husband?'—*no reply.*
'Have you been sleeping well?'—*'No, it's hard to get to sleep and I wake up early and can't get back to sleep.'*
'How is your appetite?'—*'I have no appetite.'*
'Have you been having any bad or negative thoughts?'—*'Like what?'*
'How do you feel about Kamala?'—*'I don't feel anything about her. I don't feel any love or maternal instincts. I hate it when she cries—it must mean I'm a bad mother if I don't feel anything for her. Sometimes I feel as if I want to hurt her to make her quiet!'*
'How do you feel about yourself? Have you had any thoughts of hurting yourself?'—*'Sometimes I just want to die—I feel like a bad mother. No normal mother would feel these things.'*
'Have you tried hurting yourself or the baby?'—*'No.'*
'Have you told anyone about these feelings?'—*'No.'*
'Are you hearing any voices telling you bad things?'—*'No.'*

What are your conclusions and concerns from this interview?

Clearly, Anula has significant postnatal depression. Perinatal mood disorders have a strong association with adverse outcomes for both mothers and their babies, so this is a very serious situation. You call her husband Ranjit and ask him to come up to the surgery. He brings Kamala, who does indeed cry for the entire time they are both there. You explain to both Anula and Ranjit that she has severe postnatal depression, and that you are worried about her. You feel that she and Kamala need supervised care and that she herself needs specialist psychiatric treatment.

> Postnatal depression is common, affecting about 13% of women; the peak period of onset is 4–6 weeks postpartum but it can occur at any time in the first year of the infant's life. About 80% of women will experience mild mood lability and anxiety (the 'baby blues') on the third or fourth postpartum day; this is best managed by sympathetic support and anticipation of the condition in antenatal classes, and is self-limiting. Postpartum psychosis is rare, affecting 1–3 women per 1000.

What practical measures do you take?

Managing postnatal depression can be challenging, as in many places resources are scarce. You telephone the local maternity hospital to explain the diagnosis and need for specialised psychiatric assessment, and the hospital arranges for Anula and Kamala to be admitted immediately. During her admission, Anula is assessed by a multidisciplinary team and commenced on selective serotonin reuptake inhibitor (SSRI) antidepressants. She remains in the hospital for three weeks. At the end of that time, you receive a call from the nursing staff to ask that you follow her up in the next few days. You ring Ranjit to arrange an appointment to see the entire family in 2 days' time.

> Many cities have special mother-and-baby units within psychiatric departments. These are ideal for the treatment and observation of mothers and babies, although waiting lists may be long. In smaller centres such services may not exist, but it is important to ensure that the mother and baby remain together if possible, and that they are both safely supervised.

Antidepressants may take up to six weeks to be effective, and mood may deteriorate within that interval. It is in this time that self-harm or harm to the baby is a strong possibility. SSRIs and tricyclic antidepressants are both generally thought to be safe for breastfeeding women.

The third consultation

Two days later, you meet the entire family, and Anula looks more like her old self. Her mood seems much better, and she is able to smile once or twice. She clearly adores Kamala, who seems much calmer too, and cuddles her throughout the consultation.

She now says, 'Thank you for looking after me, doctor. I felt so alone and frightened. I couldn't talk about this to anyone because I didn't want them to think I was mad, or evil. I was so scared about hurting Kamala.'

Is Anula now at risk of harming herself or her baby?

You can see that this is now a less likely scenario, which is also the psychiatrist's opinion. You institute the follow-up plan suggested by the psychiatrist, and make sure Anula knows she has someone to call if she is concerned. You reiterate this point to Ranjit as well. Relieved that all appears well, you make arrangements with Anula to perform her long-delayed 6-week baby check and CST.

 CLINICAL PEARLS

- Postpartum depression is common, affecting about 13% of women, and may have profound and long-lasting effects on the woman, her child and her family as a whole. Early detection and ongoing supervision are essential to achieve the best possible outcome for all involved.
- Sometimes women feel as if they have 'failed' if they have not had a perfectly normal, uncomplicated birth. About 30% of women having a first baby will have a caesarean section or instrumental vaginal birth. It is important to emphasise that a healthy mother and baby are the desired outcome, and that this cannot and does not have to be achieved through a spontaneous vaginal birth for every woman. Feelings of worthlessness and failure are common and should be actively addressed. It is most important to explain the reasons behind the decisions which led to the intervention,

continued

105

continued

and reassure the woman that she must not blame herself and has not failed at motherhood if a vaginal birth did not eventuate. Sometimes, a debriefing session with the hospital or obstetrician who was involved may be worth considering.

References and further reading

O'Hara MW, Wisner KL. Perinatal mental illness: definition, description and aetiology. *Best Pract Res Clin Obstet Gynaecol.* 2014;28(1):3–12.

Rodriguez-Cabezas L, Clark C. Psychiatric emergencies in pregnancy and postpartum. *Clin Obstet Gynecol.* 2018;61(3):615–27.

Case 16
Emma comes for a postnatal check. . .

Emma is a 30-year-old woman who gave birth to a healthy daughter, Bess, 4 months ago. Bess is currently fully breastfed, and Emma commenced the low-dose progestogen-only pill while still in the hospital after the birth. As well as returning to see you for a routine postnatal visit, Emma seeks contraceptive advice. Bess's birth was an uneventful spontaneous vaginal delivery after an uncomplicated pregnancy. Emma has recommenced sexual activity with her partner but reports some discomfort with intercourse; otherwise she is well and delighted with the arrival of her baby.

What further information do you need from Emma's history?

You will make specific inquiries about bowel and bladder, whether the postnatal lochia has resolved and how she is coping with her baby. Asking about her support at home is also important. Since postnatal depression is common, this is an appropriate time to check for postnatal depression, perhaps with an instrument such as the Edinburgh Postnatal Depression Scale. It is also important to offer a cervical screening test if this is due.

On looking through Emma's notes, you recall that at the age of 28, Emma had treatment (a loop diathermy excision of the cervix) for a high-grade intraepithelial abnormality (HSIL in the current nomenclature, CIN 2 in the former classification; see Table 2.1). Emma was advised to complete test of cure surveillance to confirm her treatment was successful. Test of cure surveillance is a co-test (human papillomavirus (HPV) and liquid-based cytology (LBC)) performed 12 months after treatment, and annually thereafter, until the woman receives a negative co-test on two consecutive occasions (Table 16.1). Because of her pregnancy, it is now 15 months since the last co-test, which was reported as negative.

What examination do you perform for Emma?

After admiring Bess and handing her into the care of one of your practice nurses, you carry out a short general physical examination for Emma, including taking her blood pressure and performing an abdominal examination. The uterus has completely involuted and no masses are palpable. You proceed to vaginal examination and attempt to pass a speculum but this causes marked discomfort and inspection shows the vaginal walls to be reddened and atrophic in appearance.

Table 16.1 Terminology for reporting cervical cytology for squamous abnormalities

Terminology	Abnormality
Possible low-grade squamous intraepithelial lesion (pLSIL)	Non-specific minor squamous cell changes. Changes that suggest but fall short of HPV/CIN 1
Low-grade squamous intraepithelial lesion (LSIL)	HPV effect, CIN 1
Possible high-grade squamous intraepithelial lesion (pHSIL)	Changes that suggest, but fall short of CIN 2, CIN 3 or SCC
High-grade squamous intraepithelial lesion (HSIL)	CIN 2, CIN 3
Squamous cell carcinoma (SCC)	Squamous cell carcinoma

What is the cause of this appearance?

You explain to Emma that lactation suppresses ovulation and this, combined with her use of the low-dose progestogen-only pill, has caused a state of atrophic vaginitis: this is the cause of her dyspareunia (pain during sexual intercourse). You also explain that taking a co-test at this visit may yield a scanty and unsatisfactory specimen unsuitable for interpretation. A small dose of topical oestrogen twice weekly is likely to improve the vaginitis and reduce dyspareunia, so you provide a prescription for this.

In recent times, CO_2 laser therapy has been suggested for treatment of vaginal atrophy but there is currently inadequate evidence to support its use; topical oestrogen remains the gold standard.

Emma tells you that she wishes to continue breastfeeding until Bess is 6 months old, at which time she will be returning to work. She will continue the mini-pill, which is otherwise satisfactory, and then change to a combined oestrogen/progestogen formulation after weaning Bess. You explain that small doses of topical oestrogen will not interfere with breastfeeding nor pose any risk to the baby. You arrange to see Emma in 4 weeks' time for further examination and a test of cure.

How do you manage the following visit?

When Emma returns for the next visit, she reports a great improvement in her symptoms, which she admits had been interfering somewhat with her relationship with her partner. You repeat the vaginal examination and on this occasion the vagina appears pink and well oestrogenised. You perform a test of cure. It is negative for HPV and dysplasia.

Emma asks you about the etonogestrel implant, which she is considering as a form of contraception once she stops breastfeeding. Being so busy caring for a small baby, she remarks, 'I'm often afraid I'll forget to take the pill.' She wants to know about the implant and wonders whether vaginal dryness and discomfort might be a potential problem for her if she has an implant inserted.

What is your response to her question?

The progestogen-only pill contains a small dose of oral progestogen without oestrogen. It acts by causing both a thickening of the cervical mucus and an atrophic endometrium, thereby inhibiting both sperm mobility and implantation. It has no effect on lactation (oestrogen in the combined pill may inhibit lactation) and is also useful for women in whom the COCP is contraindicated. It is highly effective, with a Pearl Index of 0.5. It is only likely to be associated with atrophic vaginitis during lactation due to the very low levels of oestrogen associated with breastfeeding.

The etonogestrel implant is a Silastic rod about the size of a matchstick that releases a steady dose of etonogestrel over a period of 3 years. (Towards the end of this time, blood levels of this synthetic steroid may decline.) Etonogestrel acts by suppressing the luteinising hormone (LH) surge, so that early follicular development and oestradiol production occur without ovulation. The endometrium is thin but not atrophic and this results in amenorrhoea in most women, although spotting and unpredictable bleeding can occur in up to 20% of users. Because follicular development still occurs, sufficient oestrogen is usually produced to avoid the symptoms of atrophic vaginitis and dyspareunia that Emma has experienced on the progestogen-only pill during lactation. The implant needs to be inserted and removed by a medical practitioner with appropriate training; occasionally when the device has been incorrectly placed, surgical removal under ultrasound scanning is needed. The etonogestrel rod provides very effective contraception, with a Pearl Index of 0.09 and few side effects, apart from the bleeding already mentioned.

You provide Emma with written material about contraceptive options to consider over the following months until she ceases breastfeeding, and make another appointment to discuss contraception with her.

Other methods of administration of progestogens for contraception include 3-monthly depot medroxyprogesterone acetate (DMPA) injections and the levonorgestrel-releasing intrauterine device (LNG-IUD), which has a life span of 5 years. Both of these usually induce complete amenorrhoea, although spotting and light unpredictable bleeding are side effects, especially in the first few months of use. Although levels of oestradiol may fall to the low normal range in women using DMPA, symptoms and signs of hypo-oestrogenism (such as vaginal dryness and dyspareunia) are not a common side effect of either long-term method of progestogen-only administration. There is the possibility that osteoporosis may develop with long-term DMPA use—this may be assessed with serial bone mineral density measurements. Both methods are also suitable treatments for dysfunctional uterine bleeding, whether contraception is desired or not.

 CLINICAL PEARLS

- Always check the whole person as well as the pelvic organs.
- At a postnatal visit, consideration of a change of contraceptive method from that used before pregnancy may be appropriate.
- It is important to screen for postnatal depression and a screen for family violence may also be pertinent.

References and further reading

Cancer Council Australia Cervical Cancer Screening Guidelines Working Party. National Cervical Screening Program: guidelines for the management of screen-detected abnormalities, screening in specific populations and investigation of abnormal vaginal bleeding. Sydney: Cancer Council Australia, 2020. https://wiki.cancer.org.au/australia/Guidelines:Cervical_cancer/Screening

Cox JL, Holden JM, Sagovsky R. The Edinburgh Postnatal Depression Scale. 1987. www.blackdoginstitute.org.au/wp-content/uploads/2020/04/edinburgh-postnatal-depression-scale.pdf

Phillips SJ, Tepper NK, Kapp N, et al. Progestogen-only contraceptive use among breastfeeding women: a systematic review. *Contraception*. 2016; 94(3):226–52.

Case 17
Jamie-Lee needs to know about safe sex. . .

Jamie-Lee is a 16-year-old teenager who has been a patient of your practice since her birth. Both her parents are also well-known to you. Jamie-Lee is requesting contraceptive advice; in particular, she would like to start taking the COCP. She states that she will tell her mother when she does start taking the pill, and does not believe her mother will object; however, she has not discussed this with her yet, and would feel embarrassed doing so.

How do you manage this consultation?

As well as addressing Jamie-Lee's specific request, you should assure yourself about her general health. From previous records you know that Jamie-Lee has enjoyed good health, although she has asthma and uses salbutamol when required for this. On questioning, she tells you that her periods began when she was 12; they are now regular and she does not have any dysmenorrhoea. Her last period finished a week ago. She also volunteers that she has been sexually active for the past 6 months.

What further history should be taken?

A full sexual history should be taken and Jamie-Lee made aware of the advantages and disadvantages of various forms of contraception. It is important also that you make sure that Jamie-Lee is aware of the need to practise safe sex, and how to do so—in particular, she should be aware of how and where to obtain condoms and how to use them. You should discuss cigarette smoking, and also ensure that no other health problems are overlooked, particularly any conditions that may be contraindications to prescribing the COCP.

Jamie-Lee tells you that she has had two sexual partners. She has been with her current boyfriend for 4 months and believes that the relationship is exclusive for both of them. She is aware of the need to use condoms except in relationships where both partners are monogamous. She tells you that her first sexual partner was reluctant to comply with condom use and on several occasions she had intercourse without protection. She smokes cigarettes at parties only, less than five per week—your strong advice to her is to quit altogether. There is nothing else she is aware of in her own medical history that might affect her suitability for the COCP.

What examination is required for Jamie-Lee?

Jamie-Lee is able to consent to examination herself, although a chaperone should be present. Her blood pressure should be taken and a check of her heart and lungs and an abdominal examination performed. Since she has had unprotected sex, she should have a vaginal examination and endocervical swabs taken; you explain the reasons for this to her.

You also advise Jamie-Lee about how cervical cancer screening is done, when to start screening and how often screening should be performed, following national guidelines (see Case 2).

You carry out a full examination for Jamie-Lee, including vaginal examination, and note nothing remarkable. You take swabs for chlamydia and gonorrhoea—both of these are taken from the endocervical canal just inside the external os. You prescribe a monophasic COCP, which Jamie-Lee can start immediately. You explain very clearly that she must not rely on this for contraceptive protection until she has taken seven active pills. You also emphasise the need for safe sex and the use of condoms unless both partners are exclusive in their sexual relationship.

> A first-catch urine specimen can be used for screening for chlamydia and gonorrhoea rather than endocervical swabs, although the test is not as sensitive as endocervical sampling.

CLINICAL COMMENT

Precautions for women taking the COCP

- Remember to take the pill at the same time every day.
- If a pill is missed, take that pill as soon as you remember—barrier contraception will be needed until you have taken a further seven active tablets.
- Gastrointestinal upsets may result in ineffective cover—barrier contraception and the 7-day rule apply.
- A regular check of blood pressure should occur when obtaining a repeat prescription.
- Common and usually self-limiting side effects include breast tenderness, nausea and headaches.

What follow-up do you arrange for Jamie-Lee?

You ask Jamie-Lee to return in 3 months' time to see how she is progressing with the pill but assure her that you are available to see her sooner if problems arise. You recommend that she tell her mother she is taking it but emphasise that your consultation with her is strictly confidential.

Three days later, you receive the results of Jamie-Lee's swabs. The chlamydia PCR is positive. No other pathogens have been detected. Your receptionist is able to contact Jamie-Lee directly on her mobile phone and make another appointment. She presents looking extremely anxious and teary.

How do you manage this consultation?

You explain that chlamydia is a common infection. Certainly, it is a sexually transmissible infection but it is treatable. In women, chlamydia can be symptomless but it can cause infertility through salpingitis and subsequent tubal blockage. Chronic pelvic inflammatory disease (PID) that commences with a chlamydia infection is a common cause of chronic ill health in women.

> '*Who did I get it from?*' she wants to know.

You reply that it is probably impossible to know the answer to this question at this stage, repeating that this is a common problem and really just requires correct management now. She should contact all recent sexual partners and tell them of the diagnosis. She is upset at this and says that she could not face doing such a thing. She then admits to unprotected sex with her current partner. You strongly advise alerting him to her diagnosis so that he can seek attention from his own doctor. You explain that your practice nurse or local sexual or public health unit can do the contact tracing or there are websites that will help her send an anonymous email or text message (e.g. www.letthemknow.org.au). She looks at a website with you and decides to send a text.

You prescribe azithromycin for Jamie-Lee and arrange to see her again in 2 weeks' time for a further swab. You also recommend a fuller STI screen, including syphilis and HIV screening, which she agrees to.

113

Table 17.1 Summary of some common sexually transmissible infections—symptoms, signs, investigations and treatment in women

Infection	Symptoms	Signs	Investigations	Treatment
Gonorrhoea	Purulent vaginal discharge, urethral discharge, dysuria, abdominal pain, pharyngitis, septic arthritis	Fever, abdominal tenderness, purulent cervical discharge	Swabs from endocervix, urethra, rectum, pharynx First-catch urine for PCR	500 mg ceftriaxone IM plus azithromycin 1 g PO stat in uncomplicated cases
Chlamydia	Often asymptomatic Abdominal pain, vaginal discharge	Abdominal and pelvic tenderness, vaginal/cervical discharge	Swabs from endocervix, urethra, rectum, pharynx First-catch urine for PCR	Azithromycin 1 g in uncomplicated cases Prolonged doxycycline for PID
Herpes simplex (HSV-1 and HSV-2)	Skin tingling, blisters, painful ulceration, neuralgia, myopathy Primary infection may be asymptomatic	Fever, rashes, vesicles, blisters, ulceration (genital and oral)	PCR of a swab from the lesion; viral culture	Oral aciclovir, valaciclovir, famciclovir for treatment and prophylaxis IV aciclovir for complicated disease (e.g. with meningitis) Local treatment with lignocaine gel, ice packs, salt baths for symptom relief
Syphilis	Chancre, rashes, enlarged tender lymph nodes in the early stages The latent phase is symptomless Late disease includes cardiovascular, neurological and psychiatric symptoms	Primary: chancre (hard, painless genital nodule) Secondary: maculopapular rash, condylomata lata Latent: symptomless (positive serology only)	RPR, VDRL tests screening for *Treponema pallidum* haemagglutination antibody (TPHA), fluorescent treponemal antibodies (FTA-AbS) tests—note: once positive, always positive	Benzathine penicillin IM

	Symptoms	Signs	Diagnosis	Treatment
Trichomoniasis	Often asymptomatic; may complain of discharge and/or odour	Frothy greenish-grey discharge with 'fishy' odour	Direct microscopic examination of wet preparation	Metronidazole or tinidazole
Human immunodeficiency virus (HIV)	Flu-like illness within 2 weeks of infection; malaise, fever, enlarged lymph nodes. Later, weight loss, fever, malaise, fatigue, diarrhoea, enlarged nodes	Asymptomatic carrier state possible for many years. Fever, wasting, lymphadenopathy, specific infections (e.g. pneumonia) and malignancies (e.g. lymphoma)	HIV antibodies appear 3 months after infection. Once positive, always positive	Specific antiretroviral treatment. Lifestyle management—diet, exercise, avoiding smoking and recreational drugs, avoiding or treating other STIs. Treat intercurrent malignancy or premalignancy (e.g. cervical intraepithelial neoplasia)
Genital warts	Warts in anogenital region, discharge, pain/discomfort	Visible warts on vulva, perineum, perianal area, cervix	Usually clinical examination only. Biopsy if concern a lesion may be malignant	Local applications of podophyllin, 5-fluorouracil, imiquimod. Ablation using diathermy, cryotherapy or laser. Warts may disappear spontaneously

CLINICAL PEARLS

- When one STI is diagnosed it is essential that a full STI screen, including screening for HIV, is offered together with contact tracing and appropriate counselling.
- Chlamydia infection is common and mainly asymptomatic among young sexually active women. It has long-term implications for fertility and future health. Screening should be offered opportunistically when performing CST and well-woman checks.

References and further reading

Gibson EJ, Bell DL, Powerful SA. Common sexually transmitted infections in adolescents. *Prim Care.* 2014;41(3):631–50.

Lewis D, Newton DC, Guy RG, et al. The prevalence of *Chlamydia trachomatis* infection in Australia: a systematic review and meta-analysis. *BMC Infect Dis.* 2012;12:113.

Oliphant J. Adolescent sexual health and STIs. *O&G Magazine.* 2017; 19(3 Spring). www.ogmagazine.org.au/19/3-19/adolescent-sexual-health-stis/

Ong JJ, Chen M, Hocking J, et al. Chlamydia screening for pregnant women aged 16 to 25 years attending an antenatal service: a cost effectiveness study. *BJOG.* 2016;123(7):1194–202.

Case 18
Miranda fears she may be pregnant. . .

Miranda is a 19-year-old student who is a long-time patient of your practice. Her family is also well-known to you. Miranda arrives the moment the practice doors open at 8 am on the Tuesday following a long weekend and asks for an urgent appointment. She appears anxious and distressed to your reception staff so, despite a heavy schedule, you agree to squeeze her in—your first booked patient has not arrived. You take a quick look at Miranda's notes and see that one of your partners last saw her 6 months previously for a prescription for the COCP. Otherwise, apart from common childhood illnesses, Miranda has been in good health.

Miranda sits down in your consulting room and bursts into tears.

'I've been really stupid,' she says. 'I went away for the weekend with some friends, not expecting to have sex, but that's what happened. I stopped the pill 2 months ago because I broke up with Chris so I didn't use anything. Now I've got this discharge and burning; I'm afraid I've got something awful and I could be pregnant.'

How do you deal with this situation?

You explain calmly that these are common situations and there are solutions that can be offered. First, you need to take a history from Miranda. Her LMP was 3 weeks previously. She has had three periods since discontinuing the COCP, including the withdrawal bleed immediately following the last active tablet. Her cycle seems to be reestablishing with 4 days of bleeding every 27 days.

Miranda has had unprotected intercourse with a new partner on the Saturday evening and Sunday and Monday mornings of the previous weekend. The first episode was about 10 pm on Saturday, that is, about 58 hours prior to your consultation. She assures you that she has not been otherwise sexually active for more than 2 months.

Since Sunday evening, she has been experiencing vaginal burning and now has a white vaginal discharge.

What other history do you take from Miranda?

Miranda has never had an STI previously and she has never been pregnant. She takes no medications, has no allergies and has no other relevant medical history.

What do you now tell Miranda?

You explain to Miranda that emergency contraception (EC) is readily available to her—in fact, it can be obtained over the counter from pharmacists without a prescription. You explain that two forms of oral EC are available: 1.5 mg tablets of levonorgestrel (LNG), which has been available in Australia for many years, and 30 mg tablets of ulipristal acetate (UPA), which has been more recently licensed in Australia. Although oral EC can be taken up to 120 hours after exposure, it becomes less effective as time passes, so you suggest that she goes to the adjacent pharmacy immediately after the consultation. You advise her that reliable studies have shown that UPA is more effective than LNG and you recommend UPA; you write the name down for her.

> *'Is it 100% effective?'* she asks, *'and are there any side effects?'*

If LNG is taken within 72 hours of unprotected intercourse, you tell Miranda, 2% of women will still become pregnant; with UPA, this is 1%. However, you also point out that at the time of the first intercourse, Miranda would have been on day 19 of her cycle, about 6 days postovulation in what is probably another 27-day cycle, so that her chances of pregnancy are thereby reduced. The risk of conception is greatest when unprotected sexual intercourse occurs in the 6 days up to and including ovulation.

Emergency contraception will not dislodge or abort an established, implanted pregnancy. Neither LNG or UPA are teratogenic—if a pregnancy has occurred from an earlier act of unprotected intercourse, there is no additional risk to the fetus. It is also likely that UPA, an anti-progestogen, may not only inhibit ovulation when taken as directed but also have an endometrial effect contributing to its effectiveness as EC.

Some pharmacists may refuse to supply EC; GPs and other doctors providing women's healthcare should try to be aware of such practices in their areas so that women are not subject to embarrassment and are able to safely obtain their medication in a timely fashion.

Another form of emergency contraception

Copper IUCD

Insertion of a copper-bearing IUCD within 5 days of unprotected inter-course will be effective at preventing pregnancy, with a failure rate of 1%. There is the advantage of a continuing contraceptive effect; however, it is not the contraceptive method of first choice in a young nulliparous woman, particularly when there is the possibility of a concurrent STI.

What further advice do you give Miranda with regard to the possibility of pregnancy?

You tell Miranda that her period may occur earlier than expected and that the subsequent cycle may be longer than normal. If she does not get her period by the expected date, she should have a pregnancy test, which she can do herself with an over-the-counter kit or by returning to your surgery. You point out that she is unlikely to be pregnant but that if she has a positive pregnancy test she should return as soon as possible to discuss her options.

You also discuss future contraception. She tells you that the encounters of the weekend may develop into an ongoing relationship. She has a supply of the COCP at home but would also like information about other hormonal forms of contraception.

You explain to Miranda that one component of the COCP (the progestogen) may interfere with the effectiveness of the UPA and that she cannot commence the pills until five days after taking UPA. She will also need to allow 7 days of COCP taking before relying on this for contraception (9 days for Qlaira); you strongly advise her to use condoms in this period.

You also explain to her the details of the progestogen-only contraceptives (apart from the mini-pill) that are currently available and suitable for Miranda: medroxyprogesterone acetate injections and the etonogestrel implant. You also mention the levonorgestrel-releasing IUCD, which could be inserted in 5 days' time.

You must also consider Miranda's second concern, the vaginal discharge, and her fear that she may have contracted an STI. How do you deal with this question?

You should conduct an examination for Miranda and offer a full STI screen. You find Miranda to be generally well and abdominal examination shows no abnormality. You proceed to vaginal examination and pass a speculum, which will allow you to sample the cervix. There is a curdy white discharge suggesting candidiasis and some reddening of the vaginal mucosa. Otherwise, the vagina and cervix appear unremarkable. You take a swab from the reddened area for HSV PCR; a high vaginal swab from the upper vagina for candidiasis and trichomoniasis; and a swab from the endocervical region for chlamydia and gonorrhoea.

As PCR testing for chlamydia and gonorrhoea does not usually become positive until 14 days after exposure, you arrange for repeating testing. You also arrange for Miranda to have both initial and follow-up serological screening for syphilis, HIV and hepatitis B and C.

Causes of vaginal discharge

Physiological
Cervical mucus and secretions from Bartholin's and other small glands opening close to the vagina normally keep the vagina lubricated, with a discharge that may be clear or white, with a pH of 3.8–4.5. Ovulation is accompanied by increased amounts of clear mucus.

Foreign bodies
For example: a forgotten tampon

Pathological

Infections of the lower genital tract
- Candidiasis (moniliasis, commonly called 'thrush')—thick, curdy white discharge adherent to vaginal walls, which may be asymptomatic or cause burning and itching
- Trichomoniasis—frothy green discharge, possible fishy odour
- Gonorrhoea—cream or yellow colour, odourless
- Chlamydia—green, yellow, malodorous
- Bacterial vaginosis—thin, greyish, fishy odour

Cervical or vaginal lesions
For example: polyps, cervical cancer

Disease of the upper genital tract
Acute or chronic pelvic inflammatory disease (in both of these, discharge may be due to ascending secondary infection from bowel or vagina); endometrial polyps or cancer.

You give Miranda a further appointment in 7 days' time for the results of her first tests but suggest that meanwhile she buy an over-the-counter topical preparation for thrush (candidiasis), as you feel that this is the most likely cause of her symptoms. A single-dose regimen (e.g. clotrimazole) is likely to be highly effective. Alternatively, she could have a single over-the-counter dose of oral fluconazole.

What other advice do you give Miranda?

You take the opportunity to remind Miranda of the importance of safe sex. Using condoms, you tell her gently, not only greatly reduces the chances of pregnancy, it also can prevent or reduce the chances of transmission of STIs.

Condoms—use and effectiveness

- A condom should be applied before any penile penetration occurs.
- Only water-based lubricants should be used with condoms.
- The air should be squeezed out of the tip before and while the condom is being put on, to reduce the risk of breakage.
- During withdrawal, the condom should be grasped by the base, to avoid slippage.
- Following ejaculation and withdrawal, the condom should be removed by holding the rolled rim and drawing it carefully from the erect penis before detumescence occurs.
- Condoms can deteriorate and may be ineffective if brittle or sticky. Condoms should never be reused.
- Condoms are highly effective if used properly and consistently, with a Pearl Index of 3. Effectiveness is increased if they are used with spermicides.
- The female condom, if used correctly, is equally effective and also protects more fully against STIs.
- Both male and female condoms should be disposed of safely.

CLINICAL PEARLS

- Information about condom use should be supplied opportunistically in all consultations dealing with contraception and STIs.
- Condoms provide effective contraception and effective protection against STIs if used appropriately and consistently.

References and further reading

Black K, Hussainy S. Emergency contraception: oral and intrauterine options. *Aust Fam Physician.* 2017;46(10):722–6.

Cameron S, Li H, Gemzell-Danielsson K. Current controversies with oral emergency contraception. *BJOG.* 2017;124(13):1948–56.

Levy SB, Gunta J, Edemekong P. Screening for sexually transmitted diseases. *Prim Care.* 2019;46(1):157–73.

McCormack D, Koons K. Sexually transmitted infections. *Emerg Med Clin North Am.* 2019;37(4):725–38.

Case 19
Tammy is unexpectedly pregnant. . .

Tammy is a 34-year-old woman, well-known to your practice, who comes to see you in some distress, late one Friday afternoon. Tammy has essential hypertension that has at times been difficult to control. She is currently on an angiotensin-converting enzyme (ACE) inhibitor. Tammy has two children and both pregnancies were eventful: both were complicated by severe preeclampsia during the third trimester and the need for urgent delivery by caesarean section. Both infants required several weeks of care in the neonatal nursery and Tammy herself was in the high-dependency unit for some days. The younger child is now 12 months old. Since his birth, you have had a number of conversations with Tammy and her partner Joe about contraception. Tammy understands that there is a high probability that another pregnancy is likely to follow the same course, and she feels that her family is probably complete, but both she and Joe have been reluctant so far to commit to an irreversible sterilisation procedure.

What kinds of contraception are medically suitable for Tammy?

Tammy understands that with her hypertension, she is not a suitable candidate for the COCP and she has decided against a progestogen-releasing intrauterine contraceptive device after reading adverse postings on the internet, although you have reassured her that she is an excellent candidate. Prior to her second pregnancy, she had 3-monthly injections of depot medroxyprogesterone acetate (DMPA) and since the birth of her second child, has been taking the progestogen-only pill. Recently, she has had several sleepless nights with both her children ill and had forgotten to take the pill regularly: the result is a positive home pregnancy test. Other forms of contraception she could have considered are the 'morning-after pill', either the single-dose levonorgestrel emergency contraceptive pill (LNG-ECP) that can be used up to 3 days (72 hours) after unprotected sex, or a single dose of ulipristal acetate (UPA) that can be used up to 5 days (120 hours) after unprotected sex.

How do you deal initially with Tammy's presentation?

You ask Tammy how she herself feels about the pregnancy. Tammy tells you that she and Joe have been discussing the situation for 3 days now. Joe will go along with what Tammy wants to do, but he is worried about her health and the possible adverse effects of another pregnancy. Tammy herself has realised that she does not want to go through another pregnancy complicated by severe preeclampsia, with risks to herself and the child. She is aware of the needs of her two existing children and feels she is incapable of properly caring for a third child. Tammy is now requesting termination of the pregnancy and sterilisation.

Despite the lateness of the hour, you take time to look at the possible options with Tammy. You outline the various scenarios, which Tammy and Joe have already considered themselves. She can be referred for excellent antenatal care in the local hospital and assisted with the care of her existing children throughout the pregnancy. However, Tammy feels that she must consider the needs of her other children, and of her partner, first. She is also aware of the potential for teratogenic effects of ACE inhibitors in later pregnancy. She asks to be referred back to the specialist obstetrician and gynaecologist who cared for her during her pregnancies with a view to both termination and sterilisation. She asks whether the two procedures can be done under the same anaesthetic.

What is your response, and how do you advise Tammy?

You agree that this can be done, but urge caution because decision-making can be difficult when dealing with an unexpected shock. Tammy must be sure that she will not change her mind in future even should something befall one or both of her existing children, or Joe. As she is clear about the decision to end the pregnancy, her options would be the following:

1. Undergo the abortion procedure first and then return for her sterilisation procedure to be performed by laparoscopy as an interval procedure. This will give her more time to think about any future pregnancy. As her pregnancy is still early (6 weeks), the abortion may be brought about medically, avoiding the need for an anaesthetic (sedation or general anaesthetic) and surgery.
2. Surgical termination of pregnancy combined with laparoscopic sterilisation at the same time. The sterilisation may be performed by the application of clips to occlude the fallopian tubes or by salpingectomy.

You explain that subsequent reversal of sterilisation can be performed with success rates of up to 90% in terms of successful full-term pregnancies when the sterilisation has been carried out using clips (Fig. 19.1). However, such reversal procedures need to be considered as major surgery

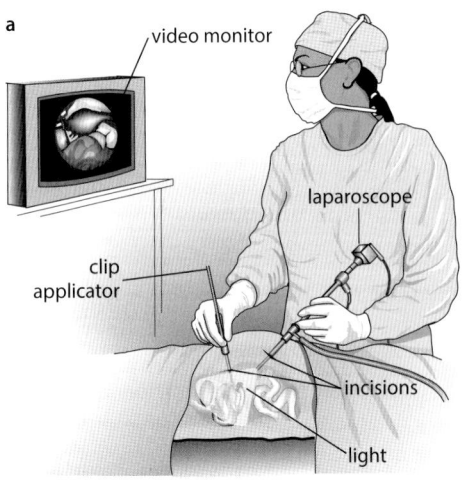

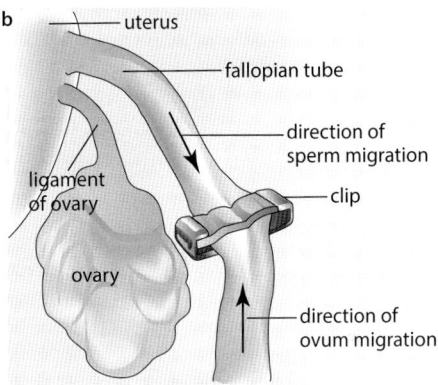

Figure 19.1 Laparoscopic sterilisation: (**a**) overview (**b**) close-up showing how the clip occludes the tube

requiring laparotomy or laparoscopy, so sterilisation must be regarded as irreversible. There is growing evidence that high-grade serous tumours of the ovary and peritoneal surface epithelium (the most common histologic subtype of epithelial ovarian cancer) may originate in the fallopian tubes. Furthermore, there is no known benefit for retaining fallopian tubes in the postreproductive period, and removal of the fallopian tubes does not appear affect ovarian function. Hence, bilateral salpingectomy should be discussed with the patient during the informed consent process for Filshie clip tubal occlusion. The other option for pregnancy after a sterilisation would be IVF treatment, and in fact this is increasingly becoming the choice of couples in this situation; however, IVF is a major and expensive medical procedure. Tammy also needs to understand that sterilisation does not carry a 100% guarantee of prevention of pregnancy—around 2 or 3 women in 1000 will become pregnant following laparoscopic clip sterilisation (figures from studies vary, and some report higher pregnancy rates). If pregnancy occurs after sterilisation, there is an increased risk of ectopic pregnancy, as the fertilised ovum lodges in a damaged but not completely occluded or removed tube.

Does Tammy meet the legal requirements for induced abortion?

Tammy meets the legal requirements for abortion in all states and territories in Australia, New Zealand and the United Kingdom, since continuing the pregnancy clearly carries a serious risk to Tammy's physical and mental health (see also Case 27). Tammy's last menstrual period was about 6 weeks ago. You discuss with her the possibility that she may feel upset about terminating the pregnancy. She acknowledges that this is so but states that she feels she is making the right decision for herself and her family. You mention that she will need a general anaesthetic for the combined procedure and that there are small but definite risks with both laparoscopy and suction curettage of the uterus. These risks include anaesthetic complications, haemorrhage, infection, damage to abdominal organs and thromboembolism. In rare cases, laparotomy may need to be performed if it is not possible to perform the sterilisation laparoscopically, especially in light of her two previous caesarean sections. Tammy needs to be aware of all these risks before she consents to the procedures.

CLINICAL COMMENT

Points for counselling prior to sterilisation

- The permanence and irreversibility of the sterilisation procedure must be clearly explained and understood.
- Other forms of contraception, including vasectomy, should be discussed.
- Time must be allowed for reflection before a decision is made.
- The failure rate of the method of sterilisation must be explained and recorded in the patient notes (this varies from 2–3 per 1000 women immediately following laparoscopic sterilisation to almost 1 in 200 women when performed in conjunction with caesarean section).

- Potential complications (see below) and the possibility of conversion to laparotomy must be discussed and documented.
- Not infrequently, even after a detailed and unambiguous explanation and advice, women assume that this is an easily reversible procedure with full return to fertility. A clear explanation is essential, and the discussion must be comprehensively recorded.
- It is helpful to use patient information sheets and procedure-specific consent forms.

Risks of surgical sterilisation

General (i.e. can occur with any surgery)
- Chest infection
- Thromboembolism
- Cardiac arrest, stroke, death
- Risks are greater in obese patients and smokers.

Specific risks of laparoscopy
- Infection—urinary tract, incision site
- Bleeding—can be severe and life-threatening if damage to major blood vessels occurs
- Damage to other organs—bladder, ureter, bowel, blood vessels
- Laparotomy may be required if there is visceral or vascular damage.
- Blood transfusion may be required.
- Wound hernias and scarring
- Carbon dioxide embolism is a rare and potentially fatal complication of laparoscopy.
- Failure of the procedure

CLINICAL COMMENT

Techniques of early abortion

- Early medical abortion (EMA) (up to 63 days' or 9 weeks' gestation) may be performed using mifepristone 200 mg orally, followed by misoprostol buccally 1–2 days later. In New Zealand, the misoprostol is usually administered, and the abortion process takes place, in a clinic; in the United Kingdom and Australia,

continued

continued

these processes generally take place in the woman's home, in the presence of a support person. These various regimens result in expulsion of the products of conception in up to 98% of cases. If the process is to take place in the woman's home, she must have adequate support and access to 24-hour emergency care if needed. Complications include heavy bleeding, infection and incomplete expulsion of the pregnancy with the need for surgical evacuation in about 2% of cases.

- In Australia, EMA is now offered via telemedicine consultation to women in rural areas who have difficulty travelling for a face-to-face consultation. If the woman requests EMA and meets the medical and legal requirements in the jurisdiction where she lives, the drugs required for EMA, mifepristone and misoprostol, will be mailed to her. However, the same provisos of adequate support and access to 24-hour emergency care still apply.

- Surgical abortion is usually by suction curettage using sedation (general or local anaesthesia) and may be safely performed in a hospital or clinic in women up to 13 or 14 weeks of pregnancy; it can be performed later in pregnancy but risks increase with increasing gestation. Risks include uterine perforation, haemorrhage and infection.

 CLINICAL PEARLS

Abortion law reform and decriminalisation in most Australian jurisdictions over the past two decades, and similar reforms in New Zealand and the United Kingdom, mean that early abortion (up to 14 weeks at least and in many cases later in pregnancy) is legally available and should be freely accessible to women requesting it from a registered medical practitioner; all women should have an appropriate consultation and investigation and give fully informed consent to the procedure. All junior doctors should be fully aware of the laws relating to abortion in the jurisdiction in which they are working.

References and further reading

NHS Choices. Overview: abortion. www.nhs.uk/conditions/abortion
Royal Australian and New Zealand College of Obstetricians and Gynaecologists. Abortion. RANZCOG Statement C-Gyn 17. Melbourne: RANZCOG: 2019. https://ranzcog.edu.au/

Royal Australian and New Zealand College of Obstetricians and Gynaecologists. Female sterilisation by Filshie clip tubal occlusion. RANZCOG Statement C-Gyn 22. Melbourne: RANZCOG; 2014. https://ranzcog.edu.au/

Royal Australian and New Zealand College of Obstetricians and Gynaecologists. Managing the adnexae at the time of hysterectomy for benign gynaecological disease. RANZCOG Statement C-Gyn 25. Melbourne: RANZCOG; 2017. https://ranzcog.edu.au/

Royal College of Obstetricians and Gynaecologists. The care of women requesting induced abortion. Evidence Based Guideline No.7. London: RCOG; 2018. www.rcog.org.uk /en/guidelines

Case 20
Daniela has a molar pregnancy. . .

Daniela is a 25-year-old woman who has occasionally visited your practice. She has been trying to conceive for more than a year and has now succeeded. Her LMP was 10 weeks previously. She has irregular cycles and did not perform a home pregnancy test until 2 weeks previously—this was positive. However, she is now very anxious: this afternoon, she noticed some slight vaginal bleeding, which has now increased in amount. She also reports almost constant nausea since the diagnosis of pregnancy was made.

What is your first step in the management of Daniela?

You take a history from Daniela. This is her first pregnancy. She has always had quite irregular menstrual cycles since her menarche at 12. Apart from her presenting complaints, she is well. In the past, she has had mild asthma requiring intermittent salbutamol, but she has no other medical or surgical history, takes no other medication apart from folate and has no allergies. She has been planning for a pregnancy for the past six months. Daniela is of South-East Asian origin, as is her partner, Lee. Her mother has diabetes but there is no other relevant family history. Daniela has had a recent negative cervical screening test.

What examination do you make for Daniela?

A general physical examination should be performed. Her BP is 110/70 mmHg, her pulse rate is 70 bpm and she is afebrile. She does not exhibit any pallor. Heart sounds are normal. Examination of the abdomen shows some lower abdominal tenderness in the midline and a mass arising centrally from the pelvis, about the size of a 12-week pregnancy.

Do you perform a vaginal examination for Daniela?

Yes—you should visualise the cervix and perform a bimanual examination. Through the speculum you see a slightly open cervix with some dark blood trickling through the os. Bimanual examination confirms a 12-week-size uterus with the os admitting a fingertip. The uterine size is therefore greater than you would expect for Daniela's pregnancy, given the date of the LMP.

What possible explanations are there for this discrepancy?

It is possible that Daniela is wrong about the date of her last period, or that what she thought was a period was, in fact, bleeding associated with implantation of the pregnancy. It is also possible that she has a multiple pregnancy—on questioning, she tells you that her mother's brothers are twins. Much less likely is gestational trophoblastic disease, either benign (a hydatidiform mole) or, very rarely, malignant (invasive mole or choriocarcinoma).

How can you make a diagnosis here?

An ultrasound scan should be performed. You arrange this in the adjacent radiology practice, requesting that it be performed urgently, and you arrange to see Daniela again after the scan. Two hours later, Daniela returns with the films. These show that no fetus is present and that there are numerous rounded echolucent areas seen: the features are highly suggestive of a molar pregnancy. Both her ovaries are noted to be enlarged to around 5 cm in diameter and are cystic with thin internal septae. No free fluid is noted in the pelvis.

How do you explain these findings to Daniela?

You explain to Daniela that she does not have a normal continuing pregnancy. She has an unusual condition (albeit one that is more common in women of her ethnic background); in molar pregnancy, the fetus has failed to develop but there is marked proliferation of the placental tissue. For further treatment, you are going to refer Daniela for immediate consultation to your local hospital. You explain that molar pregnancy is completely treatable and that Daniela's prospects of having a subsequent normal pregnancy are high. You also explain that the ovarian cysts are a response to the high levels of hormones related to the condition and that usually they will resolve after the pregnancy has been treated. You ensure that Daniela will be taken to the hospital by her partner, who will be there to support her.

A woman having had a single molar pregnancy has a 1–1.5% risk of recurrence in subsequent pregnancies; a woman who has had two or more molar pregnancies has a 20% risk of recurrence in later pregnancies. It is not uncommon to have cystic ovaries as part of the clinical picture. These are theca lutein cysts that develop in response to the high levels of β-hCG. They are soft and oedematous cysts and no attempt should be made to remove them. These will almost always resolve once the molar pregnancy is evacuated.

'What treatment am I likely to have at the hospital?' Daniela wants to know.

Further ultrasound scanning will be performed and a quantitative β-hCG level will be measured as a baseline for treatment. The treatment of molar pregnancy is evacuation of the contents of the uterus using suction curettage. Subsequently, Daniela will need to have a careful follow-up, with β-hCG levels measured to ensure that these are dropping to normal levels and that there is no persistent trophoblastic disease present.

Suction curettage of the uterus for molar pregnancy is best done under ultrasound surveillance. Prior to the procedure, she may be given a prostaglandin preparation (such as misoprostol and prostaglandin E1 preparation) to prepare her cervix to reduce the risk of uterine perforation during dilatation of the cervix. Prolonged preparation with prostaglandins should be avoided as this may increase the risk of persistent gestational trophoblastic disease (GTD). Oxytocin may be administered once the uterus is empty to reduce the risk of bleeding. Care must be taken to avoid perforating the very soft vascular uterus that surrounds the pregnancy. Following a hydatidiform mole, trophoblastic disease can persist, and spread may be local within the pelvis and/or there may be spread via the bloodstream to liver, lungs and brain. Hence, careful postoperative follow-up is indicated. Daniela is advised to attend the early pregnancy unit for follow-up where weekly serum β-hCG is checked until three consecutive normal levels. As she had a molar pregnancy, further monitoring for β-hCG is carried out monthly for 6 months from the surgical evacuation. A rise of >10% over 2 weeks (3-weekly β-hCG levels) or a fall of less than 10% over 3 weeks (4-weekly β-hCG levels) confirms a diagnosis of persistent GTD. For persisting or metastatic disease, cytotoxics, in particular methotrexate, have excellent response rates.

Six weeks later, Daniela comes to see you again. You have received her discharge letter from the hospital. After confirmation of the diagnosis by ultrasound scan and β-hCG levels, suction curettage was performed. Histological examination of the removed material confirmed a complete hydatidiform mole. Daniela will attend for follow-up at the hospital according to the schedule above. In that time, she should avoid becoming pregnant, as β-hCG levels from a new pregnancy would make follow-up of the molar pregnancy impossible. Contraception should be discussed with her (see the Clinical Comment below). Daniela's name has been placed on the hydatidiform mole register of your state to ensure and co-ordinate her follow-up.

 CLINICAL COMMENT

Hydatidiform mole may be complete or partial. With complete mole, no fetal parts are present; with a partial mole, fetal death usually occurs followed by apparent miscarriage—often the diagnosis is made only with histological examination of the products of conception.

In the United Kingdom, New Zealand and some jurisdictions in Australia, there is a central registry for gestational trophoblast disease (GTD) and this is notified whenever a woman has been diagnosed with the disease. The registry, which is regionally based, conducts follow-up for women who have completed their initial treatment at a hospital and notifies the referring unit for further follow-up if the β-hCG levels rise unexpectedly.

Women with GTD should be advised to use barrier methods of contraception until β-hCG levels revert to normal. Once β-hCG levels have normalised, the COCP may be used. IUCDs should not be used until β-hCG levels are normal, to reduce the risk of uterine perforation. Women should be advised not to conceive until their follow-up is complete. Women who undergo chemotherapy are advised not to conceive for 1 year after completion of treatment.

 CLINICAL PEARLS

- Molar pregnancy is uncommon but should not be forgotten when a woman presents with bleeding in early pregnancy or has a uterus which is 'large for dates'.

- Persistent trophoblastic disease is most common following a molar pregnancy but may occur after any pregnancy, including both early and late miscarriage and full-term delivery.

References and further reading

Royal Australian and New Zealand College of Obstetricians and Gynaecologists. Management of gestational trophoblastic disease. RANZCOG Statement C-Gyn 31. Melbourne: RANZCOG; 2017.

Royal College of Obstetricians and Gynaecologists. The management of gestational trophoblastic disease. RCOG Green-top Guideline No. 38. London: RCOG; 2020. www.rcog.org.uk

Case 21
Ruth complains of abdominal swelling. . .

Ruth is a 42-year-old woman who attends your practice intermittently. On this occasion, she has come for a cervical screening test. You note that the last time you saw her for such testing was more than 5 years ago. Ruth also tells you that she has been meaning to come for some months because she has been experiencing increasing lower abdominal discomfort, bloating and constipation, and is convinced that her abdomen is swollen—'my clothes don't fit anymore.'

What are the important points in your history taking?

After taking details of the presenting complaint, a personal history of any cancer (breast, ovarian, bowel and endometrial in particular) should be sought. Any change in menstrual cycles, any bowel symptoms, especially constipation and rectal bleeding, and any bladder symptoms should also be inquired after. A family history of breast, bowel, endometrial and ovarian cancer should be noted.

Ruth reports unchanged regular cycles with no dysmenorrhoea and no dyspareunia. She is not experiencing any hot flushes or mood changes but the lower abdominal symptoms mean she doesn't feel quite well. There is no known family history of breast or ovarian cancer. From your records you know that Ruth has two daughters, and that she underwent a laparoscopic sterilisation 10 years ago. Ruth reports some constipation but states that this has been a recurrent problem for years. Apart from the bloating, there is no other specific bowel complaint and no other significant history.

What will be the most relevant parts of your physical examination?

You must look for signs of anaemia and lymphadenopathy, and carefully palpate the abdomen.

The conjunctivae and mucous membranes show no signs of anaemia and there are no palpable lymph nodes. Routine examination of the breasts reveals a firm, very mobile lump about 1 cm diameter in the upper outer quadrant of the left breast.

Palpation of the abdomen shows a firm cystic swelling arising from the pelvis in the midline and tending towards the right lower quadrant. The swelling is non-tender and very mobile. The liver edge and the spleen are not palpable and there is no other abnormality detectable in the abdomen.

What is your provisional diagnosis?

An ovarian cyst is the most likely explanation here. A subserous fibroid on a narrow pedicle may produce the same findings. Other causes of a pelvic mass are less likely when the swelling is so mobile and feels cystic. To be absolutely certain that Ruth is not pregnant, you perform a urine β-hCG test—this is negative.

Causes of a pelvic mass

- Pregnant uterus—if in any doubt, perform a urine β-hCG test
- Fibroids or adenomyosis
- Ovarian tumour(s)—benign or malignant
- Pyosalpinx or hydrosalpinx or tubo-ovarian mass associated with pelvic inflammatory disease (PID)
- Distended bladder—with chronic retention of urine (rare in females)
- Tumours arising from bladder or bowel

Will a vaginal examination be helpful in reaching a diagnosis?

Yes—you may be able to get a better idea of the size, consistency and anatomical relations of the mass. As well, Ruth is overdue for a CST.

You perform a speculum examination for Ruth. The vagina appears normal and well-oestrogenised; the cervix also appears healthy and you take a cervical sample. There is no abnormal discharge. You then perform a bimanual examination. This helps you decide that the mass is separate from the normally sized anteverted uterus, is definitely cystic, can be balloted between your fingers and appears to arise on the right side of the uterus. It partly balloons out of the right lateral wall of the vagina. The swelling is non-tender. It is about the size of a large grapefruit. These findings reinforce your clinical impression of a right ovarian cyst.

You explain these findings to Ruth and reassure her that everything you have felt points towards this being a benign cyst. You will arrange transabdominal and transvaginal ultrasound scan and some blood tests—FBC, urea and electrolyte levels and measurement of the tumour marker CA-125. You also arrange a mammogram and possible breast ultrasound.

It is important to look for tumour markers in any woman over the age of 30 presenting with a pelvic mass. The tumour marker most commonly associated with ovarian cancer is CA-125 (cancer antigen 125). However, remember that a negative result does not totally exclude ovarian cancer, nor does a positive result necessarily indicate malignancy—in particular, CA-125 may be elevated in endometriosis, pregnancy, pancreatitis and cirrhosis of the liver, as well as during menstruation. CASA (cancer-associated serum antigen), CA 19.9, β-hCG, α-fetoprotein, LDH (lactate dehydrogenase) and inhibin are other tumour markers associated with ovarian cancers that may be helpful in diagnosis but should not be used routinely.

An FBC is an indicator of general health, and assessment of renal function is relevant to the presentation.

How do you arrange a follow-up for Ruth?

Ruth returns to you in 2 days' time for the results of these tests. You have already made an appointment with a specialist gynaecologist, Dr Nguyen, but have asked Ruth to come back to discuss the results before that visit.

Ruth's blood test results are all within normal limits including the CA-125 level, which at 18 is well within the normal range. Her mammogram and subsequent breast ultrasound strongly suggest that the breast lump is a fibroadenoma. Arrangements are in place for her to attend the breast clinic the following day, when a fine-needle aspiration will be performed. Her pelvic ultrasound scan shows a normal-sized uterus and left ovary; the right ovary appears to have been completely replaced by a 9-cm cyst, which is loculated and in some places, contains solid material. The risk of malignancy index (calculated by the ultrasonologist reading the scan) is 54, well below the threshold value of 200 for malignancy—the risk of malignancy index (RMI) and the risk of malignancy algorithm (ROMA) are both methods that combine ultrasound and biochemical information to give a risk score for a particular patient.

There is no free fluid in the pouch of Douglas. You reassure Ruth about these findings but explain that it will be necessary to remove the cyst surgically, both to make a definitive diagnosis and as treatment. The following week, Ruth has a consultation with Dr Nguyen and arrangements are made for laparoscopy or laparotomy.

> A large ovarian cyst, especially one with solid components, must be removed with caution to prevent rupture of the cyst during the operation and the possible spill into the abdomen of malignant cells. If done using a laparoscopic approach, the cyst is often placed in a bag then brought to the abdominal wall for drainage to allow delivery.

What is Ruth's subsequent progress?

You receive a discharge summary from Dr Nguyen. The complete cyst and small amount of residual ovarian tissue has been removed laparoscopically. The capsule was smooth and unbroken. The left ovary was inspected and appeared normal, as did the uterus; these organs were conserved. Histological examination of the cyst has shown it to be a serous cystadenoma with no evidence of malignant change. Ruth has made an uneventful recovery.

Cytology of the breast biopsy obtained by fine-needle aspiration indicates that the lump is a fibroadenoma, and Ruth's CST is reported as negative. Six weeks postoperatively you see Ruth again—she is well and symptoms have largely disappeared. You remind her of the importance of regular CSTs!

 CLINICAL PEARLS

- Tumours of the ovary, including ovarian cancers, commonly present late unless they are hormone-producing (rare) or undergo complications (e.g. haemorrhage, leaking or torsion).
- Bloating, swelling and vague abdominal discomfort are common presentations; such symptoms should always be taken seriously.
- In considering the causes of a pelvic mass, it is helpful to remember the five F's—fat, flatus, faeces, fetus and fluid.
- Women with a family history of ovarian or breast cancer should be offered genetic counselling.
- Simple cysts of 5 cm diameter or less that are clearly defined on ultrasound as having no suspicious features, and are asymptomatic, may be treated expectantly; in the vast majority of cases, these resolve spontaneously.

References and further reading

Biggs W, Marks ST. Diagnosis and management of adnexal masses. *Am Fam Physician.* 2016;93(8):676–81.

Royal College of Obstetricians and Gynaecologists. Management of ovarian cysts in postmenopausal women. RCOG Green-top Guideline 34. London: RCOG; 2016. www.rcog.org.uk

Royal College of Obstetricians and Gynaecologists. Management of suspected ovarian masses in premenopausal women. RCOG Green-top Guideline 62. London: RCOG; 2011. ww.rcog.org.uk

Case 22
Konstantina complains of an itch. . .

Konstantina is a woman of 65 who comes to see you in general practice, accompanied by her daughter. Konstantina has been a patient of your practice for the past 20 years, but it has been difficult to persuade her to attend regularly for visits that might require an intimate examination. On this occasion, she has come because her daughter Ophelia has insisted on it. Ophelia also helps with translation.

Konstantina has always enjoyed good health and her only real problem has been with a chronic vulvar itch. This first developed when she was 47, about the time she first missed her periods and had occasional hot flushes. Examination at that time, according to the notes of your predecessor, Dr Phillips, showed some slight vulvar and vaginal atrophic changes, and she prescribed a course of topical oestrogen cream, which settled the symptoms.

A year later, when Konstantina came along for her routine well-woman check (prompted by Ophelia), on questioning, she admitted to continuing intermittent itch and on examination, there were areas of white atrophic skin noted anteriorly on both the labia majora and around the clitoris. There were no reddened or suspicious-looking areas and vaginal examination was otherwise unremarkable.

What was the clinical diagnosis here and how was the condition managed?

After some persuasion, Konstantina attended a local gynaecologist who made a clinical diagnosis of lichen sclerosus but also took a small punch biopsy for histological examination, which confirmed the clinical impression. Daily application for 2–4 weeks of a high-dose corticosteroid cream in the form of betamethasone, followed by a maintenance application of a lower dose of the same preparation twice weekly, was recommended and for some years has kept her symptoms under control.

What follow-up has Konstantina had?

Konstantina has been invited to have annual checks of the area ever since the initial diagnosis at your practice. While her compliance has been less frequent than recommended, follow-up has been performed on several occasions. There has been a gradual increase in the amount of skin involved and the slow development of fusion of the labia anteriorly. The appearances, as documented by several of your colleagues, have always been of whitened skin with no reddened areas. On questioning, Konstantina has reported no dysuria or dyspareunia and has found that varying the application of the creams, together with occasional salt baths, has kept her symptoms under control. Her periods stopped completely by the age of 49, the associated menopausal symptoms were minimal and she did not wish to use any systemic hormone replacement. She has had cervical screening performed opportunistically and breast checks, her blood pressure has always been in the normal range and there have been no other health problems. She does not smoke cigarettes.

Lichen sclerosus is a chronic inflammatory condition provoking epidermal thinning, causing the vulval skin to become pale, thickened and split or fissured; loss of the normal architecture, with fusion of the labia minora and of these to the labia majora, is common. The clitoris may be completely obscured by such fusion and by chronic oedema of the clitoral foreskin; dyspareunia and associated psychological symptoms may be a consequence. Pruritus (itch) is the most common presenting complaint. In a small number of women (less than 5%), an affected area may develop squamous cell carcinoma; hence the condition must be kept under surveillance.

Six months ago, Konstantina's husband suffered a stroke and so, in fact, she has not had a check for more than 18 months. Today, on questioning, she tells you that she has noticed some slight bleeding and pain on the left side of the vulva. (She had not mentioned this to her daughter, who remonstrates with her, telling her that her mother's health is as important as her father's.)

On examination, the lichen sclerosus is evident bilaterally. On the anterior aspect of the left labium is a reddened, slightly ulcerated palpable nodule, about 8 mm in diameter.

What are your concerns with this change in Konstantina's history and how do you investigate her complaint?

You complete the vaginal examination, including a cervical screening test, which is both due under the routine schedule, and indicated by the vulvar findings. You have already performed an abdominal examination and found nothing remarkable but you now return to the abdomen and palpate the inguinal regions for enlarged lymph nodes—there are none. You tell Konstantina that you are concerned about the vulvar lesion and will be arranging an early gynaecological consultation. You reassure her, and Ophelia, that although this may be an early malignancy, the fact that she has come along early, that it is small and on the skin, are all good signs.

What other information may be relevant to Konstantina's situation?

You need to be aware of her home conditions as she herself may require admission to hospital. You inquire about her husband's health and find that he is recovering well. He is home from the rehabilitation unit and if Konstantina has to go to hospital, her daughter and the families of her three sons will care for him.

The following Wednesday, you receive a telephone call from the gynae-cologist, Dr Smith. He tells you that the lesion has been shown to be a squamous cell carcinoma on biopsy, and wide local excision has been scheduled for the following Monday with a gynaecological oncologist.

 CLINICAL COMMENT

> Early vulvar cancers are usually treated with wide local excision, often with sentinel lymph node biopsy; full dissection of the inguinal lymph nodes is only performed if there is more than 1 mm of invasion of the primary tumour. CT, PET/CT and MRI of the pelvis and inguinal regions may be helpful in detecting the extent of disease. For larger lesions, adjuvant radiation and chemotherapy are commonly used; they are also indicated where there are lymph node metastases. Laser ablation may also be used for extensive or multifocal lesions. Radical vulvectomy with bilateral inguinofemoral lymphadenectomy is a very disfiguring procedure and is now not often performed. Lymphoedema can complicate groin node dissection.

Staging of vulvar cancers uses the T (tumour), N (nodes), M (metastases) system: the tumour is measured and involvement of the vagina, urethra or anus, or further spread to bladder, rectum or bone is noted; groin nodes if removed are examined postoperatively and may be free of tumour or may contain tumour on one or both sides; there may or may not be evidence of distant metastases.

What follow-up should be arranged for Konstantina?

Six weeks later, Konstantina comes to see you postoperatively. She is well. Examination shows that the operation site is well-healed, although there is still some stiffness and numbness in the area. You reassure her that these symptoms will settle down and suggest gentle massage with a vitamin E cream. Dr Smith's report states that sentinel node biopsy was negative, so prognosis is good with a 95% chance of 5-year survival. Konstantina will be attending him regularly for follow-up over the next 5 years; this will include examination of the operation site, of the lungs and abdomen and of distant lymph nodes.

Konstantina remarks that one thing that is now completely cured is the itch!

CLINICAL COMMENT

Important points about vulvar cancer

- Most vulvar cancers are squamous cell cancers (VSCC); melanoma is the next most common vulvar malignancy.
- Vulvar cancer is most common in postmenopausal women but is increasing in frequency in all age groups.
- There is growing evidence for two major types of vulvar intraepithelial neoplasia (VIN) corresponding to two distinct pathways to VSCC: high-grade squamous intraepithelial lesions (HSIL), previously referred to as uVIN (usual type), which is HPV-driven and occurs in younger women; non-HPV-associated dVIN (differentiated type) affects older women and often presents on a background of lichen sclerosus or other chronic inflammatory dermatoses. Low-grade squamous intraepithelial lesions (LSIL) of low malignant potential also occur on the vulva.
- The introduction, currently in progress, of vaccines effective in protecting against HPV will hopefully reduce the incidence of VIN and vulvar cancer, as well as that of cervical cancer. Cigarette smoking should also be actively discouraged in all women and this measure should contribute to a decrease in squamous cell genital cancers.

Common causes of vulvar pruritus

- Contact dermatitis due to soaps, detergents, spermicides etc.
- Allergic dermatitis
- Drug reactions
- Infections, most commonly candidiasis
- Lichen sclerosus
- Lichen planus
- Generalised skin conditions also affecting the vulva (e.g. psoriasis)

Persistent itch and skin changes are concerning features, and the patient should be referred to a gynaecologist or dermatologist, as malignancy can easily be overlooked in these patients.

 CLINICAL PEARLS

Lichen sclerosus is a common condition in older women and symptoms are usually lifelong. Since up to 5% of women with lichen sclerosus may develop vulvar cancer, regular inspection of the vulva should be performed annually.

Older women from certain more conservative ethnic backgrounds may be reluctant to present with genital tract symptoms; well-woman checks and CST may be offered opportunistically to such women.

References and further reading

Lien NH, Park KJ, Soslow RA, Murali R. Squamous precursor lesions of the vulva: current classification and diagnostic challenges. *Pathology.* 2016;48(4):291–302.

Tan A, Bieber AK, Stein JA, Pomeranz MK. Diagnosis and management of vulvar cancer: a review *Am Acad Dermatol.* 2019;81(6):1387–96.

Weinberg D, Gomez-Martinez R. *Obstet Gynecol Clin.* 2019;46(1):125–35.

Case 23
Patricia complains of hot flushes. . .

Patricia is a 49-year-old legal secretary who comes to see you, concerned about hot flushes. These are worse at night, and she has difficulty sleeping and is tired and moody during the day. She tells you she is finding it hard to concentrate on her work and, as she is responsible for managing a busy office, this is causing her considerable anxiety.

What is the likely cause of her symptoms and what else do you need to ask?

Patricia is in the climacteric (the perimenopause), approaching her menopause, her final menstrual period. Decreasing and fluctuating hormone levels are responsible for her symptoms. However, these may be exacerbated by other events or stresses in her life, or intercurrent medical conditions—none of these possible factors should be overlooked. You need to take a full history from Patricia.

Her presenting symptom, the flushes, have worsened over the past 2 months, waking her at night. She finds it difficult to get to sleep again, and begins to worry over problems that seem easily solved in daylight hours. On further questioning, you find that her father has recently died of a stroke. Her mother has had surgery for bowel cancer and is currently very dependent on her daughter. Patricia is the sole parent for two teenage boys, having been divorced for the past 5 years. Her older son is taking his final school examinations and is also learning to drive, two things that cause her concern. She admits to feeling depressed much of the time.

What further history do you take from Patricia?

You take a full menstrual history. Periods, she says, have become lighter over the past year but recently there have been episodes of bleeding between them; in fact, she's often not sure what's a period and what's not. She has kept a menstrual calendar over the past 2 months and when you examine this you see that Patricia has had bleeding for 2–3 days every week for the past 7 weeks. She also admits to some mild pelvic pain. Patricia has not been sexually active since her divorce. She has never had an STI. From her notes you see that she last had a Pap smear in your practice 7 years previously, and she says she is sure she has not had one elsewhere in that time—'since the divorce I've tended to forget about sex and things like that,' she tells you. She also tells you she has never had a mammogram.

In the past, Patricia had two full-term deliveries. She has had no significant illnesses. Apart from the removal of a thyroid cyst in her 20s, after which she did not require thyroxine therapy, she has had no surgery, takes no medications apart from a multivitamin preparation and is allergic to penicillin only. She does smoke 20 cigarettes a day and drinks three or four glasses of wine each night. On specific questioning, she admits to drinking up to six cups of black coffee each day—'I need it to get through the day.' 'What about regular exercise?,' you ask. She tries to get to the gym on Saturdays but doesn't always do so.

What examination do you make for Patricia?

You carry out a general examination first. Patricia looks tired and drawn but otherwise well. She is slim, with a BMI of 24. Her blood pressure and examination of the heart and lungs are all within normal limits, inspection and palpation of the breasts is unremarkable and there is no lymphadenopathy. Abdominal examination reveals no abnormality.

You then proceed to a vaginal examination and pass a speculum in preparation for a cervical screening test. To your surprise, you see the strings of an IUCD protruding through the cervix. You tell Patricia of your finding and she is equally surprised. 'Good heavens,' she says, 'I thought I had that out years ago, when my marriage was breaking up. Could that be the cause of the bleeding?' 'Indeed it could,' you reply, and recommend removing the device, to which she agrees. You perform the planned CST prior to removing the IUCD so that bleeding does not contaminate the specimen. You also take swabs from the endocervical canal for microscopy and culture in case some mild infection is contributing to the bleeding. You then remove the IUCD without difficulty, identifying it as a copper-bearing device, and you also take swabs from this.

Bimanual examination shows a slightly tender normal-sized uterus and you recommend to Patricia a course of oral antibiotics (metronidazole and cephalexin), as clinically, she appears to have a degree of endometritis.

Intrauterine contraceptive devices

- IUCDs are safe, highly effective methods of contraception (Pearl Index 1 for the copper-bearing IUCD, 0.1 for the levonorgestrel-releasing IUCD).
- Copper-containing devices interfere with sperm motility, sperm and ovum transport, fertilisation and implantation; regular menstrual cycles continue and periods may be heavier than previously.
- Levonorgestrel-releasing devices thicken cervical mucus, decrease sperm motility and cause endometrial atrophy; oligomenorrhoea or amenorrhoea occurs in most women but may be preceded by several months of irregular spotting.
- Pelvic inflammatory disease (PID) is an uncommon complication of copper-bearing IUCDs, usually arising at the time of insertion; PID is rare with levonorgestrel-releasing IUCDs.
- Pain occurs in 1–2% of women, necessitating removal of the IUCD. Spontaneous expulsion occurs in 2–5% and may be unnoticed by the woman.
- It is important to remember that if pregnancy occurs in conjunction with the presence of an IUCD, it may be ectopic. If the pregnancy is intrauterine, there is a risk of septic miscarriage. The IUCD should be removed if it is easy to do so, to prevent miscarriage.

What is the next step in the care of Patricia?

You explain that normally with irregular bleeding around the time of the menopause you would refer her to a gynaecologist for full investigation. However, it seems likely that the retained IUCD was the cause of the bleeding, in which case removing it and giving antibiotics should improve the situation. You plan to send her for a transvaginal pelvic ultrasound scan to obtain a good view of the uterine cavity. You also order blood tests—FBC, FSH, TSH and LFTs (in view of her alcohol consumption) and give her information about breast screening.

> FSH is the only hormone that needs measuring for the diagnosis of the climacteric (perimenopause), but confirmatory blood testing is not always essential as in many cases the diagnosis can be made on history alone.
>
> While anti-Müllerian hormone (AMH) levels decline in the perimenopause, measurement of these is not recommended for diagnosis.

What else should be discussed with Patricia?

You explain that you believe that the approach of the menopause is the main cause of Patricia's problems but that her lifestyle and family commitments are undoubtedly contributing to her anxiety and insomnia. You also explain that short-term hormone therapy is a safe and sensible solution for her hot flushes but that until the cause of the irregular bleeding has been diagnosed, prescribing this is contraindicated. You tell her that until her next consultation, which you schedule for a week's time, a mild hypnotic such as temazepam may be helpful. You would prescribe this only until she is established on hormone therapy and sleeping well again. You also suggest that she cut down on coffee, especially in the afternoons and evenings, and reduce her alcohol intake. She should also look at a suitable program for quitting cigarettes, which she should start once the immediate problems are solved. Regular exercise and diet also get a mention.

> Patricia is happy with all this, says she is very relieved by what you have told her and agrees to return in a week.

You supply her with written information about hormone therapy.

How do you manage the second consultation?

At this consultation you immediately notice that Patricia looks brighter and less tired. She tells you that she is sleeping better and has had no further vaginal bleeding but still has significant hot flushes during the day. You now have copies of all her results. The FBC and TSH are within the normal range, as are the LFTs; however, you take the opportunity to emphasise that her alcohol intake is above that considered safe for women. The FSH level is 60 mmol/L—well into the postmenopausal range. USS of the pelvis shows a thin endometrial strip 2 mm thick and no fibroids or polyps; the ovaries are small and show no abnormality. Swabs from the IUCD and cervical canal have shown a light growth of *Streptococcus faecalis*, which is sensitive to cephalosporins. Her CST has been reported as normal.

You explain to Patricia that there is no obvious abnormality in the uterus and that almost certainly the cause of the bleeding was the continued presence of the IUCD. You can safely prescribe hormone therapy, which she would like to try. She has no family history of breast cancer, but has also made an appointment for a mammogram. She is not overweight, and has no history of thromboembolism or coronary heart disease.

Patricia has read through the written material you provided her and after some discussion with her about her options you start her on a cyclical oral preparation of oestrogen and a progestogen and arrange to review her in 2 months. You warn her that she may have some slight breakthrough bleeding on this for the first few months but that this should settle down and she should have light withdrawal bleeds subsequently. She may also experience some nausea or headache, which should be self-limiting. It will take up to 4 weeks for the hot flushes to subside completely; in this time, she will stop the temazepam.

> Patricia returns to see you in 2 months' time. She is now looking extremely well and happy.

What are the important points in this consultation?

Patricia tells you that she has had only slight withdrawal bleeding since commencing the hormone therapy. The lower abdominal pain that she had been experiencing has also completely disappeared, as have her hot flushes. Her mammogram showed no abnormality. Work is now manageable, her son has passed his driving test and seems to be acting responsibly and her mother has gone on a cruise to Fiji with a friend. Life is looking good.

> *'How long can I stay on the hormones?'* she asks.

You explain that it is safe to continue with hormone therapy in the short term (up to 5 years) to deal with the period of time in which the hot flushes and other menopausal symptoms are most debilitating. She can be switched to continuous therapy if she wishes in view of the scanty withdrawal bleeds and her elevated FSH. She may continue longer than 5 years under medical supervision but will need to be aware of a slightly increased incidence of breast cancer on combined HT. The short-term risk is low.

You explain that there is no increased risk of cardiovascular disease to Patricia with short-term use of hormone therapy, and only a slightly increased risk of stroke. The risk of thromboembolic incidents is slight for a woman of Patricia's BMI. Studies have not shown any cardiac benefit from use of HT but it does protect against osteoporosis, and this protection may continue for some years after stopping the therapy. After publication of a very large study into long-term hormone therapy (the Women's Health Initiative), there was a tendency not to prescribe it, but the pendulum has now swung back and it may be useful in some women in the long-term. Transdermal hormonal preparations have even lower risks than oral preparations, and Patricia might consider one of these if she wishes to continue with hormone therapy. Meanwhile, she can continue with her preparation quite safely, returning for a further checkup in a year's time and reporting back if she has any problems, particularly vaginal bleeding.

Patricia also tells you that she has taken up a Pilates class three times a week, and has joined a church group dedicated to quitting smoking.

 CLINICAL PEARLS

- Hormonal therapy should be tailored to the particular requirements of the individual woman and may be modified as a woman passes from the perimenopausal to the postmenopausal period.
- Lifestyle factors may be important in exacerbating symptoms and should always be inquired about. Weight loss, attention to diet, regular exercise, stopping smoking, reducing alcohol and coffee intake and taking measures to reduce stress may all improve a woman's sense of well-being at this time of life.

References and further reading

Australasian Menopause Society. Menopause treatment options. www.menopause.org.au/hp/management/treatment-options

Delamater L, Santoro N. Management of the perimenopause. *Clin Obstet Gynecol.* 2018;61(3):419–32.

National Institute for Health and Care Excellence. Menopause: diagnosis and management. NICE guideline 23. London: NICE; 2019. www.nice.org.ak/guidance/ng23

Case 24
Debbie presents with some irregular bleeding. . .

Debbie is a woman of 48 who is referred to you by the women's health nurse who conducts well-woman checks in small towns in your region. Debbie has not had a cervical screening test (CST) for 12 years. She was divorced when she was 40 and has been sexually active only infrequently since that time. She believed that she did not need cervical screening if she was not having regular sex. She presented to the women's health nurse because she had some bloodstained discharge. The nurse was concerned by the appearance of Debbie's cervix on speculum examination.

What is your first step in the management of this case?

Take a full history. Debbie tells you that her periods seemed to have stopped when she was 47. She had some hot flushes at that time, which soon settled. Then she began to have slight irregular bleeding, which she decided was part of 'the change'. More recently, she has had a bloodstained discharge that has been offensive at times and she felt that this was not normal. There has been no pain associated with the bleeding or discharge.

What further information do you need from Debbie?

Debbie informs you that she has had five children with three different partners—all normal pregnancies and deliveries. She has been married and divorced twice. She lives on her own, all her children having left home. She works as a waitress in a country pub and lives on the job. She smokes 30 cigarettes a day and drinks socially. She had her appendix removed at the age of 14. In the past 10 years, she has had a cholecystectomy and a hospital admission for low back pain—she states that on neither occasion was a CST suggested. She takes occasional analgesics for backache but no other regular medications and has no allergies. Her mother died from breast cancer at age 60 and she has had several mammograms since the age of 40 as she has been concerned about getting breast cancer herself.

You take the opportunity to counsel Debbie about the effects of cigarette smoking on her health and offer her help with giving up cigarettes.

Nearly all cervical cancers are caused by a human papillomavirus (HPV) infection. HPV is a common virus that is spread by genital skin-to-skin contact during sexual activity. It is so common that many people have it at some point and are never aware of this as there are usually no symptoms. If the body's immune system does not clear a HPV infection, it can cause changes to cells in the cervix, which in rare cases can develop into cervical cancer. This usually takes 10 to 15 years.

Other risk factors for cervical cancer are smoking, lack of regular cervical screening tests and long-term use of the COCP in women who have HPV infection.

What examination do you perform for Debbie?

General examination is performed first. Debbie is a rather underweight woman who looks generally well but with some moist sounds on auscultation of her chest. Her BP is 120/85 mmHg, her pulse is 68 bpm and she is afebrile. There is no lymphadenopathy in the cervical, supraclavicular or inguinal nodes.

Examination of the abdomen shows the scars expected from her surgery. There is no hepatomegaly or splenomegaly. There are no intra-abdominal masses and no tenderness.

What is your next step?

You perform a vaginal examination. Speculum examination shows a fungating growth about 3 cm in diameter on the anterior lip of the cervix. This bleeds on touch with the brush you use to take a co-test. On bimanual palpation, the lesion is firm and nodular and anteriorly reaches forward towards the vaginal wall. The uterus itself is mobile and anteverted.

It is important that whenever a CST is taken that the cervix is completely and carefully inspected. CSTs may fail to make the diagnosis in the presence of frank cervical cancer because much of the surface epithelium around the cancer is necrotic.

> Debbie is now very worried, and asks you if she has cancer. What do you tell her?

It is important to tell Debbie the truth in as detailed a way as you think appropriate. You explain that the women's health nurse has correctly noticed an unusual growth on the cervix. You feel that, yes, this is possibly an early cervical cancer. You will be referring Debbie promptly to a gynaecologist in the nearest large town who will take over investigations and subsequent management if the diagnosis is confirmed. You will also help Debbie make whatever social and work arrangements are needed while she undergoes investigation and treatment.

> 'What kind of investigations?' Debbie asks.

There will be an initial history and examination as already performed by you. The next steps will include blood tests (FBC, UECs, LFTs), ultrasound scan (USS) of her pelvis and kidneys, chest X-ray, examination under anaesthesia (EUA) and biopsy of the cervical lesion, cystoscopy and possibly CT or magnetic resonance imaging (MRI). All of these, you explain, will be to determine whether the cancer has spread. Debbie can then expect to have the results of all these tests explained to her in detail and treatment offered.

 CLINICAL COMMENT

Cervical cancer

There are 2 main types of cervical cancer named after the type of cells they originate from. Squamous cell carcinoma is the most common type (about 80% of all cases) and starts in the squamous cells of the cervix. Adenocarcinoma is less common and develops from the glandular cells. Cervical cancer spreads directly to the vagina, bladder and rectum (rarely to the ovary), by the lymphatics (iliac nodes then para-aortic nodes) and by the bloodstream (to liver, lungs, bones). Cystoscopy provides information about bladder involvement. MRI is increasingly being used to measure tumour volume and size; CT scanning is used for the assessment of pelvic lymph nodes.

> 'Will I need an operation?' Debbie asks.

It is likely that Debbie will be recommended a radical hysterectomy with resection of the pelvic lymph nodes. If investigations show that the primary tumour is larger than 4 cm diameter, then a combination of radiotherapy and chemotherapy as the primary treatment will be more appropriate.

Women diagnosed with cervical cancer have a 74% chance of surviving for 5 years. But this depends on stage at diagnosis and treatment regimen. Five-year survival after treatment of early stage cancer is >80% but this reduces to 30% for women with lymph node involvement.

 CLINICAL PEARLS

- All women receiving medical care for any condition whatsoever (including gall bladder disease and low back pain!) should be offered cervical screening opportunistically or, if this is not feasible, reminded of the importance of regular screening. Cervical cancer is one of the few cancers that, if detected in its premalignant or early stages, has close to a 100% cure rate.
- All women who smoke cigarettes should receive advice about the effects of smoking on health, and be offered help with quitting on every occasion on which they present to healthcare providers.
- All women with irregular vaginal bleeding, whether premenopausal, perimenopausal or postmenopausal, should have prompt examination and investigation to rule out malignancy.

References and further reading

Australian Institute of Health and Welfare. Cervical cancer. Sydney: AIHW; 2020. www.canceraustralia.gov.au/affected-cancer/cancer-types/cervical-cancer

Bhatla N, Berek JS, Cuello Fredes M, et al. Revised FIGO staging for carcinoma of the cervix uteri. *Int J Gynaecol Obstet.* 2019;145:129.

Yamashita H, Okuma K, Kawana K, et al. Comparison between conventional surgery plus postoperative adjuvant radiotherapy and concurrent chemoradiation for FIGO stage IIB cervical carcinoma: a retrospective study. *Am J Clin Oncol.* 2010;33:583.

Case 25
Alex presents with annoying menstrual bleeding. . .

You are in the gynaecology outpatient clinic and read the referral letter from a local general practitioner (GP) for your next patient. Alex is a 25-year-old man with bothersome menstrual bleeding. You learn that he is a transgender male (assumed female at birth) and has been on hormone replacement therapy with injectable testosterone for the last 12 months. You go out to the waiting room and call 'Alex?' A casually dressed young man stands up and follows you.

You introduce yourself and ask Alex what name and pronouns he prefers'. He visibly relaxes and says that he prefers 'Alex' and prefers 'he/him'. You ask him to tell you about the reason he is here. He explains that he commenced hormone replacement with testosterone injections about a year ago and that he was looking forward to his periods stopping on this treatment. Unfortunately, though, they have now become somewhat irregular—when they were previously regular and lasted 4–5 days in a 28-day cycle—and accompanied by some premenstrual and perimenstrual cramping. He needs to wear menstrual pads several days a month.

He really dislikes having menstrual bleeding and experiences a lot of dysphoria as a result. He is otherwise well and works as a sales assistant in retail. He does not smoke at all and drinks socially when out with friends. He has no relevant past medical history of note and takes no medications apart from testosterone (125 mg testosterone enantate every 3 weeks), prescribed by his GP.

He is not in a relationship currently, and usually has casual sex with cisgender males—he has a few regular 'friends with benefits' he catches up with now and again. He does not generally use condoms, and has both 'frontal' (i.e. vaginal) intercourse as well as oral and receptive anal sex.

You know that most trans men on testosterone replacement therapy will be amenorrhoeic within weeks of starting treatment, as testosterone works to produce both endometrial and vaginal atrophy. You are also aware that continued bleeding can produce significant dysphoria for many trans men, and that depressive symptoms and self-harming behaviours can peak during episodes of bleeding. One study showed that over 90% of trans men had no periods 6 months after starting testosterone.

You ask Alex if he would be comfortable with your performing a gynae-cological examination on him. You realise that this is a delicate question to ask, given the dysphoria many transgender individuals have with regards to their genitals. Although somewhat nervous about it—he has never had a vaginal examination before—Alex lets you know that he was expecting to be examined and that he is happy to consent to an examination. You outline the examination and let him know what to expect, and he again agrees.

On examination, he has a somewhat atrophic vagina and an inflamed-looking cervix with some mucoid discharge. There is also some blood at the cervical os and in the vaginal vault. On bimanual examination, the uterus is normal-sized and there are no masses palpable, nor tenderness on rocking the cervix. You take swabs and perform a cervical screening test, knowing that Alex fits the criteria and that transgender men are less likely to be screened than are cisgender women.

While Alex is getting dressed, you collect your thoughts and formulate a management plan. When Alex sits down again, you explain your examina-tion findings to him and let him know you would like to order some tests.

Q: What are the likely causes of menstrual bleeding in a transgender male?

1. The most likely cause is low testosterone levels. Alex is currently on a low dose of testosterone. The usual dose would be 250 mg given every 2–3 weeks, and he is only on half this dose.
2. Coagulation defects
3. Thyroid disease
4. Structural abnormalities (e.g. endometrial polyps)
5. Infection, trauma or pregnancy

Q: What are some of the problems that need addressing for Alex?

1. Unwanted menstrual bleeding in a transgender man.
2. STI risk and cervicitis, possibly caused by an STI such as gonorrhoea, and/or chlamydia and/or *Mycoplasma genitalium*.
3. Pregnancy risk.

Q: What tests do you think are appropriate?

Alex's main concern is menstrual bleeding while on testosterone replace-ment therapy. Appropriate blood tests would include:

- Hormone screen—serum testosterone, serum oestradiol, luteinising hormone (LH)

- Full blood count (especially looking at haemoglobin level and platelet count)
- Clotting profile
- Thyroid function tests
- β-hCG (to rule out pregnancy)

Given Alex's history of unprotected sexual intercourse with cisgender males, a full sexually transmissible infection (STI) screen would be appropriate. *The Australian sexually transmitted infection and HIV testing guidelines for asymptomatic men who have sex with men* can be found at https://stipu. nsw.gov.au/wp-content/uploads/STIGMA_Guidelines2019_Final-1.pdf/.

Tests for Alex would include:

- Hepatitis A and B serology
- HIV serology
- Syphilis serology
- NAAT (nucleic acid amplification tests)/PCR swabs for *Chlamydia trachomatis* and *Neisseria gonorrhoeae* at 3 sites: throat, low vaginal (or cervical if the clinician is doing a speculum examination) and rectum. You have already taken swabs during your examination of Alex, but in other circumstances all 3 can be self-collected by sending the patient to the toilet with suitable instructions.
- Given cervicitis is present, a NAAT/PCR for *Mycoplasma genitalium* is also recommended.

If Alex is considering HIV PrEP (pre-exposure prophylaxis)—which certainly should be recommended to him—further testing for creatinine clearance and hepatitis C serology should be offered as per guidelines.

Along with the risk of STIs, Alex is potentially at risk for pregnancy. Becoming pregnant while taking testosterone replacement is possible, though fertility *is* reduced. There are potential significant harms to a female fetus from testosterone, however. You talk this over with Alex and he asks about contraception.

What contraception options would be good for Alex?

1. The hormonal intrauterine device (LNG-IUD) is ideal as it usually results in amenorrhoea, and also provides excellent protection against pregnancy. It contains levonorgestrel (the higher dose IUCD, Mirena, is preferred due to its effects on stopping periods) and will not interfere with Alex's testosterone therapy. The downside

for trans men usually revolve around the insertion—which can be more uncomfortable due to vaginal and cervical atrophy induced by testosterone—and can sometimes be problematic due to dysphoria at having a vaginal speculum inserted. The etonorgestrel implant is also suitable and may reduce vaginal bleeding also.

2. The combined oral contraceptive pills and vaginal ring, containing oestrogen and progesterone, are generally not considered suitable as the oestrogen may interfere with the masculinising effects of testosterone.

3. Condoms will prevent pregnancy and some STIs if used consistently and correctly, though will not, of course, reduce menstrual bleeding.

4. Hysterectomy is another potential option that would solve both the problems of menstrual bleeding and potential unwanted pregnancy and is an option that can be considered, providing the person is sure they do not wish to bear a child in the future. There are also the usual risks of major surgery.

Alex thinks the IUCD may be the best option for him and says he would like to have one inserted as soon as possible. You print out some information about IUCDs and their insertion and give him a consent form to take home with him to read. You arrange for an appointment in 2 weeks' time to give him the results of his tests and to insert the IUCD as an office procedure. You also suggest he use a vaginal oestrogen cream for one week prior to the IUCD insertion in order to reduce the discomfort associated with the speculum examination—Alex is happy to take you up on this suggestion.

You also offer him treatment for cervicitis with 500 mg ceftriaxone IMI plus 1 g azithromycin orally, both as a single-dose treatment—this will cover treatment of both gonorrhoea and chlamydia, pending the results of the NAAT/PCR tests.

Two weeks later

Alex returns to see you. His test results are all back and the results are as follows:

- Serum testosterone = 7 nmol/L (the recommended range for a transgender male is 10–15 nmol/L); serum oestradiol = 225 pmol/L (normal follicular level for a cisgender woman of reproductive age); LH = 4.2 U/L (normal for adult cisgender woman)
- Full blood count (especially looking at haemoglobin level and platelet count)—haemoglobin = 145 g/L (normal level for cisgender male); platelet count = 380×10^9/L (normal)

- Clotting profile—normal
- Thyroid function tests—normal
- β-hCG (pregnancy test)—negative
- Hepatitis A and B serology—hep A IgG—non-reactive; hep BsAg—non-reactive, hep BcAb—non-reactive, and hep BsAb—88 IU/L—consistent with protection via vaccination
- HIV serology—non-reactive
- Syphilis serology—non-reactive
- Cervical screening test—negative for HPV subtypes
- NAAT/PCR (cervical swab) for *Mycoplasma genitalium*—negative
- NAAT/PCR for *Chlamydia trachomatis* and *Neisseria gonorrhoeae*
  - Throat—*Neisseria gonorrhoeae* detected
  - Cervix—*Chlamydia trachomatis* detected
  - Rectum—*Chlamydia trachomatis* and *Neisseria gonorrhoeae* detected

Working diagnosis list after test results:

1. Menstrual bleeding likely due to low level of serum testosterone—this is the commonest cause of bleeding in a trans man on testosterone treatment.
2. Gonorrhoea and chlamydia infections, leading to asymptomatic cervicitis.
3. Susceptibility to hepatitis A and HIV infection.

You talk over the results with Alex and answer his questions. You recommend increasing his testosterone dose and let him know you will write a letter to his GP including this suggestion, along with a suggestion to consider hepatitis A vaccination and prescribing HIV PrEP for Alex, as he is at risk of HIV given his sexual activities. You also discuss partner notification given his gonorrhoea and chlamydia infections.

After a positive chlamydia or gonorrhoea result, an IUCD can be inserted if the person is asymptomatic and has completed antibiotic treatment. In a person with asymptomatic chlamydia in an emergency situation, the IUCD can be inserted on the same day as treatment is instituted.

The procedure to insert the IUCD goes well and the vagina looks significantly less atrophic after Alex used vaginal oestrogen for a week—he asks if he can use this regularly to make vaginal intercourse more comfortable and you let him know he can do this but will only need to use it twice weekly. You reassure him this will not interfere with the masculinising effects of his testosterone treatment. He thanks you for all the effort you have gone to and for being so accepting and helpful. You arrange an appointment for a review in one month's time but are confident that with an increased dose of testosterone and the effect of the levonorgestrel-containing IUCD, his vaginal bleeding should cease soon.

Practice points

- When first meeting a transgender patient, ask what name and pronouns they prefer, and model appropriate behaviour for other health staff.
- The most common cause of menstrual bleeding in a transgender man is an inadequate dose of testosterone.
- Hormonal IUCDs are a very good contraceptive for transgender men and are likely to also control bleeding.
- Don't make assumptions about your patient's sexual contacts—a transgender person may be heterosexual, homosexual, bisexual or asexual, and this may change over time.
- Intimate examinations for a transgender person may cause significant anxiety and need to be handled very sensitively.

References and further reading

Australasian Society for HIV, Viral Hepatitis and Sexual Health Medicine. PrEP [communiqué]. Sydney: ASHM; 2020. www.ashm.org.au/HIV/PrEP

Australian Sexual Health Alliance. Australian STI management guidelines for use in primary care. Sydney: Australasian Society for HIV, Viral Hepatitis and Sexual Health Medicine (ASHM); 2020. http://sti.guidelines.org.au/

Cheung AS, Wynne K, Erasmus J, et al. Position statement on the hormonal management of adult transgender and gender diverse individuals. *Med J Aust*. 2019;211(3):127–33.

Clinical Effectiveness Unit of the Faculty of Sexual and Reproductive Healthcare. FSRH CEU statement: contraceptive choices and sexual health for transgender and non-binary people. Edinburgh: FSRH; 2017. www.fsrh.org/standards-and-guidance/documents/fsrh-ceu-statement-contraceptive-choices-and-sexual-health-for/

Nakamura A, Watanabe M, Sugimoto M, et al. Dose–response analysis of testosterone replacement therapy in patients with female to male gender identity disorder. *Endocr J*. 2013;60:275–81.

STIs in Gay Men Action Group. Australian sexually transmitted infection & HIV testing guidelines: for asymptomatic men who have sex with men. Sydney: STIGMA; 2019. https://stipu.nsw.gov.au/wp-content/uploads/STIGMA_Guidelines2019_Final-1.pdf/

Transhub [digital information and resource platform for all trans and gender diverse (TGD) people in NSW, loved ones, allies and health providers]. Sydney: ACON; 2020. www.transhub.org.au

Weyers S, Garland SM, Cruickshank M, et al. Cervical cancer screening in transgender men: a review. *BJOG*. 2021;128(5):822–6.

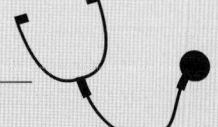

Part 3
Clinical cases
in obstetrics

Case 26
Melissa has persistent vomiting in pregnancy. . .

Melissa is a 22-year-old woman you are first called to see one Saturday afternoon in the emergency department. She has been referred by a local medical centre at 8 weeks of pregnancy because of persistent vomiting. The referring doctor also noted that Melissa appears very pale.

When you arrive in the emergency department you find Melissa leaning over a bowl, retching and spitting up bile-stained fluid. Her partner, Nat, and 1-year-old son are with her. You observe that she does, indeed, look pale and her skin is very dry.

Nat tells you that she has been vomiting increasingly frequently for the past 2 weeks. She has not eaten any solid food in this time. Initially she was able to tolerate fluids, mostly flat lemonade and water, but since yesterday he has not seen her drink anything. Over the past 2 weeks she has tried ginger tablets and antihistamines with no success. Nat also tells you that Melissa suffered nausea and vomiting during her last pregnancy but not to the current extent.

> Nausea and/or vomiting are common symptoms of early pregnancy, particularly between 6 and 14 weeks. Although often referred to as 'morning sickness', symptoms may occur at any time and be provoked by various foods and other factors and relieved by a variety of measures. The condition is poorly understood; it has been attributed to the rapid rise in β-hCG and oestriol levels in early pregnancy, but psychological factors are probably also involved.

How do you proceed in this situation?

First you take a history from Melissa. She is sure of the date of her LMP. She was taking the COCP but missed 'a couple'. She had a pregnancy test performed at the medical centre 2 weeks ago and the result was positive. She was shocked to find that she was pregnant and is not sure how they will cope. They are currently living in a caravan park and Nat is unemployed.

Her son Josh was born by caesarean section for failure to progress in labour. He was not breastfed and she commenced the COCP 6 weeks after his birth. She is not on any medications, has no other relevant medical history and has no allergies. Melissa smokes 15 cigarettes a day.

What examination do you make of Melissa?

A good general examination is indicated. Melissa's conjunctivae, mucous membranes and nail beds are pale. Her BP is 90/60 mmHg and pulse is 100 bpm. She feels dizzy standing up. Her skin on closer inspection is very dry and her tongue dry and furred. Examination of the respiratory and cardiovascular systems and the abdomen is unremarkable.

What is the next step in your management of Melissa?

Melissa needs blood taken for FBC, urea and electrolytes and LFTs. She needs rehydration, which will need to be done intravenously. She needs antiemetic therapy. You explain all this to Melissa and Nat, including the fact that Melissa requires admission to hospital. You also offer to arrange for a social worker to speak to the couple on the following Monday for assistance with their accommodation and financial problems.

Melissa is admitted to the ward and given Hartmann's solution 1 L 6-hourly for fluid replacement and prochlorperazine 10 mg 6-hourly IM as required for vomiting. Initially she is given nothing by mouth.

What further investigations are indicated?

An MSU should be performed to exclude a urinary tract infection as a cause of vomiting. An ultrasound scan should be performed as soon as possible to rule out multiple pregnancy and trophoblastic disease as causes of hyperemesis.

Melissa's investigations show no evidence of a UTI. Electrolytes are within the normal range, as are LFTs. Ultrasound shows a single fetus with a crown–rump length consistent with 8 weeks of pregnancy. The haemoglobin level is 90 g/L, despite the haemoconcentration associated with dehydration. A blood film shows hypochromic microcytic anaemia. Iron studies are ordered and low serum iron levels confirmed.

What is Melissa's subsequent progress?

As in most cases of hyperemesis Melissa settles quickly on this regimen. Within 12 hours she is tolerating oral fluids. You prescribe pyridoxine 50 mg twice daily for ongoing nausea.

What follow-up do you arrange for Melissa?

Melissa is well and discharged home in 3 days' time with an appointment for follow-up in the antenatal clinic and arrangements for accommodation having been made by the social work department. She is tolerating an oral iron-folate preparation and has been advised to have frequent small meals of bland food. She has had a consultation with the hospital dietitian to discuss healthy eating habits for herself and her family.

Treatment of severe hyperemesis of pregnancy

- Doxylamine po.
- Pyridoxine po, if symptoms are prolonged.
- Parenteral prochlorperazine (IM or rectally) or promethazine (IV or IM); metoclopramide (IV or IM) is an alternative but is usually less effective.
- Ondansetron, as a tablet, a sublingual wafer or an IV injection, may be considered in resistant cases. Ondansetron is a B3 category drug in pregnancy, which means that although no adverse effects are known in humans, it should only be used as second-line therapy. It is also expensive.
- Steroids (e.g. dexamethasone), after discussion with your consultant.

 CLINICAL PEARLS

Psychological and environmental factors may contribute to the onset and severity of nausea and vomiting of pregnancy, and may require as much attention as clinical management of the condition.

References and further reading

Lowe S, Armstrong G, Beech A, et al. SOMANZ position paper on the management of nausea and vomiting in pregnancy and hyperemesis gravidarum. *Aust N Z J Obstet Gynaecol.* 2020;60(1):34–43.

Tan A, Lowe S, Henry A. Nausea and vomiting of pregnancy: effects on quality of life and day-to-day function. *Aust N Z J Obstet Gynaecol.* 2018;58(3):278–90.

Case 27
Klara has been referred to discuss prenatal diagnosis. . .

Klara is a 36-year-old gravida 2 para 1 woman who has been referred by her general practitioner to the antenatal clinic in your hospital to discuss prenatal diagnosis. She attends the clinic with her partner, Hans, who has been with her for 12 years.

Klara is currently 13 weeks and 5 days' gestation and her pregnancy to date has been uncomplicated. This was a planned pregnancy. Her gestation by dates was confirmed by an ultrasound scan at 12 weeks, arranged by her general practitioner as part of a combined first-trimester screen. This test combines serum analytes such as PAPP-A with an ultrasound measurement of the nuchal translucency, and a computer algorithm estimates the chance of trisomy using the mother's age. The test result suggested an increase in her chance of trisomy from her age-related chance of about 1 in 300 to an adjusted chance of 1 in 80.

What are your first steps?

You take an appropriate history, including a family history of any genetic conditions. You also ensure that her dates are correct and that this has been confirmed by her scan at 12 weeks' gestation. Her first child is 3 years of age and is healthy. Her previous pregnancy was uncomplicated and her first-trimester screen then did not show any increased chance of aneuploidy. You also confirm that her blood group is O Rh(D)-negative. Hans also keeps good health and both are nonsmokers.

How would you counsel her?

You explain that Down syndrome—where three copies of chromosome 21 are present rather than two—is a congenital condition associated with a number of health issues for the baby, including the possibility of developmental delay and heart conditions. With medical treatment and social support, children with Down syndrome will usually grow up in good health and with a reasonable quality of life.

You explain to Klara and Hans that the combined first-trimester test is a screening test and that her result has shown that there is a greater than expected chance that her baby might have a chromosomal abnormality like Down syndrome.

Antenatal screening for fetal abnormalities

1. Combined first-trimester screening
   - This is carried out between 11^{+6} and 13^{+6} weeks' gestation, and involves an ultrasound examination of the fetus and blood biochemistry, typically for PAPP-A and free hCG levels. The results are combined in an algorithm that uses the age of the mother and calculates the chance of the commoner trisomies— trisomies 21, 18 and 13. Major conditions such as abdominal wall defects and neural tube defects may be detected but a number of other abnormalities might not be detected.
   - A nuchal translucency measurement is an ultrasound assessment of the soft tissue thickening behind the neck of the fetus.
   - High thickness measurements are associated with an increased chance of chromosomal conditions, and also major heart conditions.

2. Cell-free DNA-based screening
   - From about 10 weeks of pregnancy, it is possible to use a maternal blood specimen to obtain free DNA from the placental cells. Using comparative genomic hybridisation (CGH, or 'next-generation sequencing'), it is possible to obtain a great deal of information about the genome of the fetus.
   - This can be used at any stage in the pregnancy after 10 weeks—there commonly is too little free DNA in the maternal blood for accurate analysis before this—to obtain not only information about the chance of trisomy but also an increasing number of single-gene conditions and other genetic information.

3. The 18–20 week morphology ultrasound scan
   - It is now part of routine practice to offer a morphology USS from 18–20 weeks' gestation to screen for fetal structural abnormalities.
   - Most major anatomical abnormalities may be detected but tertiary-level scans will still be needed to confirm or exclude a suspected abnormality.

> Klara wishes to know what tests are available to exclude a
> chromosomal abnormality.

In the first instance, it is important to ascertain what Klara and Hans would wish to do if they found out that the baby was affected by Down syndrome. Some women and couples will wish to end the pregnancy, others will seek further information and support and continue. Each couple is different and careful counselling is required.

You explain that there are two options—the first is to undertake a non-invasive cfDNA screening test using another blood sample from Klara. This is very accurate but is still not certain. If the cfDNA result showed a low chance of aneuploidy, then because a thickened nuchal translucency may still be associated with a cardiac malformation, careful examination of the baby's heart by ultrasound later in pregnancy would be important. The second option is to move to an 'invasive test'—either chorionic villus sampling (CVS) or amniocentesis.

CVS is performed from around 11 weeks' gestation. An ultrasound scan is always performed at the same time to guide a fine needle into the placental bed where small amounts of chorionic villi (usually 10–20 mg) are removed for chromosomal studies. You explain that this procedure carries a miscarriage risk of up to 1%. This procedure is usually carried out transabdominally, as transvaginal CVS carries a higher risk of miscarriage.

Amniocentesis is usually performed from 15 weeks' gestation onwards and involves the introduction of a fine needle into the amniotic sac under ultrasound control. A small amount (usually around 15 mL) of amniotic fluid is removed. You explain that the risk of miscarriage from amniocentesis is around 0.5% (1 in 200).

As Klara is Rhesus (D) negative, she would need to have an injection of anti-D (625 IU) after the procedure to reduce the risk of sensitisation—developing antibodies against a fetus whose blood group may be Rh-positive.

After further discussion, Klara decides to undergo a cfDNA blood screen, and you make these arrangements. The results will take approximately one week.

> One week later, Klara and Hans return to the clinic to discuss the
> results.

The cfDNA screen has shown a high chance of trisomy 21 and you explain this to Klara and Hans. They ask for guidance on what to do next—you explain that, although the cfDNA screen is very accurate, it is still a screening test and the result would need to be confirmed. They request an amniocentesis. Because the cell-free DNA in maternal blood comes from the placenta and not the fetus, there is a possibility of genetic mosaicism in the placenta. Thus CVS is not helpful and should not be performed—amniocentesis will sample cells from the fetus. You arrange for an ultrasound-guided amniocentesis at 15 weeks and an urgent result using fluorescence in situ hybridisation (FISH) for the common trisomies as this returns a rapid result, with an 'extended karyotype' which will take 2–3 weeks.

The FISH result confirms a diagnosis of trisomy 21, so you meet to discuss options. Klara and Hans are considering continuing with the pregnancy but want further information to evaluate the baby for other major anatomical anomalies that might influence their decision making. You arrange a specialised fetal ultrasound with focus on the heart.

This test reveals that the fetus is affected by a severe and complex cardiac abnormality. After a long discussion, Klara and Hans feel that the prospect of major neonatal corrective cardiac surgery and the possibility of significantly reduced quality of life in childhood mean that they do not wish to continue with the pregnancy. This has been a profound and difficult decision for them to make.

You explain what is involved in termination of pregnancy in the late second trimester. You explain that the most common method would be to induce the abortion by means of medication. In the first instance, the antiprogesterone mifepristone (RU-486) is administered, then about two days later a course of misoprostol (a prostaglandin E1 analogue) is commenced to induce the onset of labour.

The decision is put to a hospital multidisciplinary ethics group who confirm the request. Klara and Hans are also seen by the maternity unit's grief counsellor to be provided with further support.

Having had the mifepristone administered orally, Klara is admitted two days later for administration of misoprostol and goes on to expel the fetus and placenta completely that evening. She is given an injection of anti-D. She agrees to a postmortem examination for her fetus. She goes home the same night after arrangements for her to be seen for a review in the clinic and an appointment to see the genetic counsellor to discuss future pregnancies. She is also given medication to suppress lactation.

Late termination of pregnancy (therapeutic TOP)

Therapeutic TOP is legal in Australia, New Zealand and the United Kingdom. It is governed by different sets of legislation in each country. In Australia, the legislation governing TOP is different in each state and territory.

Australia

While each state and territory has its own laws permitting TOP to be carried out, it is legally permitted in all to protect the life and health of the woman. This includes the psychological and physical health of the woman. The upper limit of gestation for late abortion also varies by state and territory, and in many jurisdictions later gestations simply require more medical oversight.

New Zealand

TOP in New Zealand is legal when the pregnant woman faces a danger to her life, physical health or mental health, or if there is a risk of the fetus being handicapped in the event of the continuation of her pregnancy. The procedure has to be performed in a 'licensed institution' and has to be approved by two doctors, one of whom must be a gynaecologist or obstetrician. Counselling is optional.

United Kingdom

In England, Wales and Scotland, section 1(1) of the Abortion Act 1967 now reads:

Subject to the provisions of this section, a person shall not be guilty of an offence under the law relating to abortion when a pregnancy is terminated by a registered medical practitioner if two registered medical practitioners are of the opinion, formed in good faith

(a) that the pregnancy has not exceeded its twenty-fourth week and that the continuance of the pregnancy would involve risk, greater than if the pregnancy were terminated, of injury to the physical or mental health of the pregnant woman or any existing children of her family; or

(b) that the termination of the pregnancy is necessary to prevent grave permanent injury to the physical or mental health of the pregnant woman; or

(c) that the continuance of the pregnancy would involve risk to the life of the pregnant woman, greater than if the pregnancy were terminated

(d) that there is a substantial risk that if the child were born it would suffer from such physical or mental abnormalities as to be seriously handicapped.

CLINICAL COMMENT

Methods of late TOP

- Late termination is generally carried out after 14 weeks' gestation for the reasons outlined earlier.
- Surgical termination may be carried out but can be associated with increased risks of complications such as cervical and uterine trauma and retained products of conception. It is only carried out in certain centres by highly skilled operators.
- Medical termination is the method most commonly used for late terminations.
- In the United Kingdom, Australia and New Zealand, mifepristone (RU 486) is commonly used as the initial agent prior to administration of prostaglandin. Mifepristone is a synthetic antiprogesterone that has been shown to be an effective abortifacient when combined with a prostaglandin administered 1 to 3 days later.
- Misoprostol is a prostaglandin E1 analogue that has been widely used in combination with mifepristone to induce termination of pregnancy.
- Gemeprost is licensed for termination of pregnancy. It is seldom used nowadays as it is associated with a higher frequency of side effects such as nausea, vomiting and pyrexia.

CLINICAL PEARLS

- Screening for genetic fetal conditions is offered routinely and a number of options are available.
- This can be carried out from ten weeks' gestation.

continued

continued

- The routine 18–20 week morphology scan is the most common screening test for structural fetal abnormalities.
- It is important that women understand the implications of screening tests and that they are not diagnostic tests.

References and further reading

Carlson LM, Vora NL. Prenatal diagnosis: screening and diagnostic tools. *Obstet Gynecol Clin North Am*. 2017;44(2):245–56.

Royal College of Obstetricians and Gynaecologists. Comprehensive abortion care. Best Practice Paper no. 2. London: RCOG; 2015. www.rcog.org.uk/en/guidelines-research-services/guidelines/bpp2/

Case 28
Amy wants to try for a natural birth this time. . .

Amy comes to see you at the antenatal clinic at about 30 weeks' gestation. She is 29 years old and previously attended the midwife-led clinic at the hospital.

Her first child, Penny, is now 2 years old. Penny was in a breech presentation and an attempt at ECV at 37 weeks was unsuccessful. The baby remained in a breech presentation until 40 weeks and was felt to be large for dates. Consequently, the mode of delivery was discussed and Amy was advised to undergo elective caesarean section. This procedure was carried out and was uncomplicated. Penny weighed 4.2 kg. Amy's recovery was smooth but she was frustrated because she had her heart set on trying for a vaginal birth. She is very keen to discuss trying for a vaginal delivery this time. (The terms used here include trial of labour (TOL), trial of labour after caesarean (TOLAC) and vaginal birth after caesarean (VBAC)).

What more do you need to know?

You review Amy's shared care card. She has been relatively healthy and her blood pressure has been normal, although she had mild hypertension in her first pregnancy. Amy is a non-smoker. The second-trimester morphology USS revealed no sign of abnormality, with the placenta positioned at the fundus of the uterus. Screening blood tests, including a GTT, were normal.

Today her blood pressure is 110/65 mmHg and weight 85 kg. There is some mild ankle oedema, the symphysiofundal height is 34 cm and the fetus is in a longitudinal lie with a cephalic presentation. The fetal heart rate is normal.

What factors influence the advice you give Amy?

A number of factors may influence the chances of achieving vaginal birth after a previous caesarean section. The first important consideration is the reason for the primary caesarean section: if labour occurred but was obstructed, with failure to progress to full dilatation, then the chances of a vaginal delivery are reduced. Similarly, women who have not had a vaginal delivery in the past have a lower rate of vaginal birth when VBAC is attempted. The chances also fall with increasing birth weight of the current baby. Older women and women with other risk factors (such as obesity, gestational diabetes or other medical disorders) are less likely to achieve a vaginal delivery after a previous caesarean section. Certain types of caesarean section—for example, when a vertical ('classical') or compound ('inverse-T' or 'J-shaped') incision is made on the uterus—often mean that vaginal delivery should not be attempted, since the risk of uterine rupture is higher.

Fortunately for Amy, she is a relatively young woman with no other complications or health problems that might increase her risks, although she is overweight. The primary caesarean section was for a 'non-recurring' reason (breech presentation) and the procedure was uncomplicated. You explain that a careful assessment of the baby's size and position will be required later in the pregnancy if she is still motivated to attempt vaginal birth.

Amy comes to see you at about 37 weeks for a routine visit. She remains well, with a blood pressure in the normal range. The symphysiofundal height is 36 cm and the baby is active. The baby's back is on Amy's left side and the head three-fifths palpable in the abdomen. An ultrasound scan a week earlier reported the baby's measurements to be on the 60th centile, with a predicted birth weight at term of about 3.8 kg (range 3.5–4.0 kg).

What are the risks of attempting vaginal birth after a previous caesarean?

You explain to Amy that attempting vaginal birth after a previous caesarean delivery requires some precautions. Induction of labour is to be avoided: using prostaglandins for induction is associated with a twofold to threefold increased risk of uterine rupture. If induction is undertaken, a balloon catheter may reduce the risk of uterine hypertonus. Once labour begins, careful assessment of progress will be made, as obstruction in labour also increases the risk of uterine rupture.

Augmentation of labour with oxytocin also carries an increased risk of uterine rupture, with a quoted risk of 22 to 74 per 10 000 trials of labour. This will mean regular vaginal examinations to monitor the rate of descent of the baby's head and the rate of dilatation of the cervix. Continuous monitoring of the fetal heart rate with a CTG will also be required because an abnormal trace is the most consistent finding in uterine rupture, being present in 55–87% of cases.

Amy wishes to know the chances of achieving vaginal birth and you explain that, overall, 50–75% of women who attempt a trial of labour will achieve a vaginal delivery. There is also a slight increase in the risk of adverse outcomes for both mother and baby, when compared to a planned repeat caesarean section, but this is not a reason not to try.

The postnatal visit

Amy comes to see you, proudly showing off 6-week-old baby Jack. The hospital discharge summary reveals that Amy laboured spontaneously for a few days before her due date. She chose an epidural for pain relief (which is not contraindicated). After about 10 hours with steady progress she had a ventouse lift-out with a small episiotomy, as she was getting tired in the second stage. Jack weighed 3.9 kg at birth and was in excellent condition. There were no problems in the puerperium and both are well. You explain that she will be due for a CST once the lochia has completely ceased, and you discuss contraception with her.

 CLINICAL PEARLS

- Since primary caesarean section is common, discussions about how to deliver the next baby are also common. Avoid terms such as 'success' and 'failure' as much as possible when discussing attempted vaginal birth following previous caesarean birth.
- The best outlook for vaginal delivery occurs in younger women who have had a previous vaginal birth and where the second baby was delivered by caesarean section for 'non-recurring' reasons such as breech presentation or placenta praevia.
- A trial of labour requires careful assessment and counselling and should be undertaken in a centre with adequate facilities for one-to-one care in labour and recourse to urgent caesarean section if required. The discussions and plans should be carefully documented.

Factors associated with attempted VBAC resulting in vaginal birth

- Previous vaginal birth, particularly previous VBAC, is the best predictor for vaginal birth in attempted VBAC and is associated with an 87–90% vaginal birthrate.
- Birth weight less than 4000 g (which can only be an estimated fetal weight (EFT) antenatally).
- Systematic and summative reviews have shown an overall rate of vaginal birth of 50–75% among VBAC attempts.

Risk factors for attempted VBAC not resulting in vaginal birth

- Induced labour
- No previous vaginal birth
- BMI (pre-pregnancy) greater than 30
- Previous caesarean section for dystocia
- Gestation greater than 41 weeks
- Birth weight greater than 4000 g
- No epidural anaesthesia
- Previous preterm caesarean section
- Cervical dilatation at admission less than 4 cm
- Advanced maternal age (over 35 years)
- Less than 2 years from previous caesarean section
- Non-White ethnicity
- Short stature
- Male infant

Contraindications to a trial of labour

- Prior history of classical caesarean section (vertical incision on uterus)
- Prior history of two or more previous caesarean sections. Some women with two previous caesarean sections may still achieve a successful VBAC but they need to be carefully assessed by an experienced obstetrician and appropriately counselled.
- Previous uterine rupture
- Some types of uterine incision, such as the J or inverted-T incisions
- Large-for-dates fetus (>4000 g)

Complications of a trial of labour

Maternal complications

- Uterine rupture (22 to 74 per 10 000)
- Blood transfusion (170/10 000—an additional risk of 1% compared to the elective repeat caesarean section group)
- Endometritis (289/10 000)

There is no statistically significant difference between planned VBAC and elective repeat caesarean section (ERCS) in terms of hysterectomy, thromboembolic disease or maternal death.

Fetal complications

- Increased perinatal mortality rate (an additional risk of 2 to 3 per 10 000 of birth-related perinatal death compared to ERCS). This is related to more advanced gestation (greater than 39 weeks) and uterine rupture.
- Hypoxaemic ischaemic encephalopathy (8/10 000). The effect on the long-term outcome of the infant is unknown.

References and further reading

Royal Australian and New Zealand College of Obstetricians and Gynaecologists. Planned vaginal birth after caesarean section (trial of labour). RANZCOG Statement C-Obs 38. Melbourne: RANZCOG, 2019. www.ranzcog.edu.au.
Royal College of Obstetricians and Gynaecologists. Birth after previous caesarean birth. RCOG Green-top Guideline No. 45. London: RCOG; 2015. www.rcog.org.uk/globalassets/documents/guidelines/gtg_45.pdf

Case 29
Louise requests a caesarean section. . .

In the antenatal clinic, you are carrying out a routine consultation for Louise, a 28-year-old woman. Louise works as an accountant with a large firm; her partner, Vincent, is studying for his PhD in astronomy. They are a bright and very well-informed couple who have planned this pregnancy. Louise underwent NIPT screening that revealed her to be at low risk of a chromosomal aneuploidy. Her blood group is A positive, and all of her investigations (including a screen for GDM) have been completely normal. Louise is now 34 weeks into the pregnancy.

You inquire about her general wellbeing and fetal movements. Louise tells you she has felt increasingly fatigued and is troubled by quite unpleasant gastro-oesophageal reflux symptoms that only partly respond to antacids. This is making it difficult for her to sleep, and she wakes frequently with the need to empty her bladder. On examination, you find that Louise has gained a total of 9 kg in the pregnancy so far. There is only very mild peripheral oedema, and she has some scattered stretch marks on the abdomen and upper thighs. The fundal height measures 35 cm, and the fetus is in a cephalic presentation, with the back on Louise's right side. The fetal heart rate is about 140 bpm, and there appears to be a normal amount of liquor around the baby.

A surprising request

As you are writing in her shared care card, Louise tells you that she wants to have an elective caesarean birth.

This request comes as a surprise, as Louise had previously seemed to be highly motivated to have a vaginal birth. She has enrolled in birth classes and pregnancy yoga and sought advice from you about a 'good pregnancy book to read'. You ask her what the reasons are for her request. Louise tells you that two of her friends had long and challenging attempts at vaginal birth—one ultimately underwent emergency caesarean section, the other had a difficult forceps delivery that led to a third-degree perineal tear for the woman and a transient facial nerve injury in the baby. She has since spent a great deal of time searching the internet and various maternity chat rooms and blogs and says that, after consideration, she will refuse an attempt at vaginal birth. Since you are seeing Louise in a busy clinic, you explain that such a request will take much longer to talk through with her and arrange a further appointment for her later in the week. You suggest that she brings Vincent along with her.

Maternal-request caesarean section

When a caesarean section is performed at the woman's request, where this is no true obstetric or medical indication for the procedure, this is usually called a maternal-request caesarean section (MRCS). The available data suggest that, in Western countries, more than 5% of elective (planned) caesarean sections might be MRCS. Common reasons for such a request include 'tocophobia' (a fear of childbirth), concerns about the welfare of the baby during labour and concerns about adverse outcomes of labour, both short-term (maternal injuries such as large perineal lacerations, or injury to the baby) and long-term (prolapse, incontinence or sexual difficulties). It is important to listen to such a request sympathetically, discuss any concerns a woman might have in detail and offer further help and assistance.

Louise and Vincent return, as planned. They have downloaded a great deal of information from the internet to show you.

Your first step is to ask whether Louise thinks she faces risks over and above those of other women. She explains that her mother, who had four children vaginally, has problems with vaginal prolapse and urinary incontinence that have been treated surgically. She says that her mother put up with her symptoms for many years before seeking help. Vincent adds that some other men in his workplace have told him that intercourse with their wives is 'much less satisfying' since they had children. He tells you that, as an academic, he has helped Louise with her internet searching, and that there are many websites that have only added to their level of concern.

You listen to what they say, then explain that it is quite normal to have concerns about childbirth—most women have worries especially in their first pregnancy, even if they don't freely admit them to friends or carers. In Louise's case, where she is a healthy young woman whose pregnancy has been progressing normally, she would face no greater risk than any other woman. You explain that the most likely outcome of labour for her is a normal vaginal birth, although the majority of women having their first vaginal birth are likely to require sutures to either a perineal tear or an episiotomy. She has about a one-in-four chance of needing instrumental assistance—with ventouse or forceps—and around 20% chance of emergency caesarean birth. You direct Louise to the NICE website (www.nice.org.uk) and suggest she downloads the statement on caesarean section. A site such as this will provide unbiased information to help her with decision making.

A summary of relevant information is provided in Tables 29.1–29.5.

Table 29.1 Maternal conditions that studies suggest may be *reduced* during or after a planned caesarean section

Effects around time of birth	Magnitude of difference
Pain during birth	Much lower
Pain in immediate postpartum period	Slightly lower
Early postpartum haemorrhage	Very much lower

Table 29.2 Maternal conditions that studies suggest may be *reduced* after planned vaginal birth

Effects around time of birth	Magnitude of difference
Length of hospital stay	Slightly lower
Hysterectomy due to postpartum haemorrhage	Much lower

Table 29.3 Maternal conditions for which *no difference* is found between planned caesarean section and planned vaginal birth

Pain 4 months postpartum
Injury to the bladder or ureter
Injury to the cervix
Iatrogenic surgical injury
Pulmonary embolism
Wound infection

Table 29.4 Neonatal conditions that studies suggest may be *reduced* after a planned vaginal birth

Effects around time of birth	Magnitude of difference
Neonatal intensive care unit admission	Moderate

Table 29.5 Neonatal conditions for which *no difference* is found between planned caesarean section and planned vaginal birth

Hypoxic-ischaemic encephalopathy
Intracranial haemorrhage
Neonatal respiratory morbidity

A happy ending

After your discussion, Louise and Vincent agree to consider what you have told them, and say they will seek more information from the NICE website. You next see Louise 6 weeks later. She tells you she decided to try for a natural birth. She laboured spontaneously two days after her due date and chose an epidural for pain relief in labour. She pushed well over 90 minutes, and baby Amelia was delivered by ventouse with a resulting second-degree perineal tear. Louise explains that breastfeeding is going well, and so far her recovery has been uneventful. She says that she and Vincent are very happy with the way the labour and birth were managed. You congratulate her on the birth of Amelia, and also offer her information about future contraception.

 CLINICAL COMMENTS

In women with high levels of anxiety and/or depression, a decision for maternal-request caesarean section does not always lower these levels antenatally. However, provision of MRCS does lead to lower levels of anxiety/depression postnatally, so it may be considered a valid option.

References and further reading

D'Souza R. Caesarean section on maternal request for non-medical reasons: putting the UK National Institute of Health and Clinical Excellence guidelines in perspective. *Best Pract Res Clin Obstet Gynaecol.* 2013;27(2):165–77.

National Institute for Health and Care Excellence. Caesarean section. NICE Clinical Guideline CG132. London: NICE; 2019.

Olieman R, Siemonsma F, Bartens MA, et al. The effect of an elective cesarean section on maternal request on peripartum anxiety and depression with childbirth fear: a systematic review. *BMC Pregnancy Childbirth.* 2017;17(1):195.

Royal Australian and New Zealand College of Obstetricians and Gynaecologists. Caesarean delivery on maternal request (CDMR). College Statements & Guidelines. C-Obs 39. Melbourne: RANZCOG; 2017. www.ranzcog.edu.au

Case 30
Kahlia's baby seems small. . .

Kahlia is an 18-year-old woman whom you meet for the first time in the antenatal clinic at 33 weeks of pregnancy. She has not booked or had any prior antenatal care apart from a scan at 9 weeks, which was done in a hospital in another town when she presented with a threatened miscarriage. The pregnancy was not intended and had been a surprise for her. At the time she was in difficult circumstances and could not access an abortion although this had been her first thought. Kahlia comes to the clinic with a supportive female friend with whom she is 'couch surfing', but says that she no longer has any contact with the baby's father or with her own parents, who live in another state. She has just recently moved to your area to be with her friend.

What further history do you take from Kahlia?

Kahlia had regular periods from the age of 13. She became pregnant at the age of 16 and had a medical abortion with mifepristone at that time. Her periods subsequently became infrequent. Kahlia explains that she was a regular user of cannabis in various forms, and used this to help with morning sickness, but has done her best to cease use later in her pregnancy on the advice of her friend (Table 30.1). She does, however, still smoke up to a packet of cigarettes a day. She is on no regular medications and has no allergies of which she is aware. Kahlia has not had a recent STI check nor, indeed, any formal antenatal care until this point.

What examination do you make for Kahlia?

First, you perform a general examination. Kahlia weighs just 45 kg and you calculate her BMI at 18 kg/m^2. You see that she has a number of tattoos, and scars on her arms suggesting self-harm in the past, but no recent needle tracks. Her blood pressure is normal, and examination of the cardiovascular and respiratory systems shows them to be within normal limits. Examination of the abdomen shows no enlargement of the liver or spleen or

Table 30.1 Effects of recreational drugs in pregnancy

Drugs	Risks in pregnancy	Risks to infant	Management in pregnancy	Remarks
Cannabis	Health risks not clearly established—possible respiratory, mood and psychological problems. Neonate may experience mild withdrawal symptoms in second week of life.	Possible effects on memory and higher cognitive processes in childhood; possible increased hyperactivity and inattention disorders in childhood.	Encourage counselling and psychological treatment for cannabis dependency. Encourage smoking away from infant. No contraindications to breastfeeding.	Cannabis is frequently used in conjunction with tobacco, and cannabis users are often heavy tobacco users as well. Advice and assistance with quitting tobacco should be offered.
Heroin	Apart from the risks of harm to the mother associated with injecting drug use, maternal withdrawal from heroin and other opiates is associated with miscarriage, fetal death in utero, IUGR, preterm labour and fetal distress in labour.	Withdrawal symptoms in neonates.	Stabilisation on methadone; drug and alcohol counselling; psychosocial support. Women who are stable on methadone should be encouraged to breastfeed.	Infants of heroin-dependent mothers will require close monitoring postnatally, regardless of whether the mother has been stabilised on methadone or not. Close liaison with the social work team is often indicated.

continued

continued

Drugs	Risks in pregnancy	Risks to infant	Management in pregnancy	Remarks
Cocaine	Maternal complications include stroke, seizures, placental abruption, acute myocardial infarction and cardiac arrhythmias. Higher risk of miscarriage, IUGR, preterm rupture of membranes, preterm labour and stillbirth.	Possible mild withdrawal symptoms in neonates; necrotising enterocolitis in neonates; possible abnormal behavioural development in infancy.	Pregnant women using cocaine should be advised of the health risks to themselves and their infants. Counselling and psychosocial support should be offered. Early intervention for behavioural and educational problems in cocaine-affected infants have been shown to be beneficial.	Concurrent tobacco use is common among cocaine users; it may be difficult to distinguish causation in individual women. Assistance with quitting tobacco should be offered. Women who continue to use cocaine and who wish to breastfeed should be discouraged from breastfeeding for 24 hours following cocaine use.
Amphetamines	Health risks in pregnancy not clearly established; possible risk of cerebral ischaemia in the fetus; possible IUGR and placental abruption.	Possible mild withdrawal symptoms. Possible agitation and hyperactivity if amphetamines used close to time of birth.	Pregnant women using amphetamines should be advised of health risks to themselves and their infants. Counselling and psychosocial support should be offered.	Women who continue with amphetamine use should be discouraged from breastfeeding for 24 hours following use.

other masses apart from the pregnant uterus. The uterine symphysiofundal height is 29 cm. You determine that the fetus appears to be presenting by the breech, and the fetal parts are easily palpated suggesting a reduced liquor volume. The fetal heart is heard with the hand-held Doppler machine. Kahlia states that she is feeling regular and plentiful fetal movements.

What investigations do you order for Kahlia, and why?

Kahlia has with her a copy of the ultrasound report from the first hospital confirming her gestational age, so it is clear that her baby is clinically small-for-gestational age (SGA). You order an urgent USS for fetal growth, morphology, amniotic fluid index and Doppler measurements of umbilical blood flow. You also order the routine blood and urine tests for antenatal booking visits, which have not yet been performed for Kahlia. After discussing the rationale, you arrange for her to give a first-void urine specimen to perform a PCR for chlamydia and gonococcus. While she is still in the clinic you arrange a CTG—the baby's heart rate is within normal limits, reactive, with no decelerations. You arrange to review Kahlia in 2 days' time in the day pregnancy unit. You also arrange for her to talk with the hospital's medical social worker for help with more permanent accommodation and introduction to the local drop-in centre for young single mothers.

Fetal growth restriction (FGR) is a relatively common complication of pregnancy. There are a number of conditions associated with the development of FGR. These include chromosomal conditions in the baby, congenital infections such as CMV or toxoplasmosis and pregnancy complications such as pre-eclampsia or other hypertensive disorders. Smoking, illegal or recreational drug use and alcohol use in pregnancy may also play a part. A baby affected by FGR is at increased risk of adverse outcomes including stillbirth, so diagnosis is important. Managements include cessation of smoking or drug use, use of vitamin D and dietary improvement. Often there are no specific treatments and management is based on careful monitoring of the baby and timely birth.

How do you manage Kahlia's second consultation?

Kahlia's results are now to hand: there are two results of note. She is positive for hepatitis C virus (HCV). You believe she is unaware of this and this is the first time the diagnosis has been made. In addition, the ultrasound confirms your clinical suspicion of SGA. The estimated weight is 1400 g, which is on the 3rd centile for gestation. There appears to be 'head-sparing' with a greatly reduced fetal abdominal circumference but head measurements on the 10th centile. The liquor volume is reduced, with an AFI of 5.1, and Doppler scans show absent end-diastolic flow. Detailed scanning shows no anatomical abnormality. Kahlia also tells you that the baby is moving much less than previously.

What is the immediate management for Kahlia?

A CTG is performed and this shows an abnormal trace. Your consultant decides that immediate delivery is indicated, and with the compromised baby in a breech presentation, arrangements are made for a caesarean section later that day. There is no time for a course of antenatal corticosteroids for fetal lung maturation. A baby girl weighing 1380 g is delivered in fair condition, with Apgar scores of 3 at 1 minute and 7 at 5 minutes. The infant is transferred to the care of the neonatal paediatric team.

What are your ongoing concerns for Kahlia?

Kahlia needs a detailed consultation to explain the significance and long-term implications of the finding of HCV antibodies on routine screening. Fortunately, she is negative for HIV and hepatitis B. You explain to Kahlia that the rate of mother-to-baby transmission is low, probably less than 5%. Breastfeeding is not contraindicated, except with cracked or bleeding nipples, but as the baby has been born preterm and is requiring special care, feeding is likely to be with expressed colostrum and breastmilk, at least initially. This will allow time for further testing to determine the viral load that Kahlia carries. Babies born with hepatitis C infection may clear the infection in up to half of cases within the first year of life. The usual screening is using a PCR test for the baby at two months and again a month later. An antibody test is done at 18 months.

You arrange for Kahlia to make contact with a hepatology clinic for ongoing management and follow-up of her own HCV status. She is also given a referral to the social worker attached to your maternity unit for assistance with housing, financial entitlements and other support. In addition, before discharge you discuss contraception and the need for safe sexual practices in depth with her.

 CLINICAL PEARLS

> Hepatitis C infection is not uncommon among Australian women. Antenatal screening should routinely include screening for HCV infection—there are implications not only for the woman but also for her child.

References and further reading

Dunkelberg JC, Berkley EM, Thiel KW, Leslie KK. Hepatitis B and C in
pregnancy: a review and recommendations for care. *J Perinatol.*
2014;34(12):882–91.

Figueras F, Gratacós E. Update on the diagnosis and classification of fetal growth
restriction and proposal of a stage-based management protocol. *Fetal Diagn
Ther.* 2014;36(2):86–98.

ACOG Practice Bulletin no 204. Fetal Growth Restriction. *Obstet Gynecol.*
2019;133(2):e97–e109.

Baschat AA. Planning management and delivery of the growth restricted fetus.
Best Pract Res Clin Obstet Gynaecol. 2018;49:53–65.

Case 31
Maria is followed through a twin pregnancy. . .

You are conducting an antenatal clinic when you first meet Maria, 38 years old and 14 weeks advanced in her fifth pregnancy. Maria has had a diagnosis of twin pregnancy made by her general practitioner at 8 weeks. She had an ultrasound scan at 11 weeks, which has confirmed a continuing twin pregnancy. The pregnancy is dichorionic diamniotic (DCDA). The FNT has been measured for each twin and is not abnormal for either. Maria declined the option of non-invasive prenatal testing (NIPT) when she learned that the rate of test failure is quite high (5–6% in twin pregnancies). Her general practitioner has explained the possibility of chorionic villus sampling (CVS) or amniocentesis for fetal chromosomal abnormality in view of Maria's age, but after discussion with her husband Maria has decided not to have any further testing for fetal abnormality apart from the routine 18-week scan.

What further information is related to your immediate care of Maria?

Maria has been experiencing marked nausea and vomiting but this now seems to be lessening. She has had four normal full-term pregnancies in the past and four spontaneous vaginal deliveries of healthy boys. There is no other relevant medical or family history. Maria is taking an iron-folate preparation. She is as yet unaware of fetal movements.

General examination is unremarkable, with a BP of 120/80 mmHg. The uterine fundus measures just to the level of the umbilicus and fetal heart tones are audible with Doppler scan, although you explain to Maria that you cannot with certainty identify two separate heartbeats. You order her 18-week scan and arrange to see her after this.

What are the important points for following antenatal visits?

At 18 weeks Maria reports that she is well. She is feeling frequent fetal movements. Her ultrasound report confirms the dichorionic and hence diamniotic pregnancy; both fetuses are the expected size for 18 weeks and no abnormality has been demonstrated. The placentas appear fused, and they lie posteriorly and fundal, well away from the lower pole of the uterus.

You arrange for Maria to have further ultrasound scans for fetal growth at 24, 28, 32 and 36 weeks. You explain that intrauterine growth restriction is not uncommon with one or both twins, although it is more likely with monochorionic twins. In such cases and particularly with the rare monoamniotic twin pregnancy, twin-to-twin transfusion syndrome may occur because of vascular anastomoses within the two placentas.

How do you monitor progress of the pregnancy?

Maria is seen regularly from 24 to 36 weeks, and all observations are within normal limits. No vaginal bleeding or excessive discharge is reported and her blood pressure is always within the normal range. The growth scans at 24, 28, 32 and 36 weeks are performed as planned. All show growth of both babies within the 10th and 90th percentiles. At 36 weeks both babies are presenting cephalically.

> Possible complications of late pregnancy with twins include pre-eclampsia, gestational diabetes, antepartum haemorrhage, intrauterine growth restriction and the onset of preterm labour.

How and when is delivery planned for Maria?

At 36 weeks you discuss with Maria probable arrangements for delivery. She is feeling extremely tired and uncomfortable. You agree that it may be reasonable to carry out induction of labour for her at 38 weeks. Insertion of an epidural cannula in early established labour is recommended because, although both babies are cephalic, urgent operative delivery of the second twin is sometimes needed.

The following Sunday evening you are called to the birth suite. Maria has been admitted in spontaneous labour. Her husband, Renato, is with her. She reports that her membranes ruptured during family dinner. She has come straight to the hospital—in the car, her contractions became strong and regular and now she has an urge to push. The midwife in attendance, Doreen, has performed a vaginal examination and reports that the cervix is 9 cm dilated with the head of the first baby below the ischial spines. All Maria's observations, including blood pressure, pulse and temperature, are normal; external fetal cardiac monitoring is in place and both fetal heart traces are reactive. You send for anaesthetic, paediatric and further obstetric assistance; however, almost immediately with a strong contraction the head of the first twin crowns and you rapidly conduct a normal delivery of a baby boy in excellent condition.

Palpation of the abdomen now shows the second twin to be lying longitudinally with the head presenting. Over the next 10 minutes there are two short, quite feeble contractions, so you add oxytocin 5 units to the IV Hartmann's solution already in place. The fetal heart trace for the second twin is satisfactory. On vaginal examination at 12 minutes after delivery of the first twin you find the fetal head well applied to the cervix and at the level of the iliac spines. You rupture the membranes, the liquor is clear and 2 minutes later the second twin is born—a girl!

Knowing that Maria is at moderate to high risk of PPH (because of high parity and twin pregnancy) you order one ampoule of oxytocin/ ergometrine IM and an infusion of 40 units of oxytocin in 1 L of Hartmann's solution over 4 hours. The placentas are delivered and the uterus is felt to be well contracted.

Mode of birth in twin delivery

- If the first twin is a cephalic presentation, vaginal birth is possible. If the first twin is a malpresentation (breech presentation, or transverse of oblique lie), elective caesarean section is generally advised.
- Risk during birth mainly relates to the second twin and to the interval between delivery of this twin and the first delivery.
- An experienced obstetrician should be present for all twin births.
- Paediatric and anaesthetic staff should also be present.
- Continuous electronic fetal heart rate monitoring of both twins is required.
- Elective epidural anaesthesia is strongly advised—if internal podalic version (reaching for a fetal foot and bringing it down into the birth canal, followed by the second foot and subsequent breech extraction of the second twin) is performed, anaesthesia is mandatory.
- There is an increased risk of PPH due to uterine atony.
- Monochorionic twins carry the risk of twin-to-twin transfusion syndrome (TTTS), due to the shared circulation between both twins. In monochorionic twins, scanning every 2 weeks from 18 weeks' gestation is recommended to exclude TTTS.
- The risk of TTTS is non-existent in DCDA twins.
- Chorionicity is best determined before 14 weeks' gestation.

CLINICAL PEARLS

- All the minor discomforts of pregnancy and most complications of later pregnancy are more frequent in multiple pregnancy.
- Perinatal mortality is increased by a factor of 6 in twin pregnancy compared to singleton pregnancies; perinatal morbidities show similar increases.

References and further reading

Barrett JFR, Hannah ME, Hutton EK, et al. A randomized trial of planned cesarean or vaginal delivery for twin pregnancy. *N Engl J Med.* 2013;369(14):1295–305.

Asztalos E, Hannah ME, Hutton EK, et al. Twin birth study: 2 year neurodevelopmental follow-up of the randomized trial of planned cesarean or planned vaginal delivery for twin pregnancy. *Am J Obstet Gynecol.* 2016;214(3):371.e1–e19.

Royal Australian and New Zealand College of Obstetricians and Gynaecologists. Management of monochorionic twin pregnancy. College Statements and Guidelines. C-Obs 42. Melbourne: RANZCOG; 2017. www.ranzcog.edu.au

Case 32
Helen presents with raised blood pressure in pregnancy. . .

Helen is a 32-year-old woman whom you have been asked to see in the antenatal clinic. She is currently 34 weeks pregnant.

Helen has had two previous vaginal births, and a miscarriage at 8 weeks of pregnancy. Her children are now aged 8 and 10. Since her last delivery Helen has been divorced and has re-partnered; this baby will be the first child for her partner, Scott. Helen suffers from essential hypertension. When she is not pregnant her blood pressure is well controlled with the use of labetalol.

Helen has carefully planned this pregnancy, knowing the implications of her hypertension and the treatment she is usually on. She had a levonorgestrel-releasing intrauterine contraceptive device (IUD) in place for 5 years; at the time this was removed to enable her to try to conceive, which she did within 2 months, her general practitioner confirmed her dose of 200 mg labetalol twice daily as appropriately managing her hypertension. Helen also commenced folate supplements.

CLINICAL COMMENT

Classification of hypertensive disorders in pregnancy

- Chronic hypertension—blood pressure of 140/90 mmHg or greater before pregnancy or before 20 weeks' gestation; may be essential (90% cases); secondary to renal, endocrine or other disease; or 'white coat' hypertension—higher BP readings brought on by anxiety from interacting with a health professional.
- Gestational hypertension—blood pressure of 140/90 mmHg or greater without proteinuria after 20 weeks' gestation; the diagnosis may also be made when a patient has a rise of 30 mmHg systolic, or 15 mmHg diastolic, above the known pre-pregnancy or early pregnancy blood pressure.
- Pre-eclampsia—a multi-system disorder characterised by hypertension and involvement of one or more other organ

systems and/or the fetus. While significant proteinuria is common (a spot urine protein:creatinine ratio (UPC) ≥30 mg/mmol, equivalent to a 24-hour urine protein >300 mg), other evidence of renal involvement (raised creatinine, oliguria); haematological involvement (platelets ≤100 000/μL, haemolysis or disseminated intravascular coagulation); liver involvement (raised serum transaminases, epigastric or RUQ pain); neurological involvement (eclampsia, hyperreflexia with sustained clonus, persistent new headache, visual disturbances, stroke); pulmonary oedema; and fetal growth restriction may all contribute to a diagnosis of pre-eclampsia.

- Pre-eclampsia superimposed on chronic hypertension—symptoms and/or signs of pre-eclampsia occurring after 20 weeks' gestation in a woman known to have chronic hypertension.

Eclampsia is a seizure disorder following pre-eclampsia—the onset of pre-eclampsia and seizure(s) may be very sudden.

What do you need to know about Helen's previous pregnancies?

Helen's first pregnancy was complicated by moderate pre-eclampsia super-imposed on her known chronic hypertension. She required increasing doses of methyldopa to control her blood pressure and at 34 weeks developed some proteinuria and non-dependent oedema. There was a degree of intrauterine growth restriction of the fetus, which led to her having her labour induced at 37 weeks' gestation. The baby, a boy, weighed 2240 g and spent 4 days in the special care baby unit (SCBU) having jaundice treated.

In her second pregnancy Helen experienced some hypertension again, requiring increased methyldopa from 30 weeks. She was also treated with low-dose aspirin from 8 weeks' gestation. She did not develop proteinuria during the pregnancy, but there was slowing of fetal growth from 32 weeks that led to the induction of labour at 38 weeks' gestation. The baby, a girl, weighed 2500 g and required treatment for jaundice in the SCBU.

How has this pregnancy been managed?

In this pregnancy Helen was first seen at the antenatal clinic at 8 weeks of pregnancy. Apart from some mild nausea, she was feeling well. Her blood pressure at this time was 125/85 mmHg, which was 'good' for her, she said. She was then on labetalol 400 mg daily. Her last CST had been 10 months previously.

In addition to routine antenatal blood tests, Helen had tests for baseline urea, creatinine and electrolytes performed. Results of these were all within the normal range. She also underwent a 24-hour urine collection for total protein—the result of this was 183 mg of protein excreted in 24 hours, well within the normal range. She had a portable ultrasound scan (USS) performed to confirm her due date—she gave the date of her LMP as 'certain' and had a 28-day cycle. Ultrasound showed a single fetus with a crown–rump length (CRL) of 1.5 cm, as expected for 8 weeks and 2 days.

After her last pregnancy Helen underwent full thrombophilia screening; all tests were negative. However, in view of her history of pre-eclampsia superimposed on hypertension in her first pregnancy, and intrauterine growth restriction in both previous pregnancies, Helen was commenced on low-dose aspirin (75–100 mg daily) at the booking visit and has continued with this throughout the pregnancy.

What are your current concerns?

On looking through Helen's notes you see that her blood pressure has been well controlled in a range of 120/85 to 140/95 mmHg during her pregnancy. Fetal growth has been assessed with USS at 18 weeks, 28 weeks and 32 weeks of pregnancy. All parameters are within the 95th percentile and the baby is growing well and symmetrically; estimated fetal weight at 32 weeks was 1900 g, there was adequate liquor around the baby and Doppler studies showed systolic/diastolic (S/D) ratios of 2.9 (normal for 34 weeks).

What examination do you make for Helen?

You take Helen's blood pressure and find it to be 150/100 mmHg. On questioning, Helen feels well, with no headache or abdominal pain, and the baby is moving normally, but she is aware of some puffiness of fingers and feet, which you confirm on examination. On examining the pregnant abdomen you find the baby to be lying longitudinally with the head presenting; the uterine fundus measures 34 cm.

You ask Helen to move into the day pregnancy unit where blood is taken for routine tests and a CTG performed. After she has rested for 30 minutes, Helen's blood pressure is again checked and found to be 140/90 mmHg. Dipstick testing of urine shows +1 protein. Arrangements are made for Helen to perform a 24-hour urine collection for proteinuria and she is allowed to go home, to return to the day pregnancy unit in 2 days' time.

Day pregnancy units provide care for women who need assessment of pregnancy more often than regular antenatal clinics provide, but who do not need to be inpatients in hospital. They provide assessment and surveillance of women with mild to moderate degrees of hypertension, those with diabetes both preceding pregnancy and gestational, women with prolonged pregnancy and those with certain other complications of pregnancy. Day pregnancy units provide a particularly suitable environment for women found to have raised blood pressure during pregnancy—the blood pressure can be checked again after a period of rest, a CTG performed and blood and urine tests arranged. In a day pregnancy unit the opportunity can be taken by staff to discuss concerns such as contraception, sterilisation, interpersonal violence and depression. This is often more easily done in this environment than in the context of a busy antenatal clinic.

What are your conclusions and what plans do you make for Helen?

You make a presumptive diagnosis of pre-eclampsia superimposed on chronic hypertension. You note that Helen has a new partner and therefore is at renewed risk of pre-eclampsia in this pregnancy. You recall that pre-eclampsia is more common in women who have preexisting hypertension. You plan to manage Helen's condition with visits to the day pregnancy unit 3 times weekly to check her blood pressure, blood results, proteinuria and fetal movements and perform a CTG. You organise a further USS to assess fetal growth, the amniotic fluid index and umbilical blood flow and arrange to review the results of this at the day pregnancy unit in 2 days' time. Your plan is to manage Helen's pregnancy expectantly unless her pre-eclampsia worsens or the baby shows signs of intrauterine growth slowing or an abnormal CTG. You explain to Helen that expectant management will be continued to 37–38 weeks depending on her progress, and that at that stage, induction of labour will probably be advised. Helen is happy with this plan, which reflects her management in her two earlier pregnancies.

CLINICAL PEARLS

- Pre-eclampsia is more common in nulliparae or in women pregnant with a new partner, women with diabetes, women with multiple pregnancy or molar pregnancy and women

continued

continued

with chronic hypertension, renal disease, thrombophilias and connective tissue disorders.

- Expectant management of mild pre-eclampsia includes surveillance of both mother and baby—intrauterine growth restriction may occur.
- Antihypertensive therapy in mild or moderate pre-eclampsia does not modify the course of the disease and has no role.

References and further reading

Lowe S, Bowyer L, Lust K, et al. SOMANZ guidelines for the management of hypertensive disorders of pregnancy 2014. *Aust N Z J Obstet Gynaecol.* 2015;55(5):e1–e29.

Case 33
Megan develops pre-eclampsia. . .

Megan is a 26-year-old primigravida you have been called to see in the day pregnancy clinic. Megan has been having antenatal care shared between her general practitioner, Dr Khan, and the hospital antenatal clinic. She made her first visit to the clinic at 11 weeks' gestation, when she was booked for delivery in your hospital. She carries with her a hand-held patient record on which Dr Khan and the hospital doctors and midwives have made notes of all visits.

What is your first step in the care of Megan?

You take an appropriate history. Much of this comes from her shared care card. From this you learn that Megan has no previous significant medical history apart from an appendicectomy at the age of 15. Her menarche was at age 12, and she started the combined oral contraceptive pill (COCP) at the age of 15 for dysmenorrhoea; she continued it when she became sexually active at the age of 18. This is a planned pregnancy—Megan became pregnant 3 months after stopping the pill. Her cervical screening is up to date and normal.

Megan's booking blood pressure at 11 weeks of pregnancy was 110/70 mmHg. She experienced some mild nausea and vomiting in the first trimester but otherwise the pregnancy has been unremarkable; all blood pressures have been within the range 110/70 to 120/80 mmHg and until the previous day Megan has continued her work as a librarian.

Why has Megan presented to the hospital now?

Yesterday at 36 weeks' gestation in Dr Khan's practice her blood pressure was found to be 135/90 mmHg. After she had rested for several minutes it was rechecked and found to be 130/85 mmHg. Megan felt perfectly well; on questioning by Dr Khan she denied any headache, abdominal pain, visual disturbance or ankle swelling, and was feeling normal fetal movements. Examination of her abdomen showed the fundal height to measure 36 cm (the expected size for 36 weeks), the baby was in a longitudinal lie with the head presenting, and four-fifths of the fetal head was palpable above the pelvic brim. Dr Khan tested Megan's reflexes and these were not abnormally brisk, nor was any clonus present. Testing of a urine sample showed +1 of proteinuria. Dr Khan arranged for Megan to attend the day pregnancy clinic the following morning.

What are your concerns for Megan?

Your main concern is that Megan may be developing pre-eclampsia, a common condition in primigravidae in the latter weeks of pregnancy. On questioning Megan you find that she still feels quite well and the baby is moving normally. Her blood pressure is 145/90 mmHg, general physical examination is unremarkable apart from ankle oedema and her reflexes are normal with no clonus. A urine protein:creatinine ratio reveals a ratio of 32 mg/mMol indicating proteinuria. A CTG is carried out and this shows a baseline fetal heart rate of 140 bpm; the trace is normal.

You order blood tests—FBC, electrolytes, urea and urate levels and liver function tests (LFTs)—then allow Megan to go home to rest with instructions to return to the day pregnancy clinic the following day, or to telephone the birth suite if she develops headache, abdominal pain or any other symptom that concerns her overnight.

In the day pregnancy clinic the next day you find Megan's blood pressure to be further elevated at 150/100 mmHg. She states she has a mild frontal headache and she feels that her ankles, fingers and face are swollen. On examination you find the reflexes to be brisker than on the previous day but there is no clonus. The CTG shows no abnormality. The results of blood tests from the previous day show that Megan's FBC, urea, creatinine, electrolytes and liver function tests were all within normal limits but her urate level was slightly raised.

What is your management plan now for Megan?

You explain to Megan that she has developed pre-eclampsia and it seems that her symptoms are worsening, her blood pressure is rising and it is therefore important to monitor both her wellbeing and that of the fetus. You recommend hospital admission for closer observation and possible delivery of the baby. She understands and agrees to this. You reassure her that, with pre-eclampsia, the outlook for herself and her baby is excellent with appropriate care but that treatment, including delivery of her baby earlier than she had anticipated, is likely to be indicated.

CLINICAL COMMENT

What is pre-eclampsia?

The Society of Obstetric Medicine of Australia and New Zealand (SOMANZ) defines pre-eclampsia as:

> A multi-system disorder unique to human pregnancy characterised by hypertension and involvement of one or more other organ systems and/or the fetus. Raised blood pressure is commonly but not always the first manifestation. Proteinuria is the most commonly recognised additional feature after hypertension but should not be considered mandatory to make the clinical diagnosis.

Hypertension is defined as a systolic blood pressure >140 mmHg and a diastolic blood pressure ≥90 mmHg. Blood pressure should be measured in the seated position and two elevated blood pressures 4–6 hours apart are needed for the diagnosis of hypertension. Proteinuria is defined as the excretion in a 24-hour period of >300 mg of protein— a timed urine collection must be performed. However, a spot urinary protein:creatinine ratio of >30 mg/mmol indicates significant proteinuria.

Non-dependent oedema—not always present—includes oedema of the face and hands; sacral and lower limb oedema may also be present.

The underlying pathophysiology of pre-eclampsia is vasoconstriction and endothelial damage leading to 'leaky vessels', intravascular fluid depletion and oedema; however, the exact cause or 'trigger' for the condition is not yet completely understood. Delivery of the baby and placenta cures the condition.

Megan is admitted to the antenatal ward. Her blood tests are repeated and the 24-hour urine result is now available—this shows 650 mg of protein excreted in 24 hours (the normal upper limit is 300 mg). After 1 hour of bed rest in the ward, Megan's blood pressure settles to 140/95 mmHg.

It is decided after discussion with your consultant that Megan requires delivery for her evolving pre-eclampsia and that induction of labour should be carried out. Abdominal examination shows the head to be three-fifths above the pelvic brim. You perform a vaginal examination and find the cervix to be posterior, firm, 3 cm in length and closed, and the head is at –2 cm, giving a modified Bishop score of 1 (Table 33.1).

Table 33.1 Modified Bishop scoring is used to assess the cervix for suitability for induction of labour

Score	0	1	2	3
Dilatation (cm)	0	1–2	3–4	5+
Length of cervix (cm)	3	2	1	0
Station (above or below ischial spines)	–3	–2	–1,0	+1,+2
Consistency		Firm	Medium	Soft
Position		Posterior	Mid	Anterior

What is the significance of your findings?

It is not possible to proceed directly to artificial rupture of the membranes (ARM). Preliminary treatment with a synthetic prostaglandin is needed to ripen the cervix, making it possible to rupture the membranes at a later stage and also increasing the chances of the induction leading to effective labour and vaginal birth. You insert intravaginal dinoprostone to ripen the cervix.

Overnight Megan's blood pressure remains about 140/85 to 140/95 mmHg, her headache responds to paracetamol and a CTG shows normal fetal reactivity. The following morning your vaginal examination shows the cervix to be favourable enough for ARM to be performed (soft, 1 cm in length, mid-position, 2 cm dilated, at spines: Bishop score 2). An oxytocin infusion is commenced after ARM has been carried out. Blood tests are repeated—the results are unchanged and, in particular, Megan has a platelet count of 290×10^9/L, confirming her suitability for epidural anaesthesia. Her blood pressure at this time is 140/95 mmHg. Megan's partner Brad is present in the birth suite to support her.

How should Megan's labour be managed?

Megan will be under close observation by both the midwifery and the medical staff, and will have continuous fetal monitoring. Regular contractions begin within 4 hours. At this time Megan's blood pressure is noted to be 150/100 mmHg, and an epidural catheter is inserted by an anaesthetist. The blood pressure settles to 120/80 mmHg but within 1 hour has risen again to 170/110 mmHg. A urinary catheter is also inserted at this time and Megan's urine output, measured hourly, remains <30 mL per hour.

What are your immediate concerns and how do you deal with these?

Megan's pre-eclampsia is worsening and you are concerned about the possibility of a seizure; you are also concerned about the development of renal and liver complications. Megan is transferred to the high-dependency area of the birth suite where hydralazine and magnesium sulphate infusions are started. Further blood tests are ordered urgently—these show an elevated urate level of 0.55 mmol/L, but a normal platelet count at 266×10^9/L. The oxytocin infusion is continued, and Megan's contractions are regular every 3 minutes, lasting 60–90 seconds. However, her blood pressure is difficult to control, with increasing levels of hydralazine needed to keep it at 160/110 mmHg, and 4 hours after inserting the epidural your vaginal examination shows the cervix to be only 3 cm dilated.

Not all maternity units have a high-dependency area but most have at least one separate room for the management and one-to-one nursing of high-risk cases.

Complications of severe pre-eclampsia

- Renal—decreased glomerular filtration rate, proteinuria, oliguria, renal failure
- Haematological and vascular—thrombocytopenia, coagulopathy, microangiopathic anaemia, severe hypertension ($\geq$170/110 mmHg)
- Neurological—headache, visual disturbance, hyperreflexia, seizures (eclampsia), cerebrovascular accident, blindness
- Pulmonary—pulmonary oedema
- Hepatic—raised liver enzymes, subcapsular haematoma, hepatic rupture
- Fetal—restricted intrauterine growth, oligohydramnios, placental abruption, fetal hypoxia, fetal death
- HELLP syndrome—occurs in 20% of women with severe pre-eclampsia

---

HELLP syndrome—haemolysis (haemolytic microangiopathic anaemia), elevated liver enzymes, low platelets—indicates rapid deterioration in the woman's condition and the need for urgent delivery.

CLINICAL COMMENT

Control of blood pressure in severe pre-eclampsia

Aim to keep the blood pressure in the range 140/90 to 160/100 mmHg—at blood pressures >170/110 mmHg there is a significant risk of cerebral haemorrhage, at blood pressures below a diastolic of 90 mmHg placental perfusion may be compromised, resulting in adverse fetal outcomes. Continuous CTG monitoring is essential.

An antihypertensive should be administered parenterally. The most widely used is hydralazine 5–10 mg given by slow IV injection followed by an IV infusion; 80 mg hydralazine is diluted to 40 mL with normal saline and administered by syringe pump, commencing at 1 mL per hour. The rate of infusion is titrated against the blood pressure and the maximum dose should not exceed 30 mL per hour (60 mg per hour). If the maternal pulse rises above 100 bpm, a beta-blocker may be used; alternatively hydralazine should be ceased and other antihypertensives started. Labetolol, metoprolol and nifedipine have all been extensively used in this situation; however, it should be noted that difficulty controlling blood pressure usually indicates urgent need for delivery.

Patients with severe pre-eclampsia are usually but not always hypovolaemic and hypoalbuminaemic, with resulting oliguria. A urinary catheter should be inserted and output measured hourly. Colloid solutions should be given intravenously, cautiously in boluses rather than by increasing the infusion rate, with careful monitoring to avoid pulmonary oedema. In difficult cases a central venous pressure (CVP) line should be inserted and fluid replaced to maintain a pressure of 8 mmHg and urine output of ≥30 mL per hour. Iatrogenic fluid overload and pulmonary oedema must be avoided.

What is appropriate management for Megan at this point?

In view of Megan's deteriorating pre-eclampsia, a decision is made by your consultant for caesarean section. You explain this decision to Megan and Brad. Since you have already clearly explained to them everything that has happened to Megan since her admission, they understand the situation, the fact that Megan's high blood pressure endangers both herself and the baby, and that caesarean section is strongly indicated medically. Brad will accompany Megan to the operating theatre and Megan will have the operation performed under epidural. The anaesthetist comes to institute this arrangement.

The decision–incision interval is just under 1 hour. You assist at the caesarean section, which results in the delivery of a baby girl. The baby is in good condition, with Apgar scores of 8 at 1 minute and 10 at 5 minutes, and Megan and Brad are able to hold her very soon after birth.

How do you manage Megan postoperatively?

Following the caesarean section, Megan's blood pressure stabilises at 140/90 mmHg but Megan remains in the high-dependency unit for 24 hours on magnesium sulphate and hydralazine, as her reflexes remain brisk and it is well recognised that eclampsia can occur postpartum. Gradually her condition returns to normal.

CLINICAL COMMENT

Anticonvulsant therapy in severe pre-eclampsia

Magnesium sulphate 50% is the prophylactic anticonvulsant drug of choice. It is administered intravenously via a syringe pump and a peripheral line—it should not be given directly via a CVP line because sudden boluses can cause marked side effects. A 4 g loading dose (8 mL) is given over 20 minutes. The maintenance dose is 1–2 g or 2–4 mL per hour. Women should be warned of possible transient hot flushes.

Magnesium may cause muscular weakness, respiratory depression and cardiac arrhythmias, and levels of magnesium may rise with poor urinary output. Respiratory rate and urine output should be monitored hourly. Patellar reflexes should be tested 4 hourly, lung bases auscultated and the jugular venous pressure checked for signs of cardiac failure. If urine output falls, there are absent reflexes, the respiratory rate falls below 10 breaths/minute or eclampsia supervenes, then the infusion should be stopped while serum magnesium levels are monitored—1.7–3.5 mmol/L is considered therapeutic. Calcium gluconate 1 g or calcium chloride (5 mL 10% solution) can help reduce magnesium levels if toxicity occurs.

Does Megan require further postnatal follow-up?

Yes. Megan is transferred to the postnatal ward on day 2, her blood pressure settles rapidly, breastfeeding is established and Megan's postnatal course is otherwise uncomplicated. She is discharged home on day 6 to have home visits from the domiciliary midwifery service of the hospital. Handover of outpatient care to Megan's family doctor, Dr Khan, is a key part of care.

Management of eclampsia (seizures)

- Protect the patient from harm—put up the sides of the bed, use pillows.
- Secure the airway—place the patient on the left side in coma position, insert an airway.
- Administer oxygen.
- Obtain IV access if not already in place.
- Use the loading dose of magnesium sulphate to control the fit—diazepam has been associated with an increased maternal mortality rate.
- Institute magnesium sulphate IV as outlined for the treatment of severe preeclampsia.
- Institute hydralazine therapy as for severe pre-eclampsia.
- If patient is undelivered, arrange delivery once the situation has stabilised.

It is important that underlying hypertension be excluded, so 6 weeks later you see Megan in the outpatients department. She is quite well, the abdominal incision is well healed and her blood pressure is 110/70 mmHg. Breastfeeding is well established. You order a FBC, urea, electrolytes and uric acid, and all results are within normal levels. You reassure Megan that she will suffer no lasting effects of her preeclampsia, that she has a 50% chance of experiencing pre-eclampsia in a future pregnancy and that since the indication for the caesarean section was confined to that pregnancy she could anticipate a vaginal birth in her next pregnancy if she so wished. Should Megan become pregnant again, management with low-dose aspirin and calcium should be instituted from the first trimester to reduce the risk of recurrent hypertensive complications.

 CLINICAL PEARLS

- Severe pre-eclampsia requires stabilisation of blood pressure and anticonvulsant therapy followed by delivery of the baby, as the condition will not improve until after delivery, and severe pre-eclampsia threatens the lives of mother and fetus.
- Women with no underlying predisposing condition who experience pre-eclampsia in a first or subsequent pregnancy have a 50% chance of a recurrence in a later pregnancy, but the condition does not generally worsen with successive pregnancies.

- Some units use a spot urine specimen to measure the PCR. This is as accurate as the 24-hour collection of urine for quantifying proteinuria. Ranges vary and a PCR greater than 45 mg/mmol (which is equivalent to an albumin:creatinine ratio of greater than 30 mg/mmol or approximately 300 mg/g) is considered significant proteinuria.

References and further reading

Amaral LM, Wallace K, Owens M, LaMarca B. Pathophysiology and current clinical management of preeclampsia. *Curr Hypertens Rep*. 2017;19(8):61.

Lowe SA, Bowyer L, Lust K, et al. SOMANZ guidelines for the management of hypertensive disorders of pregnancy. College Statements & Guidelines. Melbourne: RANZCOG: 2014. www.ranzcog.edu.au

Case 34
Zuzanna develops diabetes in pregnancy. . .

Zuzanna has presented to you in the antenatal clinic for a visit at 28 weeks' gestation. Zuzanna has migrated from Poland and her first baby was also born there, a boy who was delivered with forceps after a 26-hour labour and weighing 4300 g. This birth was complicated by a large perineal tear and anal sphincter injury. Fortunately her recovery was complete and she has no problems with continence. For various reasons of access Zuzanna did not have a screen for gestational diabetes mellitus (GDM) in that pregnancy. In this current pregnancy—her second—the midwife at the migrant health centre has arranged a 75 g oral glucose tolerance test the day before her visit with you. This has shown a fasting blood glucose level of 5.9 mmol/L and a 2-hour level of 9.1 mmol/L, which means that Zuzanna has developed GDM.

 CLINICAL COMMENT

> Development of gestational diabetes is common, with data from Australia showing that about one pregnancy in seven is affected using current criteria for diagnosis. This is a very similar rate to that in the United Kingdom and other countries. Risk factors for GDM include diabetes in a previous pregnancy, polycystic ovary syndrome, overweight and obesity, a previous large baby and certain racial groups including women of South-East Asian and Aboriginal and Torres Strait Islander background. Screening is offered at the beginning of the third trimester—between 26 and 28 weeks—except where there is a history of previous GDM or other risk factors, in which cases it should be offered at the beginning of the second trimester (or even earlier if there is a particularly high risk). In these cases, if the screening result is negative, screening should be offered again at 26–28 weeks.

The 75 g GTT is standard; the test should be done with the woman having fasted for the previous 8 hours. Criteria for a diagnosis of GDM are a fasting glucose of greater than 5.0 mmol/L, a value at 1 hour of greater than 9.9 mmol/L or at 2 hours of greater than 8.4 mmol/L.

What will be included in your initial discussion with Zuzanna?

You need to assess Zuzanna's general health and the progress of her pregnancy so far. Zuzanna reports that she is well and feeling fetal movements, but she wants to know what her test results mean. You explain that high sugar levels in the blood can bring about accelerated growth of the baby, as glucose crosses the placenta freely while maternal insulin does not. The elevated levels of glucose in the baby's circulation provoke an insulin response which accelerates growth of the baby and can cause problems immediately following birth with low blood sugar levels. These fetal physiological changes also can impact the maturity of the baby's systems. You explain the importance of good blood sugar control for the remainder of the pregnancy, with the aim of maintaining fasting levels less than 5.1 mmol/L, and postprandial levels of less than 7.4 mmol/L. The mainstays of management of GDM are an appropriate diet, exercise and blood glucose monitoring.

Zuzanna will attend the combined antenatal diabetic clinic and be under the care of the diabetes in pregnancy team of your maternity unit. Zuzanna will be provided with education about GDM, including about the principles of dietary management and physical activity. She will be issued with a glucometer and taught how to measure her blood glucose levels and record them.

What examination does Zuzanna need at this visit?

You carry out a routine antenatal check for Zuzanna. Her blood pressure is normal; the uterine fundal height is 30 cm, a little large for dates. Zuzanna had a fetal anomaly ultrasound scan at 20 weeks that confirmed her dates and showed no fetal abnormality; the placenta was noted to be fundal. You order a further scan to assess fetal growth. The diabetes educator spends some time with Zuzanna discussing diet and explaining the use of the glucometer. Zuzanna will keep a record of blood glucose levels before breakfast and at 2 hours following each meal over the next 2 weeks, and then will have a virtual consultation with the diabetic team to assess her blood glucose readings.

What are your concerns at following visits?

Two weeks later you see Zuzanna again in the clinic. She continues to feel well—in fact, since modifying her diet with less carbohydrate and fat, she feels better than earlier in the pregnancy. However, perusal of her diabetic record book shows that many of her glucose levels, particularly the fasting readings, are above the target range. Zuzanna explains that she had a telehealth consultation that morning with the diabetes team and they plan to commence insulin treatment. The ultrasound scan report shows the baby to be close to the 97th percentile when plotted on a fetal growth chart (Fig. 34.2). On physical examination the fundal height now measures 33 cm but otherwise is unremarkable.

Over the next six weeks Zuzanna's glucose levels prove difficult to control and she is in regular contact with the team at the diabetes clinic. Her doses of insulin are increased sequentially to maintain control of her blood glucose levels. A further ultrasound for growth assessment shows the growth continuing to be above the 97th centile for gestation; Doppler studies are reassuring but the liquor volume is well above the normal range.

Diagnosis of gestational diabetes (GDM) and preexisting diabetes in pregnancy

The diagnosis of GDM includes those women with previously undiagnosed abnormalities of glucose tolerance, as well as women with glucose abnormalities related to the pregnancy alone. A definitive diagnosis of non-gestational diabetes cannot be made until the postpartum period. The Australasian Diabetes in Pregnancy Society (ADIPS) does not currently recommend the use of the term 'overt diabetes' as proposed by the International Association of Diabetes and Pregnancy Study Groups to describe marked hyperglycaemia (consistent with diabetes if detected outside pregnancy) first detected in pregnancy.

A diagnosis of GDM is made if one or more of the following glucose levels is elevated:

Fasting glucose ≥5.1 mmol/L
1-h glucose ≥10.0 mmol/L
2-h glucose ≥8.5 mmol/L

Management of Gestational Diabetes (GDM) and preexisting diabetes in pregnancy

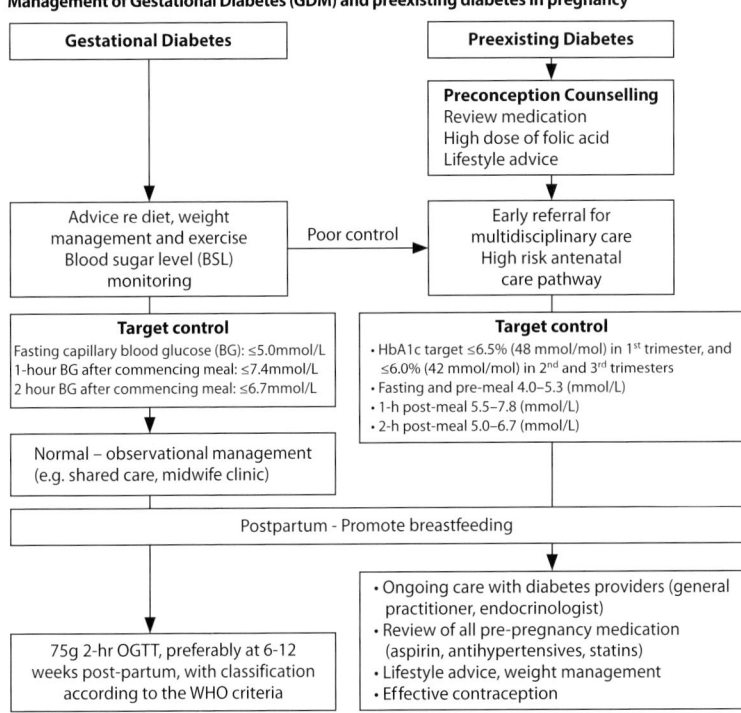

Figure 34.1 Flow chart for the management of abnormal glucose tolerance in pregnancy—75 g glucose tolerance test

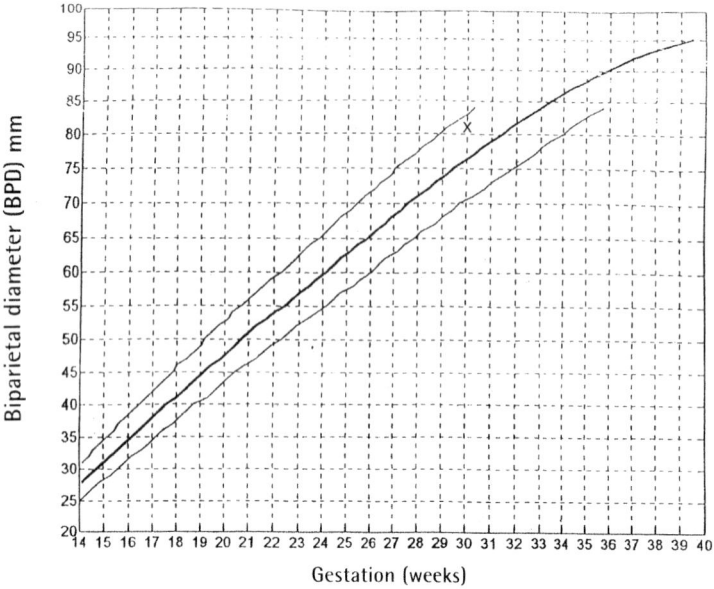

Figure 34.2 Fetal growth chart shows growth rates on the 50th percentile and 3rd and 97th percentiles on either side. The X indicates measurement of BPD at 30 weeks' gestation

At 36 weeks Zuzanna returns to the clinic, and you are contacted by the endocrinologist. She explains that Zuzanna's blood glucose levels continue to be high and that Zuzanna is requiring high doses of insulin. On examination, the fundal height is greater than a typical term size and the fetal head is not engaged and is, in fact, ballotable. At this point, you have a detailed conversation with Zuzanna about the timing and mode of birth of her baby. Zuzanna herself is very concerned about the size of her baby, which she feels is greater than that of her first child, and about her ability to have a vaginal birth. You explain to Zuzanna that given the fact that her diabetes is becoming difficult to control and the baby appears to be larger than her first, a decision will need to be made about induction of the labour. Zuzanna, naturally, is apprehensive following the anal sphincter injury she sustained with her first birth. You agree to make a decision at 38 weeks.

At 38 weeks you perform a vaginal examination to assess the cervix. The presenting part is out of the pelvis, and the cervix is long and closed. Taking all of these factors into consideration, and after a careful discussion with Zuzanna, you agree to arrange an elective caesarean section within the next couple of days. After discussion about the details and risks of a caesarean section, Zuzanna assures you she is happy with this plan.

What arrangements do you make for this procedure?

You arrange admission for the following day—Zuzanna will fast from midnight, omit her normal morning dose of insulin and come into the birth suite at 7 am. The operation is scheduled for 9 am. You order a FBC and 'group and hold' for Zuzanna. Anaesthesia is discussed with her—she requests regional anaesthesia and will bring her partner, Aleksander, as her support person in the operating theatre. You explain to Zuzanna what will happen during the surgery, the risks of caesarean section and what she can expect to feel after the operation—she will have an epidural cannula inserted for the anaesthetic, which can be left in postoperatively for analgesia, which she herself can control.

Risks of caesarean section

- Anaesthetic risks—anaesthesia is more commonly regional but women must be aware of the possibility that general anaesthesia may be required.
- Haemorrhage—consent should be obtained from all women for blood transfusion; if this is declined, this should be discussed and noted.
- Infection—of operation site, urinary tract infection, pulmonary infection related to anaesthesia, distant infection.
- Damage to adjacent organs, in particular bladder and bowel.
- Thromboembolic complications.
- Rarely, need for hysterectomy.

The following morning Zuzanna presents to the birth suite as planned. She feels well, the baby is moving normally and a short CTG strip shows a normal reactive pattern. An IV line is established and Zuzanna is commenced on infusions of glucose and insulin, with hourly BSLs. Zuzanna is then transferred to the operating suite, where a spinal anaesthetic is placed. A lower segment caesarean section is performed by your consultant, resulting in the birth of a baby boy weighing 4700 g, whom they name Szymon. The baby is in good condition, with Apgar scores of 8 at 1 minute and 9 at 5 minutes, and is handed to Zuzanna; however, after some minutes he appears to have mild respiratory distress so he is transferred to the SCBU for observation. Over the next 3 days the baby remains in the nursery, being treated for mild respiratory distress and hypoglycaemic episodes, but by day 3 he is well enough to be transferred back to the postnatal ward with his mother. Breastfeeding is establishing well.

What care does Zuzanna need postnatally?

Postnatally Zuzanna makes a very good recovery. She is able to eat soon after the birth, and her blood glucose monitoring is continued for 48 hours but her insulin requirements fall rapidly to zero. Otherwise her postnatal course is uneventful, the wound heals well, the subcuticular suture is removed on day 5 and Zuzanna is able to go home with her baby, arrangements having been made for the community midwife to call daily over the following days.

Before discharge, arrangements are made for Zuzanna to attend her general practitioner at 6 weeks and to have further glucose tolerance testing. You explain to her that she is predisposed to develop type 2 diabetes in later life.

 CLINICAL PEARLS

Tight glucose control is the key to a successful outcome in women with diabetes in pregnancy.

References and further reading

Buchanan TA, Xiang AH, Page KA. Gestational diabetes mellitus: risks and management during and after pregnancy. *Nat Rev Endocrinol.* 2012;8(11):639–49.

Nankervis A, McIntyre HD, Moses RG, et al. ADIPS consensus guidelines for the testing and diagnosis of hyperglycaemia in pregnancy in Australia and New Zealand. Sydney: Australasian Diabetes in Pregnancy Society; 2014. www.adips.org/downloads/2014ADIPSGDMGuidelinesV18.11.2014.pdf

Plows JF, Stanley JL, Baker PN, et al. The pathophysiology of gestational diabetes mellitus. *Int J Mol Sci.* 2018;19(11):3342.

Rudland V, Price S, Hughes R, et al. ADIPS 2020 guideline for pre-existing diabetes and pregnancy. *ANZJOG.* 2020;60(6):e18–e52.

Case 35
Ranji has diabetes and is pregnant. . .

In the combined antenatal diabetic clinic you carry out a booking visit for Ranji. She is a 27-year-old primigravida who has had type 1 diabetes since the age of 11 and uses an insulin pump. She now is 8 weeks advanced in this pregnancy. Prior to her pregnancy she worked hard with both her general practitioner and endocrinologist to make sure that her blood sugar levels were tightly controlled, with fasting levels at 4–5.5 mmol/L and postprandial levels at or below 7.8 mmol/L. Ranji also had baseline renal function tests, which are normal with no evidence of increased urinary protein excretion, and ophthalmological examination has shown minor retinal changes that require ongoing monitoring. She has been taking folate daily for the past 5 months and had an ultrasound scan 2 weeks ago that shows a 6-week fetus and a fetal heartbeat, all consistent with her dates. Her glycohaemoglobin (HbA_{1c}) level has been tested and is within the reference range.

How do you manage the initial visit and what plans do you make?

At the initial visit you discuss the options for first-trimester screening. These include taking no action, a combined first-trimester screen of the fetal nuchal translucency measurement and biochemistry (PAPP-A, free hCG), or a cell-free DNA test. As Ranji is young and at low risk of conditions such as trisomy 21, she opts for an ultrasound-based screen, as an increased nuchal translucency might be an indicator of a cardiac anomaly which is slightly more common in the pregnancies of women with type 1 diabetes. You stress the importance of good glucose control and discuss Ranji's case with the diabetic educator. She is commenced on low-dose aspirin to reduce the risk of pre-eclampsia developing.

You arrange for Ranji to be seen at the combined antenatal diabetic clinic regularly, to allow both the progress of the pregnancy and her diabetic control to be assessed concurrently. Clinically all goes well—her blood pressure remains within the normal range, as does clinical assessment of uterine size. At 20 weeks Ranji undergoes a careful ultrasound review of the fetal anatomy and the results are reassuring.

You explain to Ranji that glucose crosses the placenta whereas the hormone insulin does not, so high blood sugar levels in the fetal circulation provoke insulin secretion and this can stimulate accelerated truncal growth of the developing fetus. To monitor this, additional ultrasound measurements are scheduled at 26, 32 and 36 weeks. These results reveal an appropriate growth trajectory with all measurements lying between the 10th and 90th percentiles. From 28 weeks' gestation measurements are also made of the volume of liquor by calculating an amniotic fluid index (AFI), and Doppler ultrasound studies of umbilical and cerebral artery blood flow are carried out.

> The AFI is calculated by adding together the maximum amniotic fluid depths in each of the four quadrants of the uterus, as seen on ultrasound; the normal range in the third trimester is 7–25 cm. Umbilical arterial blood flow is commonly expressed as a pulsatility index or PI. This index is calculated from the maximum, minimum and mean Doppler frequency shifts during the cardiac cycle; it is a measure of the resistance to flow in the cord vessels. As placental resistance increases, diastolic flow can decrease, cease and eventually be reversed—these changes are evidence of chronic fetal hypoxia and perinatal mortality and morbidity are increased in these circumstances.

How is Ranji's diabetes managed?

Insulin requirements are managed by the endocrine team—an endocrinologist, diabetic educator and diabetic nurse—in conjunction with the obstetric service. Ranji's insulin requirements, as expected, rise during her pregnancy, but BSLs remain within the desired range; HbA_{1c} levels are assessed regularly.

Will Ranji be permitted to go past term?

Pregnancy complicated by type 1 diabetes presents increased risks during birth, and these tend to increase at and beyond term. The evidence suggests that, provided other factors are reassuring, birth should occur by 39 weeks if the dates are certain for a woman with insulin-dependent diabetes. In the presence of complications birth might need to occur earlier. Intrauterine fetal death due to variations in glucose levels is increasingly a possibility in the last weeks of pregnancy. Pre-eclampsia may be a complication of pregnancy in women with diabetes.

At 38 weeks Ranji develops some mild hypertension, headache and proteinuria and a decision is made to induce labour. Vaginal examination shows the cervix to be unfavourable for artificial rupture of the membranes (ARM), so a balloon catheter is used for cervical ripening.

The following day the cervix is suitable for ARM and oxytocin induction. A glucose-insulin infusion is commenced prior to the induction and BSLs are performed hourly during labour, adjustments to the infusion rate being made to keep the BSL within the range 4–7 mmol/L. After a 6-hour labour Ranji proceeds to a vaginal birth of a baby girl weighing 3900 g.

Postnatally Ranji is kept on the glucose-insulin infusion with hourly BSLs performed, but her insulin requirements quickly drop back to pre-pregnancy levels. Ranji's baby Priya maintains skin contact with Ranji and has regular blood sugar level monitoring by heel prick. Some of her initial blood glucose levels are low and she is given colostrum that Ranji has stored prior to the labour.

 CLINICAL PEARLS

> The causes of mortality and morbidity in the babies of mothers with diabetes include respiratory distress syndrome, hypoglycaemia, hypocalcaemia, hypomagnesaemia, jaundice and macrosomia leading to traumatic delivery. Level 3 nursery facilities may be required for the infants of such mothers, particularly when there has been poor glucose control or where delivery takes place before 36 weeks' gestation.

References and further reading

Alexopoulos AS, Blair R, Peters AL. Management of preexisting diabetes in pregnancy: a review. *JAMA*. 2019;321(18):1811–9.

Broughton C, Douek I. An overview of the management of diabetes from pre-conception, during pregnancy and in the postnatal period. *Clin Med* (Lond). 2019;19(5):399–402.

Rudland VL, Price SAL, Hughes R, et al. ADIPS 2020 guideline for pre-existing diabetes and pregnancy. *Aust N Z J Obstet Gynaecol*. 2020;60(6):e18–e52.

Case 36
Lisa presents to the birth suite at 28 weeks of pregnancy...

Lisa is a 20-year-old primigravida at 28 weeks' gestation whom you meet for the first time at 3 am in the birth suite. Lisa gives a history of painful contractions every 10 minutes.

What further history do you take from Lisa?

You need to know the earlier details of Lisa's pregnancy. You also need to know whether there is any evidence of ruptured membranes associated with her contractions, and whether there has been vaginal bleeding. Lisa denies both these things. She was woken up at midnight by the painful contractions, which are now 10 minutes apart. She has had an uncomplicated pregnancy so far and her general medical history is unremarkable.

What examination do you make for Lisa?

You need to establish whether Lisa is in labour, and determine whether there is evidence of infection. You also need to know the lie and presentation of the fetus.

Lisa is afebrile, her pulse rate is 80 bpm and her blood pressure is 120/65 mmHg. The fundal height is 28 cm and the fetal lie is longitudinal, but you are unable to confirm the presentation on palpation. A bedside ultrasound examination demonstrates a cephalic presentation. The midwife, Rhonda, tells you that she can palpate moderately strong contractions, which appear to be increasing in intensity. The CTG is normal, with no evidence of fetal distress. You perform a sterile speculum examination and the membranes are intact. The cervix appears slightly open and on digital examination you find the cervix 3 cm dilated and only 1 cm thick.

What do you conclude from your findings?

Lisa appears to be in preterm labour.

Speculum examination should be performed with full aseptic technique, avoiding contact of the cervix with the speculum. Cervical swabs should be taken for immediate bacteriological assessment. If the cervix is closed and there is no blood or amniotic fluid to be seen in the vagina, a fetal fibronectin (fFN) test should be performed if clinically indicated. Digital examination should be avoided unless there is a significant possibility of a cord presentation or prolapse.

CLINICAL COMMENT

- Preterm birth (PTB) is defined as birth at less than 37 weeks' gestation. Approximately 1 in 11 babies are born preterm in Australia. Preterm babies have a higher risk of neonatal mortality and morbidity.
- Although many factors have been associated with an increased risk of PTB, the cause of spontaneous preterm labour remains unidentified in up to half of all cases.
- 'Threatened' preterm labour (TPL) is common. TPL implies contractions that do not lead to labour (i.e. cervical effacement and dilatation). It can be difficult to distinguish between true preterm labour and TPL. Serial cervical examinations may be necessary. Some units use an fetal fibronectin (fFn) test to help distinguish between these two clinical entities. Fetal fibronectin is a glycoprotein released from the decidua and is normally present in low concentrations in the cervicovaginal secretions which rise as term approaches. A positive test does not mean that preterm labour is inevitable, but a negative test means it is unlikely. In other words, this test is useful because it has a good negative predictive value.
- The QUIPP app is a tool for predicting spontaneous PTB using the results of a fFn test and may be used to assist with management decisions.

Table 36.1 Risk factors associated with preterm birth

Maternal characteristics	Age
	Smoking
	Residing in rural and remote areas
	Indigenous
	Late or no antenatal care
	Lack of continuity of care
	Low socio-economic status
	High or low body mass index

continued

continued

Medical and pregnancy conditions	Multiple birth (twins, triplets) Short cervical length Infections including genital tract and urinary tract Vaginal bleeding Preterm prelabour rupture of membranes (PPROM) Surgical procedures involving the cervix Uterine anomalies

What is your immediate management of Lisa?

You explain the diagnosis of preterm labour and its treatment to Lisa. You further explain that attempts will be made to suppress her labour in order to delay delivery of the fetus for at least 48 hours while steroids are given to accelerate fetal lung maturation and transport is arranged for her to a tertiary hospital with appropriate neonatal care facilities. Lisa is treated with an oral nifedipine regimen to try to stop her contractions, and with betamethasone 11.4 mg IM to assist with fetal lung maturation. The dose is repeated 12–24 hours after the first dose.

You tell Lisa that you would like to administer intravenous antibiotics to reduce the risk of infection in the baby. You will also commence her on an infusion of magnesium sulphate for neuroprotection of the baby.

The best results for the baby, you tell her, follow transfer of the baby in utero and birth in a tertiary centre, rather than postnatal transfer. You also explain that long-term results for preterm babies born at or after 28 weeks are good, both in terms of survival and in regard to long-term physical and intellectual abnormalities.

Happily, contractions cease over the next hour and you arrange for Lisa to be transferred to the nearest hospital with a tertiary neonatal intensive care service.

 CLINICAL COMMENT

- The main aim of tocolysis (stopping uterine contractions) is to allow the administration of maternal steroids, which improve fetal lung maturation and outcome. Therefore, tocolysis is only used for up to 48 hours. The effectiveness of tocolytics is difficult to assess:

women who do not deliver may not have been in true preterm labour. In order not to miss true preterm labour, many women are treated who in retrospect were clearly not in preterm labour, making the diagnosis difficult.

- Maternal anxiety often causes difficulty with diagnosis.
- There are many medications that can be used for tocolysis. All are similarly effective, and most have significant fetal or maternal side effects. These medications include indomethacin, which can be administered as a suppository and is suitable for use if maternal transfer is required. It does reduce fetal renal and cerebral blood flow, and can close the ductus arteriosus in utero after 34 weeks, so this drug is not favoured by neonatologists. An oral nifedipine regimen has no fetal side effects but can cause maternal hypotension, so careful maternal observation is mandatory. Older drugs include intravenous salbutamol, which has the potential to cause serious maternal side effects, such as ketoacidosis and pulmonary oedema.
- The administration of a course of maternal steroids such as betamethasone or dexamethasone (both of which cross the placenta) has been shown to reduce the incidence of fetal respiratory distress (hyaline membrane disease) and the length of time of ventilation in a neonatal intensive care unit. There is no reduction in neonatal mortality, but morbidity has been shown to be reduced when steroids are used under 34 weeks' gestation. A course of betamethasone consists of two IM doses of 11.4 mg given 12–24 hours apart.
- Tocolysis is contraindicated in the presence of obvious infection or significant antepartum haemorrhage.

Nifedipine administration

- Nifedipine is given as an initial dose of 20 mg oral stat.
- Onset of tocolysis is within 30–60 minutes and institution of a second tocolytic should not be considered before that time.
- If contractions persist after 30 minutes the same dose is repeated up to 3 doses.
- Minor side effects include facial flushing, headache, nausea, tachycardia and dizziness.

Intravenous antibiotics

- Intrapartum antibiotics are given for the prevention of early-onset group B streptococcal disease or if there are signs of chorioamnionitis.
- Offer benzylpenicillin as the first choice for intrapartum antibiotic prophylaxis. If the woman is allergic to penicillin, offer clindamycin unless individual group B streptococcus sensitivity results or local microbiological surveillance data indicate a different antibiotic.

Magnesium sulphate for neuroprotection

- Magnesium sulphate administered shortly before birth may assist in reducing the risk of cerebral palsy and protect gross motor function.
- Give a 4 g intravenous bolus of magnesium sulphate over 15 minutes, followed by an intravenous infusion of 1 g per hour until the birth or for 24 hours (whichever is sooner).
- Monitor for clinical signs of magnesium toxicity at least every 4 hours by recording pulse, blood pressure, respiratory rate and deep tendon (e.g. patellar) reflexes.
- If a woman has or develops oliguria or other signs of renal failure:
    - monitor more frequently for magnesium toxicity
    - consider reducing the dose of magnesium sulphate.

It is critical that Lisa delivers in a hospital with tertiary neonatal intensive care facilities. Outcomes for babies are not so favourable if they have to be transferred after birth, although sometimes this is unavoidable. Certainly, a woman in active labour must not be transferred because delivery of a preterm infant in an ambulance or aircraft has a poorer outcome than delivering in any hospital.

Follow-up

Lisa is successfully transferred by road ambulance to the tertiary centre and you are contacted by the registrar on call the following day about her progress. Labour recommenced and Lisa progressed slowly but delivered a live female infant weighing 1200 g in good condition, not requiring ventilation.

C P CLINICAL PEARLS

- Maternal anxiety can make diagnosis of preterm labour difficult. A calm, clear explanation about how preterm labour is managed and the probable outcomes for the baby, by allaying anxiety, can assist with both diagnosis and management.
- Significant sepsis or antepartum haemorrhage in conjunction with threatened or definite preterm labour are absolute contraindications to tocolysis and steroid administration. Urgent delivery is required regardless of the period of gestation.

References and further reading

Australian Institute of Health and Welfare. Australia's mothers and babies: 2017 in brief. Perinatal statistics series no. 35. Cat. no. PER 100. Canberra: AIHW; 2019. www.aihw.gov.au/reports/mothers-babies/australias-mothers-and-babies-2017-in-brief

McCue B, Torbenson VE. Fetal fibronectin: the benefits of a high negative predictive value in management of preterm labor. *Contemp Ob/Gyn.* 2017; Suppl:1–6.

National Institute for Health and Care Excellence. Preterm labour and birth. NICE Guideline 25. London: NICE; 2015. www.nice.org.uk/guidance/ng25

Queensland Clinical Guidelines. Preterm labour and birth. Guideline No. MN20.6-V9-R25. Brisbane: Queensland Health; 2020. www.health.qld.gov.au/qcg

Case 37
Su San is bleeding at 31 weeks of pregnancy...

Su San is a 34-year-old multipara whom you are called to see in the birth suite one Sunday afternoon. Su San is gravida 4, para 4 and is at just 31 weeks' gestation in this pregnancy. She has had one set of twins born by caesarean section and has had two spontaneous vaginal births, one before and one after the caesarean. She presents with the history of a painless vaginal bleed about an hour previously. Su San estimated the amount of blood she lost as about half a cup, which she describes as 'running down my legs, like my waters had broken'. This, naturally, is of great concern to her.

What are your immediate concerns?

You must quickly establish what Su San's overall status is, and whether the bleeding is continuing—antepartum haemorrhage can be swift and potentially catastrophic. You also need some basic information about this and previous pregnancies.

Su San's blood pressure is 120/70 mmHg, her pulse rate is 85 bpm and she is afebrile. You insert an IV cannula and draw blood for an FBC, coagulation screen and group and hold for blood group confirmation and cross-matching, while continuing to take her history.

Su San has been having shared antenatal care with her general practitioner, Dr El Shawi, and brings her antenatal record card. At 20 weeks she underwent a detailed antenatal ultrasound that showed a 'low-lying' placenta and she is booked for a further scan to determine the placental position next week, at 32 weeks. The pregnancy, otherwise, has been uneventful. The bleeding was not postcoital and Su San has not experienced any contractions in association with the bleeding. In the past she has had two uncomplicated pregnancies ending in normal deliveries plus the caesarean section for the twins, who were both in breech presentation. All her children are healthy and well.

Although about 20% of pregnancies will be noted to have a 'low-lying' placenta in the second trimester, in more than 90% of women uterine growth and the formation of the lower uterine segment means that by term these placentas are well clear of the cervical os.

What further examination of Su San do you now carry out?

General examination shows no signs of anaemia. Su San's heart and lungs appear normal. Inspection of the abdomen shows an obvious pregnancy and a central linea nigra. There are also some striae from previous pregnancies and a Pfannenstiel scar. Palpation of the abdomen reveals a non-tender uterus with a symphysiofundal measurement of 33 cm. The uterus is soft and the fetus easily palpable, lying slightly obliquely with the head in the left iliac fossa. A CTG trace shows the fetal heart to have a baseline of 140 bpm, good reactivity and no decelerations.

Do you now perform a vaginal examination?

No! History and abdominal examination are pointing towards a diagnosis of placenta praevia; if this is the case, vaginal examination has the potential to cause further bleeding. You should inspect the vulval region and any pads used to try to assess the degree of haemorrhage but vaginal examination must not be performed.

Do not perform vaginal examination in any case of antepartum haemorrhage until you are certain that the placenta is not praevia!

What investigations can be safely performed?

In the birth suite you perform a bedside ultrasound using a portable machine. You obtain a reasonable view of the placenta, which lies below the fetal head and appears to be across the cervix. You explain this finding to Su San and the need to admit her to hospital. Bleeding appears to have settled but you order a cross-match of 2 units of blood to be kept available in view of the diagnosis. You also initiate a course of steroid injections (betamethasone 11.4 mg given twice at an interval of 24 hours) to increase surfactant production in the fetal lungs in case further bleeding necessitates urgent preterm delivery.

The following day a formal USS is performed in the medical imaging department. It shows that the placenta lies both anteriorly and posteriorly and directly across the cervix—a central placenta praevia. There is no ultrasound evidence of placenta accreta in association with the scar of the previous caesarean section. The fetus has measurements consistent with normal growth, there is adequate liquor and Doppler scans show normal umbilical blood flow.

> Placenta praevia is more common in women of higher parity and following previous caesarean section; when an anterior placenta praevia occurs in association with a prior caesarean scar, there is an increased risk of the placenta being morbidly adherent to the uterus—placenta praevia accreta. This is a very serious condition with up to 10% maternal mortality in some series.

What arrangements are now made for Su San?

You explain to Su San that the placenta blocks the passage of the baby through the lower segment and cervix and that the only safe way of delivering her baby is by repeat caesarean section. There has been no further vaginal bleeding overnight, all Su San's observations are satisfactory and the fetal heart trace is reactive. It is decided that if there is no further bleeding over the next 24 hours, then Su San may be able to return to her home, which is less than 1 km from the hospital, provided that she always has access to transport if she has further bleeding and that cross-matched blood is kept available on a weekly basis.

However, overnight Su San has a further small bleed and although this also settles it is decided that she must remain as an inpatient. While it is hoped that this can be until the fetus is close to term, i.e. 37–38 weeks, she understands that it may be necessary to perform urgent caesarean section at any time if a major haemorrhage occurs.

For several weeks the pregnancy continues uneventfully and Su San remains in hospital. At 34 weeks there is a further moderate bleed but this also settles. Serial ultrasound scans show the baby to be growing normally. A date is selected at 38 weeks' gestation for a planned caesarean section—this is in early January. Su San has to face spending Christmas in hospital and is despondent about this prospect.

> *'What about tubal ligation at the time of the caesarean section?'* Su San asks.

Tubal ligation at the time of a caesarean section, especially a repeat caesarean, is an excellent option when the woman, and her partner, have time to discuss the matter and are aware of the advantages and disadvantages of the procedure. The risks of the procedure to the woman, over and above the risks of the caesarean surgery, are minimal, whereas the alternative procedure, laparoscopic sterilisation after an interval postnatally, carries small but nevertheless significant risks. However, the failure rate of tubal ligation is slightly higher if it is performed at caesarean section—approximately 0.5–1 per 200 women. For Su San, it is important to emphasise that placenta praevia carries risks to both mother and baby—if she were to have a tubal ligation and then experience the death of the baby in the postnatal period she may have major regrets at having decided to have the procedure done. It is important to stress that this is an irreversible procedure. There is also an increased risk of an ectopic pregnancy in the rare event that she falls pregnant. After careful thought and discussion with her husband, Su San decides to have the procedure and completes the consent forms so that it can be carried out even if an emergency caesarean is required.

You have also carefully discussed the forthcoming caesarean section with Su San and completed consent forms. You have explained that she may need a blood transfusion during or after the operation and that there is a risk of her requiring a hysterectomy if there is difficulty controlling bleeding postoperatively.

At 36 weeks' gestation on Christmas Eve you are called urgently to see Su San, who is experiencing a major haemorrhage. What is your immediate course of action?

You establish IV access and order 4 units of blood to be available. You inform your consultant and the anaesthetic team. A decision is made to proceed to an urgent caesarean section under general anaesthesia. You arrange the operation with theatre staff and inform Su San's family.

You assist your consultant with a repeat lower-segment caesarean section and bilateral tubal ligation. Measured blood loss during the operation is 1600 mL and Su San is given a 4-unit blood transfusion. A balloon tamponade is used to help control bleeding from the lower segment, and a B-Lynch suture placed as a precaution. At the conclusion of the procedure vaginal bleeding has diminished and the uterus is well contracted, but you arrange for Su San to be observed overnight in the high-dependency unit of the birth suite. The baby, a girl, has Apgar scores of 4 at 1 minute and 9 at 5 minutes, weighs 2400 g and after spending the night under observation in the SCBU is transferred back to her mother on Christmas Day.

Antepartum haemorrhage due to placenta praevia may be followed by PPH, as the lower uterine segment is thinner than the upper myometrium and contracts down less well after delivery.

 CLINICAL PEARLS

- Placenta praevia is distinguished clinically from the second main cause of antepartum haemorrhage, placental abruption, by its generally painless presentation.
- A small antepartum haemorrhage may herald a catastrophic haemorrhage. Women presenting with antepartum haemorrhage require an immediate assessment in a unit in which both ultrasound scans and caesarean section can be performed and where blood bank facilities are available; women in remote areas should be transferred to an appropriate hospital setting as soon as possible.

References and further reading

Royal College of Obstetricians and Gynaecologists. Placenta praevia and placenta accreta: diagnosis and management. Green-top Guideline No. 27a. London: RCOG; 2018. www.rcog.org.uk/en/guidelines-research-services/guidelines/gtg27a

Sebghati M, Chandraharan E. An update on the risk factors for and management of obstetric haemorrhage. *Womens Health* (Lond). 2017;13(2):34–40.

Case 38
Amanda suffers a placental abruption. . .

Amanda is a 32-year-old woman you are called to see in the birth suite. Amanda is at term in her second pregnancy and has brought herself to the birth suite with a history of mild contractions every 3–4 minutes over the past 3 hours. Amanda is keen to have a water birth and after admission and checking of her vital signs by a midwife, she has entered the spa bath where she is being supported by her partner, mother and 5-year-old daughter. She has, however, now developed some constant upper abdominal pain.

What is your initial management?

To conduct an adequate examination you must ask Amanda to get out of the bath and into a hospital bed. You take a short but pertinent history, having scrutinised the antenatal notes, and determined that the pregnancy has progressed normally and that her previous delivery was a spontaneous vaginal birth at 40 weeks' gestation following a labour of 5 hours.

Fetal movements have been normal. Amanda reports the sudden onset of dull pain over the upper part of the uterus. The pain is continuous and is unlike the mild pain of contractions, which she is now experiencing more strongly. There is no associated nausea or vomiting.

Amanda's blood pressure is 120/80 mmHg, unchanged from her admission, and her pulse rate is 92 bpm. Palpation of the abdomen reveals tenderness and hardness over the fundus of the uterus. The lower part of the uterus is soft and non-tender and you are able to palpate the fetal head, of which three-fifths is above the pelvic brim.

What is your next step?

You need to check immediately on fetal wellbeing. A cardiotocograph (CTG) is performed, which shows a baseline fetal heart rate of 175 bpm with good variability, acceleration with contractions and no decelerations.

Cardiotocograph

Table 38.1 Features of a normal cardiotocograph (CTG)

Definition	Feature	Description
Normal CTG	Baseline fetal heart rate	Rate 110–160 bpm
	Variability—fluctuations around the baseline rate	6–25 bpm
	Accelerations—transient increases in the heart rate of 15 bpm lasting 15 seconds or more	Present
	Decelerations—transient decreases in the heart rate of 15 bpm lasting 15 seconds or more	Absent

What is your clinical impression?

It is likely that there has been a degree of placental abruption with some separation of the placenta from the uterine wall. This has led to fetal tachycardia and there exists the possibility that the abruption may extend, with further fetal compromise and even acute fetal distress.

How can this diagnosis be confirmed and what further steps are indicated?

Placental abruption is a clinical diagnosis and there are no sensitive or reliable diagnostic tests available. Ultrasound detection of abruption is poor, but when the ultrasound suggests an abruption, such as detecting a retroplacental clot, the likelihood of abruption is high. You also establish IV access and take blood for an FBC, coagulation screen and group and hold.

> In placental abruption of moderate to severe degree, a coagulation screen should be performed.

Do you perform a vaginal examination?

Yes. You need to know whether Amanda is established in labour and, if so, how far she has progressed. You explain to her your clinical impression and the fact that because the abruption may extend, you wish to expedite delivery. You perform the vaginal examination and find that the cervix is 4 cm dilated, fully effaced and well applied to the fetal head. To accelerate labour and to check the colour of the liquor you rupture the membranes—some fresh meconium and some bright blood are expelled. You apply a scalp electrode and continue CTG monitoring—the fetal heart rate settles to 155 bpm with good variability and no decelerations.

> Women presenting with clinical signs of placental abruption and no evidence of fetal distress may be permitted to attempt vaginal delivery under close surveillance. If there is definite fetal distress and the woman is not close to full dilatation, then caesarean section may be the most appropriate action.

How do you continue to monitor the labour?

You explain to Amanda and her family the need for continuous monitoring—she has moved from a low-risk situation to a high-risk one. If the CTG trace becomes abnormal, then fetal scalp blood pH and lactate levels can be checked to assess the baby's wellbeing. Within 10 minutes of ARM, Amanda is having stronger and more regular contractions and she begins to use nitrous oxide inhalation for pain relief. Monitoring continues for another hour with no significant abnormalities detected. At this point Amanda is feeling an urge to push.

Should Amanda have a further vaginal examination?

Yes. If she has reached full dilatation, then delivery of the baby in good time with maternal effort is desirable. If the cervix is not fully dilated Amanda should be discouraged from pushing.

Vaginal examination shows the cervix to be fully dilated with the head 1 cm below the ischial spines in the left occipito-anterior (OA) position. At this point the fetal heart rate tracing begins to show some prolonged decelerations down to 100 bpm with and following contractions, returning only briefly to the baseline of 160 bpm.

What are the implications of this change and what action should be taken?

These are 'late decelerations', decelerations that commence after a contraction has begun, with the bottom of the deceleration after the peak of the contraction, indicating fetal hypoxia and the need to deliver the baby immediately.

Immediate delivery can be achieved by vacuum extraction (Fig. 38.1). After briefly explaining the need for urgent delivery to Amanda and calling a neonatal paediatrician, you empty the bladder with a catheter. Amanda uses nitrous oxide inhalation during the catheterisation and when the vacuum cup is applied over the flexion point of the baby's scalp. The vacuum pump is employed and with the next contraction, maternal effort is encouraged and downward traction exerted via the vacuum handle. The head is rotated to the occipito-anterior position and some descent occurs. With two further contractions the head crowns and the baby is born. The baby is handed to the paediatrician. The birth is followed by a gush of fresh blood and clots.

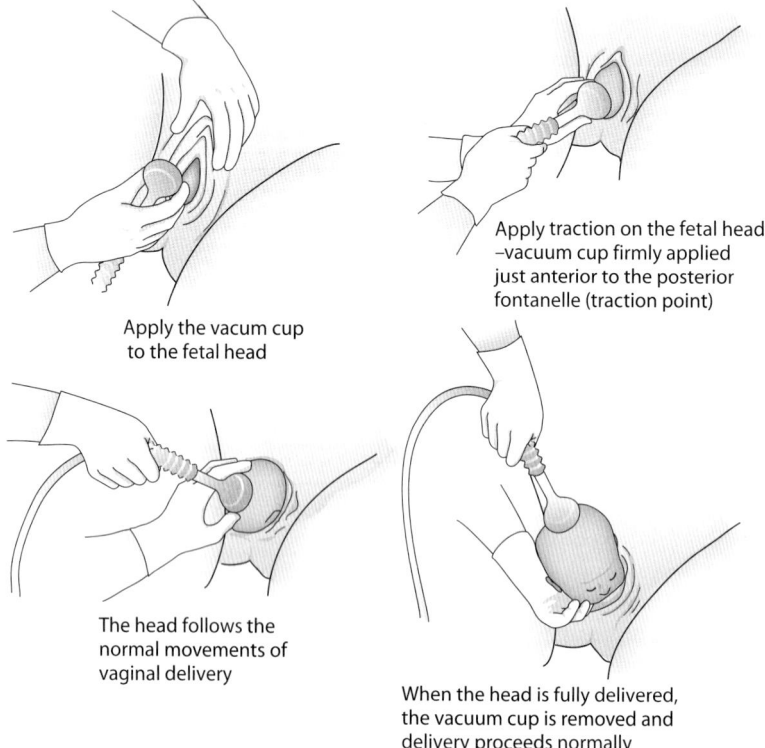

Apply the vacum cup to the fetal head

Apply traction on the fetal head, −vacuum cup firmly applied just anterior to the posterior fontanelle (traction point)

The head follows the normal movements of vaginal delivery

When the head is fully delivered, the vacuum cup is removed and delivery proceeds normally

Figure 38.1 Use of the vacuum extractor in delivery

What is your immediate concern?

Amanda is at risk of a PPH following an intrapartum haemorrhage. The abruption will have been associated with infiltration of blood among the myometrial fibres, which are thus less able to contract down postpartum.

With more major degrees of abruption, depletion of clotting factors may contribute to the development of PPH.

How do you manage this situation?

Active management of the third stage of labour is essential. You give one ampoule of oxytocin/ergometrine IM and add 40 units of oxytocin to 1 L of Hartmann's solution to be given IV. Signs of placental separation are noted and the placenta is delivered by controlled cord traction. With the placenta comes a large clot of dark blood, confirming your diagnosis. The total blood loss is estimated at 800 mL. You massage the uterus to establish a firm contraction and continue with the oxytocin infusion, 40 units over 8 hours.

 CLINICAL PEARLS

- PPH continues to be a major cause of maternal mortality and morbidity in low-income, middle-income and high-income countries. Anticipation and active prophylaxis combined with aggressive management of active haemorrhage is the key to reducing the incidence of this common problem.
- Either the vacuum extractor or forceps can be used to effect delivery rapidly when fetal distress arises and the head has descended to below the level of the ischial spines. The vacuum extractor assists with flexion and rotation of the head so that a smaller fetal head diameter is presented to the maternal pelvic outlet. Forceps add to the expulsive efforts of the mother. Forceps can only be used when the head is in or close to the OA position, whereas the vacuum extractor, because it assists with rotation, can be used with the head in positions other than OA.

References and further reading

Murphy DJ, Strachan BK, Bahl R, on behalf of the Royal College of Obstetricians and Gynaecologists. Assisted vaginal birth. BJOG. 2020;127:e70–e112.

Royal Australian and New Zealand College of Obstetricians and Gynaecologists. Management of postpartum haemorrhage (PPH). Melbourne: RANZCOG; 2017. https://ranzcog.edu.au/

Royal College of Obstetricians & Gynaecologists. Antepartum haemorrhage. Green-top Guideline No. 63. London: RCOG; 2011. www.rcog.org.uk/globalassets/documents/guidelines/gtg_63.pdf

231

Case 39
Tayla presents with herpes in pregnancy. . .

Tayla is a 17-year-old primigravida whom you are called to see in the birth suite late one Saturday night. Tayla is 33 weeks pregnant by a late ultrasound, being unsure of the date of her LMP. She booked at the antenatal clinic at about 25 weeks of pregnancy and made one subsequent visit to a general practitioner but otherwise has had no antenatal care. Tayla is accompanied by her mother but not by the child's father, with whom she says she no longer has contact.

What history do you take from Tayla?

Tayla gives a history of a sudden gush of fluid from her vagina about an hour previously. She has also been experiencing burning and tingling in the perineum and now thinks she may have some sores in the area. From her notes you see that Tayla's routine blood and urine tests done at her booking visit were all unremarkable apart from a positive urine PCR test for chlamydia—Tayla has been prescribed azithromycin for this. Tayla is allergic to penicillin. She smokes more than 20 cigarettes a day.

What examination do you undertake?

You initially make a general examination of Tayla. Her blood pressure is 110/75 mmHg, pulse 70 bpm and temperature 37.6° C. Tayla appears mildly distressed and she complains of some period-like cramps as well as the perineal pain. Examination of her abdomen shows a uterine fundus 33 cm in height with a cephalic presentation. The uterus is soft and not tender and the fetal heart trace is reassuring. Palpation over the renal angles reveals some tenderness on the right.

Inspection of the vulva shows copious clear fluid consistent with amniotic fluid draining from the vagina. The posterior aspect of the left labium is inflamed and several vesicular lesions are present, two or three of which are blistered and weeping. The lesions extend onto the perineum as far as the anal margin. The appearance is typical of herpes genitalis (HSV) infection.

What are your concerns and how are these managed?

You explain the probable diagnosis to Tayla. 'Have you had previous episodes of herpes?' you ask. She denies this firmly. She is well aware of what herpes is. 'Will it affect my baby?' she asks. You answer that primary infections in the mother carry a high risk of infection of the baby if a vaginal birth occurs—50% develop encephalitis or generalised infection with major organ involvement and death. You ask about prodromal symptoms and Tayla admits to feeling some burning and tingling in the perineum for several days, but she had simply related this to the pregnancy. She is anxious about her baby's wellbeing, and asks if a caesarean section will be safer for the baby. You answer that you have discussed her case with your consultant, and caesarean section is indeed recommended. While you have been talking with Tayla she has had two quite strong uterine contractions that were moderately painful and with each there has been a further gush of fluid from the vagina.

How do you proceed to a definite diagnosis of HSV?

You take swabs from two of the vesicular lesions after pricking each with a sterile needle. You explain to Tayla that it will be some time until you can get the results of these to confirm the diagnosis of herpes, but that on the basis of the appearance of the lesions and the fact that she is becoming established in labour, you recommend caesarean section as soon as it can be arranged. You will also commence her on a course of aciclovir and the baby will be given aciclovir after birth. You assure her that with caesarean delivery the baby's outlook is excellent.

> Preterm labour and birth (before 36 completed weeks of pregnancy) is associated with teenage pregnancy, underweight mothers, cigarette smoking, little antenatal care and maternal infection, including urinary tract infection and bacterial vaginosis.

What other clinical problems does Tayla appear to have?

You also explain that she has signs of a urinary tract infection involving especially her right kidney, and that this may be what has precipitated early labour. A short general physical examination shows that her throat and lungs are clear and there is no mastitis or generalised lymphadenopathy and no tenderness or swelling of her calves. You obtain a midstream urine

(MSU) specimen and after establishing an IV line prescribe cephalothin IV 6-hourly, observing her closely after the first dose to make sure there is no allergy to cephalosporin. You then make arrangements for an emergency caesarean section, obtaining consent, contacting the anaesthetist and paediatrician, taking blood for an FBC and group and hold and inserting a urinary catheter. Tayla's mother will accompany her to the operating theatre.

 CLINICAL COMMENT

Urinary tract infection in pregnancy

- Urinary stasis and vesico-ureteric reflux associated with progesterone and other pregnancy hormones, and short female urethral length, predispose to urinary tract infection, by faecal organisms in particular.
- Asymptomatic infection can occur, usually in the bladder. It may become symptomatic and may ascend to involve the kidneys.
- Urinary tract infection is a major predisposing cause of preterm labour.
- Recurrent infections may need prophylaxis for the remainder of the pregnancy; full urinary tract investigation postpartum is recommended.

A routine caesarean section is performed without incident and a baby girl delivered, weight 2200 g and Apgar scores of 7 at 1 minute and 10 at 5 minutes. The baby, Trinity, is transferred to the SCBU for observation.

> The principal risks to the baby from preterm birth are: respiratory distress syndrome due to relative deficiency of surfactant; intraventricular haemorrhage; hyperbilirubinaemia and jaundice with the risk of kernicterus; infection owing to the poorly developed immune system; and hypoglycaemia, as the preterm infant has relatively low glycogen stores.

What is your ongoing plan for Tayla and her baby?

Trinity progresses well over the ensuing few days, there is no evidence of neonatal herpes and breastfeeding is established. Results of the investigations you ordered antenatally are now received—PCR testing on swabs from the vulval lesions is positive for HSV2, and the MSU shows growth of *Escherichia coli* sensitive to cephalosporins. In view of her age and single status you arrange for Tayla to be seen by the hospital's adolescent team social worker and for appropriate support to be provided on discharge. You also refer Tayla to the sexual health clinic for follow-up and management should she experience recurrent episodes of genital herpes and for possible contact tracing. You discuss various appropriate methods of contraception with Tayla. She wishes to breastfeed her daughter for several months, so you suggest either the progestogen rod implant or medroxyprogesterone, but you also emphasise the importance of using condoms to reduce the chances of contracting further STIs if she is not in a mutually monogamous relationship. You also discuss ways of reducing cigarette consumption, which Tayla has indicated she wishes to do. You stress how important it is for her infant daughter to avoid passive smoking and explain that the baby was smaller than expected possibly because of Tayla's cigarette smoking during pregnancy. Tayla seems keen to follow your advice.

 CLINICAL COMMENT

Acquisition of HSV in pregnancy occurs in 0.3–3% of women, depending on the population surveyed. Primary infection in the first half of pregnancy may cause miscarriage. Primary infection later in pregnancy may be associated with intrauterine growth restriction (IUGR) and/or preterm labour. Primary infections in pregnancy may be safely treated with aciclovir. Neonatal herpes occurs as a direct result of contact of the baby with maternal lesions during delivery; the risk is highest from primary infections. It is probable that maternal antibodies cross the placenta and protect the fetus, so that in subsequent infections the risk of fetal infection is greatly reduced (from 50% to 3–5% of cases). Caesarean section is therefore recommended only for primary infection and in subsequent infections where extensive vulval or perineal involvement makes protecting the infant from lesions difficult. Caesarean section should be performed within 4 hours of rupture of the membranes. In women with recurrent herpes infections, prophylaxis using aciclovir or valaciclovir from 36 weeks has been shown to significantly reduce the incidence of recurrent infection. (Further information about HSV infection in pregnancy can be found in Case 12.)

ⓒⓟ CLINICAL PEARLS

Preterm birth occurs in 5–10% of all pregnancies and this figure has changed little in the past 30 years despite the more frequent use of tocolytics. Previous preterm birth is a positive predictor of a similar problem in a future pregnancy; education about quitting cigarette smoking, promoting a healthy lifestyle and prompt treatment of any infections during pregnancy may contribute to prevention.

References and further reading

Groves MJ. Genital herpes: a review. *Am Fam Physician.* 2016;93(11):928–34.

Schneeberger C, Geerlings SE, Middleton P, Crowther CA. Interventions for preventing recurrent urinary tract infection during pregnancy. *Cochrane Database Syst Rev.* 2015;2015(7):CD009279.

Smaill F, Vazquez JC. Antibiotics for asymptomatic bacteriuria in pregnancy. *Cochrane Database Syst Rev.* 2019;11:CD000490.

Case 40
Julia has a breech presentation. . .

Julia is a 32-year-old primigravida whom you meet for the first time in the antenatal clinic at 36 weeks' gestation. Julia has booked for a homebirth with an independent midwife, Thalia, who has been providing her antenatal care. Julia has made one visit to book in your antenatal clinic, as the hospital requires such a visit if women are to be referred in later pregnancy or labour. That visit, at 7 weeks, revealed Julia to be a healthy woman with no relevant medical or surgical history. Julia runs her own media relations company and is extremely well informed about birthing options and patient rights.

What history do you take from Julia?

You need to establish why Julia has been referred to the antenatal clinic at this point in her pregnancy. At 34 weeks Thalia has queried whether the presentation is breech. Two days ago at Julia's 36-week visit she was still uncertain, but yesterday afternoon ultrasound confirmed that the baby is lying with the breech presenting and legs fully extended along the body. The placenta is posterior, and not low-lying. The ultrasound estimate of fetal weight (at 36 weeks) is 3900 g. Thalia has referred Julia to the hospital clinic and she has come along with her partner Damian, her mother and a friend, Kathleen.

How do you proceed with this consultation?

You check Julia's shared care card, which shows that there has been no abnormal bleeding during the pregnancy, her blood pressure has always been within normal limits and the fundal height has been increasing as expected. You ask about fetal movements; they are being felt as usual. You outline to Julia and Damian why Julia has been referred and she states that even if the baby remains in breech position she wants to try for a homebirth.

You suggest to Julia that you recheck the baby's presentation and she agrees. Abdominal palpation reveals a very prominent head easily felt in the right upper quadrant but to be certain you use bedside ultrasound to demonstrate the breech presentation to all present.

With a diagnosis of breech presentation late in pregnancy, you take the opportunity to explain further about the issues that should inform decision making about the birth. In fewer than 1 in 25 pregnancies the baby presents by the breech at term. Over time fewer vaginal breech births are attempted, meaning that expertise in the specialised manoeuvres required for breech delivery is decreasing. Indeed, many more recently qualified obstetricians and midwives may never have participated in a planned vaginal breech birth. Although some specialised breech birth services are available in Australia, the outcomes are guarded. A planned vaginal breech birth is more likely to lead to adverse outcomes for both baby and mother, and systematic reviews confirm that a planned caesarean birth for breech reduces the risk of perinatal or neonatal death of the baby, and of serious neonatal morbidity.

Julia explains that she has been researching breech birth on the internet and points out that many breech babies have been successfully born vaginally. Julia's mother intervenes to say that her own sister had two breech deliveries quite safely; one of those children is now successful in insurance and the other is a wife and mother. Kathleen also has a friend who successfully birthed her third child as a breech.

What is your response to these comments?

You agree with all this but point out that, currently, there is no reliable way of determining in advance which babies will be successfully born as breeches. There is therefore a greater risk for Julia's baby if she attempts vaginal delivery with the baby in a breech presentation than there would be with a cephalic presentation. Furthermore, in a home delivery without ready access to experienced obstetric care, the risks are much greater should a problem arise. Already the baby weighs close to 4000 g and by term could be expected to be well above 4000 g, which poses an additional risk. As this is Julia's first baby there is not the comfort of knowing, as one might with a multipara, that she has previously safely delivered an infant of weight greater than 4000 g as a cephalic presentation.

What other options are available to Julia?

You further explain that, while elective caesarean section is a definite safe option, there is also the possibility of attempting external cephalic version (ECV). This could be done the following week after confirming that the baby is still breech and performing a CTG to check fetal wellbeing. You tell Julia that there is approximately a 40% chance that her baby will be turned to a cephalic presentation and that there is a small risk of harm to her baby, placenta or cord that may necessitate immediate caesarean section. You also tell her that there is a possibility that the baby will turn spontaneously to a cephalic presentation any time up until labour starts, although because this is her first baby and the baby lies with the legs splinted along the body (frank breech) this is less likely than with a baby with the legs flexed (complete breech) in a multiparous woman.

Details and risks of external cephalic version (ECV)

- ECV should be performed at about 36–37 weeks—before this the baby may turn spontaneously; after this the chances of success are reduced.
- It should be performed with facilities close by for emergency caesarean section if needed, although the need for this is rare.
- Contraindications are antepartum haemorrhage, hypertension in pregnancy, uterine scar and multiple pregnancy.
- The fetus should be monitored before and after the procedure.
- A tocolytic is usually given 30 minutes before attempting the procedure.
- Risks include direct damage to the baby, cord entanglement and placental abruption.
- The procedure involves gently dislodging the buttocks and/or legs and feet of the baby from the mother's pelvis and 'somersaulting' the baby into cephalic presentation.
- Rhesus-negative women should be given anti-D prophylaxis.

Damian asks, *'Why is the baby a breech?'*

You explain that the reasons for breech presentation aren't always well understood—sometimes there can be an obstruction low in the pelvis, such as a placenta praevia or a cervical fibroid or ovarian cyst, although this is not the case for Julia; sometimes there can be minor variations in the shape of the uterus—again this is not obvious in Julia's case as there is no evidence of a uterine septum or separate horn. Some babies seem to prefer this position and to remain in it to term, although many babies in breech position in earlier pregnancy (25% at 28 weeks) do turn spontaneously by 36–37 weeks. Congenital abnormalities are also higher in breech presentations, and as Julia chose not to have an 18-week anomaly ultrasound, this possibility cannot be excluded (Fig. 40.1).

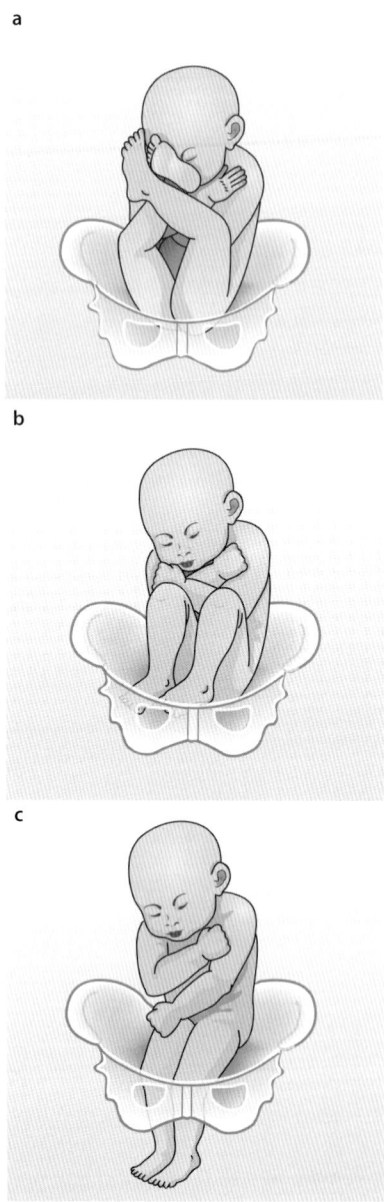

Figure 40.1 Types of breech presentation: (**a**) frank breech (**b**) complete breech (**c**) footling breech

> Julia then asks about the details of caesarean section.

You explain that an elective caesarean section would be done at about 39 weeks to try to avoid Julia going into labour early, thus avoiding an elective procedure becoming a semi-emergency, although you emphasise that this can be safely dealt with, as the facilities for caesarean section are always available in the operating theatre. You outline the procedure for an elective caesarean: regional anaesthesia will be offered so Julia will be awake, the surgery will occur at a planned time with Damian present, she will be able to see the actual delivery and to hold and nurse her baby very soon after the birth. Only one support person will be allowed into the operating theatre but others can remain close by outside and see the baby as soon as feasible. It should also be possible for Julia to go home within 24 hours if mother and baby are well and there is adequate support at home. Thalia can also come into the operating theatre for the surgery and then be available for support postoperatively and at home postnatally. You explain that one lower-segment caesarean section does not mean that future babies also need caesarean delivery—if a later child is in a cephalic presentation, then a trial of labour (TOL), hoping for a vaginal birth after caesarean section (VBAC), can safely be attempted with a good chance (60–70%) of vaginal delivery.

How do you conclude this interview?

You explain that you understand that attempted ECV and a possible caesarean section are very far from the couple's preferred option for the pregnancy. However, you ask them to think about what you have told them, which they are agreeable to, and to return the following day.

The following consultation

Julia now tells you that her main concern is the health of the baby. She and Damian consider the risks of ECV too high and she wishes to be booked for caesarean section, although if the baby turns spontaneously she will continue with her plans for a homebirth. You reiterate that ECV is a safe and evidence-based procedure, but respect their wishes.

What information must you give Julia about caesarean section?

Julia must be well informed about the risks of caesarean surgery. Having outlined these risks and given Julia an information leaflet about the surgery, you complete consent forms with her for the surgery in 2 weeks' time and arrange blood tests—FBC and group and hold—and an anaesthetic consultation. You assure Julia that the presentation of the baby will be assessed by ultrasound just prior to surgery to be certain that there has not been any last-minute change. The couple are happy with this plan.

> The risks of caesarean section to the woman include anaesthetic risks (e.g. allergic/anaphylactic reactions to medications, unsuccessful regional anaesthesia and aspiration pneumonia) and the risks of the surgery itself (haemorrhage, infection, damage to adjacent organs and thromboembolism). There is a small risk that the woman may die (about 2 per 10 000 primary elective caesarean operations). There is also a small increase in the incidence of placenta praevia in subsequent pregnancies.

Two weeks later Julia presents for admission and you confirm the breech presentation and presence of the fetal heart. Julia is transferred to the operating theatre, where epidural anaesthesia is performed. You assist your consultant in an uneventful lower-segment caesarean section, after which Julia returns to the maternity ward and the following day is discharged home to the care of her midwife.

One week later, you are called to see Julia in the emergency department, where she has presented on the advice of her midwife. She complains of feeling feverish and generally unwell, and has pain in her left breast. On examination her temperature is 38°C, pulse 90 bpm and blood pressure 110/70 mmHg. Her chest is clear, the abdominal wound is clean and healing well and there is no tenderness over the loins or calves. The right breast appears normal but the left is swollen and reddened, especially over the upper outer quadrant. It is hot and tender on palpation but there is no fluctuation; the overlying skin is shiny.

What is your clinical impression?

You make a diagnosis of mastitis and explain to Julia that although she can continue breastfeeding she should complete a full course of antibiotics to prevent the infection developing into a breast abscess. Knowing that the most likely causative organism is *Staphylococcus aureus*, you prescribe a 10-day course of dicloxacillin, recommend a paracetamol-codeine combination for pain relief and also suggest the use of warm packs. You arrange follow-up for Julia with both her midwife and her general practitioner.

Causes of postpartum pyrexia

- Urinary tract infection
- Endometritis
- Wound infection—at site of caesarean section, episiotomy or vaginal tear or cannula insertion for regional anaesthesia
- Basal atelectasis and pneumonia after general anaesthesia for caesarean section
- Mastitis
- Deep venous thrombosis
- Incidental—influenza, chest infections, meningitis, endocarditis—always examine the whole woman!

CLINICAL PEARLS

- Breech babies may turn spontaneously to cephalic at any time up until the start of labour. Always check the presentation immediately before performing a caesarean section when the indication is breech presentation.
- Women and their partners should be included as fully as possible in all decisions about pregnancy intervention, particularly elective caesarean section. Women's perceptions of involvement in decision making greatly influence their physical and emotional wellbeing postpartum.

References and further reading

Carbillon L, Benbara A, Tigaizin A, et al. Revisiting the management of term breech presentation: a proposal for overcoming some of the controversies. *BMC Pregnancy Childbirth*. 2020;20(1):263.

Hannah ME, Hannah W, Hewson SA. Planned caesarean section versus planned vaginal birth for breech presentation at term: a randomised multicentre trial. Term Breech Trial Collaborative Group. *Lancet*. 2000;356(9239):1375–83.

Hutton E, Hannah M, Ross S, et al. The early external cephalic version (ECV) 2 trial: an international multicentre randomised controlled trial of timing of ECV for breech pregnancies. *BJOG*. 2011;118(5):564–7.

Case 41
Lucy's long labour leads to further problems. . .

Lucy is a 27-year-old primigravid woman who presents to the birth suite one Sunday morning about 7 am. She is 41 weeks pregnant and you are called to the birth suite to assess her on admission.

What is your first step?

You need to take an appropriate history. This is made easier by the fact that Lucy has been having shared care with her general practitioner, Dr Cameron, and she brings with her the shared care card she has been carrying (Fig. 41.1). You see from this that Lucy has always enjoyed good health, with no medical or surgical history of note apart from an appendicectomy. She takes no medications, has no allergies, her cervical screening is up to date and normal and she has attended antenatal classes with her partner, Alice. The treasured pregnancy was the happy result of fertility treatment using anonymously donated sperm.

Further information about investigations during the pregnancy is also noted on this card. Lucy's initial blood and urine tests were all within normal limits—her blood group is A Rh (D) positive and no antibodies were detected. Throughout the pregnancy her blood pressure has been in the range of 110/70 to120/80 mmHg, the uterine fundus has had an appropriate height and fetal movements have been felt. Lucy was certain of the due date due to the nature of the conception. She had undergone pre-pregnancy reproductive carrier screening—for cystic fibrosis, spinal muscular atrophy and fragile X carrier status—that was negative. Her DNA-based first-trimester screen was normal, and the fetal anomaly ultrasound at 20 weeks was reassuring.

Lucy reports that she has been having mild, irregular lower abdominal pains since 10 pm the previous night, although she has been able to get some sleep. At 6 am she was awakened by a gush of fluid from her vagina and she wonders if her waters have broken. There are normal fetal movements.

LMP: **CYCLE:**   **AGREED EDC:**
INVESTIGATIONS: **ULTRASOUND:** Date: Weeks:
BOOKING: Date
BLOOD GROUP   ANTIBODIES   Hb   RPR   HEPB   HEPC   RUBELLA
HIV   MSU
24–28 WEEKS: Date   **34–36 WEEKS:** Date
Hb   Antibodies   Hb   Antibodies   RPR
40 WEEKS: Date
Hb   Antibodies

ANTENATAL VISITS   **DISCUSSIONS**   **Comments**

DATE	B.P.	Oedema	GEST Calc	Size	Pres	1/5 Palp	Liquor Volume	F.H.S.	F.M.	Return
										Sig.
										Sig.
										Sig.
										Sig.
										Sig.
										Sig.
										Sig.
										Sig.
										Sig.
										Sig.
										Sig.
										Sig.
										Sig.
										Sig.
										Sig.

Discussions checklist:
☐ Ultrasound
☐ Exercise
☐ Pelvic floor exercise
☐ Optimal fetal positioning
☐ Perineal massage
☐ Signs of labour
☐ When to come in
☐ Hospital access
Pain management
☐ Non-medicated
☐ Medicated
☐ 3rd stage
☐ Vitamin K
☐ Hep B vaccination
☐ Length of stay
☐ EMS
☐ Breastfeeding
Special requests for birth

Figure 41.1 Shared care card for use by pregnant women; increasingly such cards are being replaced by electronic medical records accessible to all practitioners providing antenatal care to a particular woman

What examination is made for Lucy?

Lucy's temperature, pulse rate and blood pressure are all normal and a short cardiotocograph (CTG) trace is also normal with a baseline of about 140 beats per minute (bpm) with a reactive pattern. While being admitted by midwife Nerissa, Lucy has found that the contractions have become stronger, longer and more regular. Nerissa reports that Lucy is, in fact, contracting every 3 minutes, the contractions lasting 60–90 seconds. Lucy is in moderate discomfort.

What further examination do you perform for Lucy?

After explaining what you are about to do and obtaining her permission, you inspect and palpate Lucy's abdomen. The fundal height measures 42 cm and you see that Dr Cameron has written 'big baby' on the shared care card. The presentation is cephalic, with four-fifths of the head above the pelvic brim and the baby's back far out on the mother's left side. You conclude that the baby is probably lying in a left occipito-posterior position. Since Lucy appears to be in established labour you perform a vaginal examination after scrubbing and donning sterile gloves. You find that the cervix is very soft, almost completely effaced, posterior and 4 cm dilated. The forewaters are still intact, although a little fluid is draining vaginally. Through the membranes you can feel that the baby's head is loosely applied to the cervix, at a level 3 cm above the ischial spines, and you can just make out the sagittal suture line running diagonally in relation to the maternal pelvis, although you are unable to palpate either fontanelle. Your findings confirm that Lucy is in established labour and support your impression of a left occipito-posterior position.

What information do you now give to this couple?

You explain your findings to Lucy and Alice, including the information that occipito-posterior positions are common with first babies and that sometimes this can make progress in labour slower as the baby's head has to rotate anteriorly through 135°. You encourage Lucy to mobilise as much as possible in labour and discuss pharmacological options for pain relief, which include gas and air (Entonox, a combination of nitrous oxide and oxygen), opiates and epidural. Lucy has been well informed about epidural analgesia during her antenatal classes but you give her an information leaflet to refresh her memory. For the moment Lucy feels able to cope with the contractions and she plans to get back under the shower to benefit from the warm water, which she found soothing. You reassure Lucy and Alice that all is well, explain that labour will be observed but that there is no indication for further assistance at this point and leave her in the care of Nerissa. A partogram (Fig. 41.2) is started to record and assess the progress of Lucy's labour, and warning and action lines are drawn.

```
..............................HOSPITAL          SURNAME_____U.R. No._____

                                                Given Names_____

            PARTOGRAM                           Sex_____        D.O.B._____

                                                    (Affix Patient Identification Label Here)
```

1 DATE:_____ TIME:_____

VAGINA

CERVIX: EFFACEMENT_____
      CONSISTENCY_____
      DILATATION_____
      APPLICATION OF P.P._____
      MEMBRANES_____
      LIQUOR AMNII_____

PRESENTING PART
    NATURE_____   A
    LEVEL _____
    SUTURES_____
    FONTANELLES_____ R   L
    POSITION_____
    CAPUT_____
    MOULDING_____   P

PELVIC ASSESSMENT

PROCEDURES & RECOMMENDATIONS

  SIGNATURE_____

2 DATE:_____ TIME:_____

VAGINA

CERVIX: EFFACEMENT_____
      CONSISTENCY_____
      DILATATION_____
      APPLICATION OF P.P._____
      MEMBRANES_____
      LIQUOR AMNII_____

PRESENTING PART
    NATURE_____   A
    LEVEL _____
    SUTURES_____
    FONTANELLES_____ R   L
    POSITION_____
    CAPUT_____
    MOULDING_____   P

PELVIC ASSESSMENT

PROCEDURES & RECOMMENDATIONS

  SIGNATURE_____

3 DATE:_____ TIME:_____

VAGINA

CERVIX: EFFACEMENT_____
      CONSISTENCY_____
      DILATATION_____
      APPLICATION OF P.P._____
      MEMBRANES_____
      LIQUOR AMNII_____

PRESENTING PART
    NATURE_____   A
    LEVEL _____
    SUTURES_____
    FONTANELLES_____ R   L
    POSITION_____
    CAPUT_____
    MOULDING_____   P

PELVIC ASSESSMENT

PROCEDURES & RECOMMENDATIONS

  SIGNATURE_____

4 DATE:_____ TIME:_____

VAGINA

CERVIX: EFFACEMENT_____
      CONSISTENCY_____
      DILATATION_____
      APPLICATION OF P.P._____
      MEMBRANES_____
      LIQUOR AMNII_____

PRESENTING PART
    NATURE_____   A
    LEVEL _____
    SUTURES_____
    FONTANELLES_____ R   L
    POSITION_____
    CAPUT_____
    MOULDING_____   P

PELVIC ASSESSMENT

PROCEDURES & RECOMMENDATIONS

  SIGNATURE_____

247

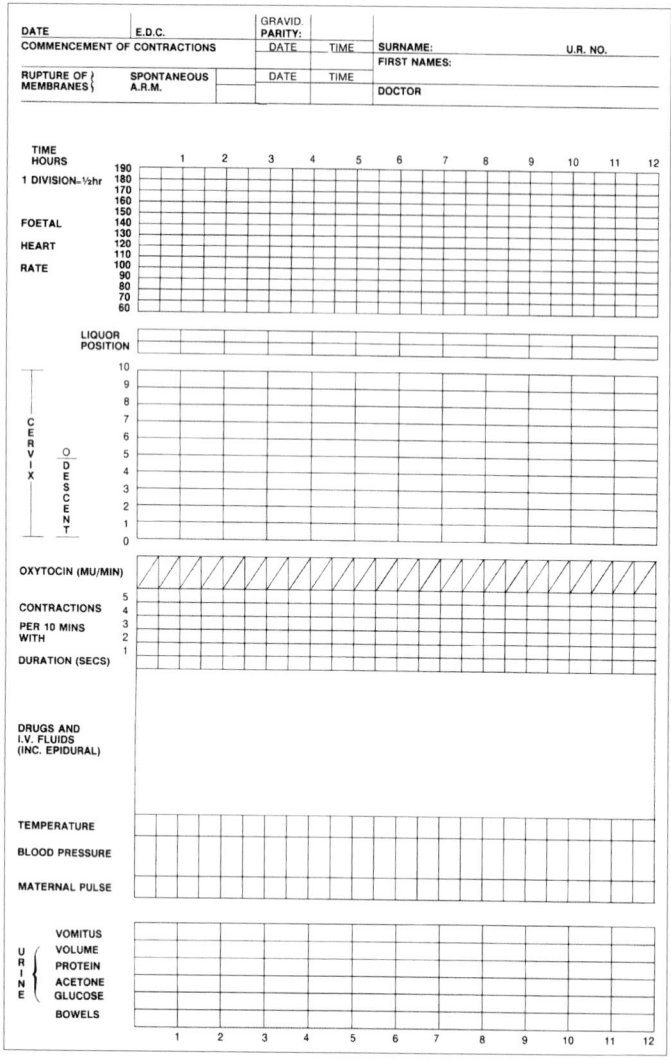

Figure 41.2 A partogram is commenced when a woman enters a birth suite and labour is established. This is defined as the cervix being at least 3 cm dilated with associated regular painful contractions of 3–4 in 10 minutes (protocols may vary between units). Warning and action lines are drawn 2 hours and 4 hours, respectively, to the right of the projected cervical dilatation rate of 1 cm per hour. Delay in labour is suggested when the warning line is crossed and diagnosed when the action line is reached. This is a trigger for appropriate management such as augmentation of labour

How is Lucy's labour monitored?

Four hours later you are requested to see Lucy again. Contractions have continued to be regular every 2–3 minutes and are moderate to strong. Initially, Lucy coped well without analgesia but 2 hours ago she asked for an injection of morphine. This was effective for some time but now Lucy is complaining of severe back pain and requesting an epidural.

How should you proceed?

You re-examine Lucy, but because of her pain it is difficult to ascertain on abdominal palpation whether there has been any abdominal descent of the head. However, on vaginal examination you find that the cervix has changed very little since the previous examination—effacement is complete but there has been no further dilatation or rotation or descent of the head. You explain that Lucy has, in fact, crossed the action line on the partogram and you must decide on a plan of action. After discussing the situation, Lucy and Alice request an epidural anaesthetic and you call the anaesthetist to arrange this for Lucy. She is happy for you to rupture the membranes (ARM): this may enable the head to be more closely applied to the cervix and bring about the production of increased amounts of natural prostaglandin. You use an amnihook to rupture the forewaters: the liquor is clear and the fetal heart following the procedure is within the normal range. At the time of ARM you also insert an indwelling urethral catheter. The anaesthetist explains the epidural procedure to Lucy, who signs a consent form, then inserts a combined spinal-epidural anaesthetic (Fig. 41.3) and Lucy gains effective pain relief from the block. You commence Lucy on continuous electronic fetal monitoring.

Continuous electronic fetal heart rate monitoring is not used routinely in normal labour in most centres: only 'at-risk' pregnancies are continuously monitored in labour. Continuous CTG monitoring during labour is associated with a reduction in neonatal seizures, but not with significant differences in the incidence of cerebral palsy or with decreased perinatal mortality rates. Furthermore, continuous monitoring has been shown to be associated with increased rates of interventions including caesarean sections and operative vaginal delivery. Fetal scalp blood sampling (for pH or lactate measurement) used in conjunction with continuous monitoring can reduce the incidence of false-positive diagnosis of fetal distress, and hence of unnecessary intervention. Fetal ECG wave form

continued

continued

analysis is used in some units for detection of fetal compromise during labour but requires an internal (scalp) electrode after membrane rupture. Indications for continuous CTG monitoring include preterm labour, prolonged labour, suspected fetal compromise (e.g. meconium-stained liquor, fetal heart rate abnormalities noted on auscultation), the use of oxytocin infusions, epidural analgesia, previous caesarean section, multiple pregnancy and any condition that led to antenatal CTG monitoring.

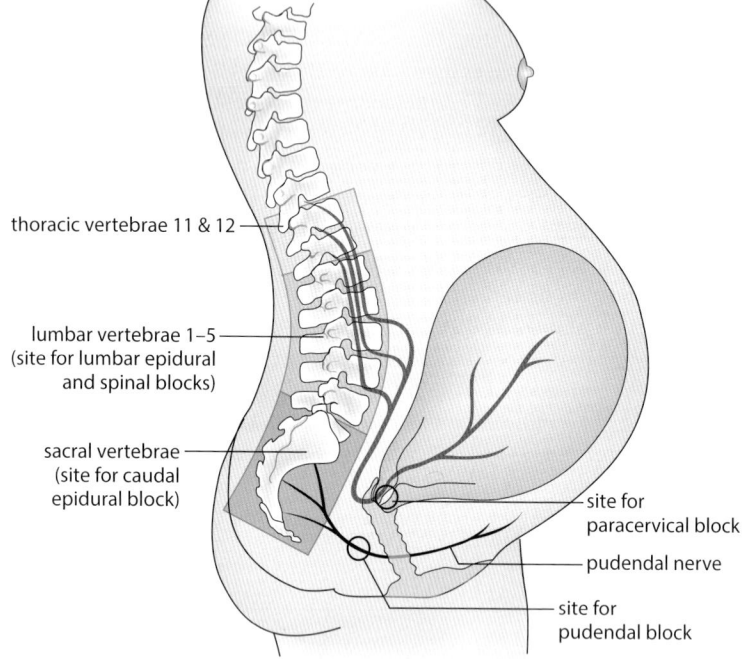

thoracic vertebrae 11 & 12

lumbar vertebrae 1–5
(site for lumbar epidural
and spinal blocks)

sacral vertebrae
(site for caudal
epidural block)

site for
paracervical block

pudendal nerve

site for
pudendal block

Figure 41.3 Sites for regional anaesthesia, including epidural sites

About four hours later, at 4 pm, you come to assess Lucy again. Although tired she is quite comfortable and has been able to sleep. Abdominal palpation shows only two-fifths of the head above the brim now; vaginal examination shows the cervix to be 6 cm dilated with a well-applied head in the left transverse position 1 cm above the spines. However, her contractions over the past hour have been weaker on palpation and much less frequent, about every 5–6 minutes. The CTG trace has been satisfactory throughout the previous 4 hours.

Risks of epidural analgesia

- Maternal motor blockade, which can limit or prevent movement
- Loss of bladder sensation, leading to need for urinary catheter
- Need for continuous electronic fetal monitoring
- Possible maternal hypotension
- Slight increase in the overall length of labour
- Slight increase in operative vaginal delivery rates
- Small risk of postnatal headache

What is your next step?

The partogram shows that, although Lucy has made some progress, she is still well to the right of the action line. You conclude that Lucy's labour needs augmenting. You explain this to her and arrange an oxytocin infusion; she has already had an intravenous cannula inserted when the epidural was performed.

 CLINICAL COMMENT

To institute an oxytocin infusion for induction or acceleration of labour, a main-line infusion of Hartmann's solution or normal saline is commenced, with a T-connector inserted between the intravenous (IV) cannula and the IV tubing; this infusion is run slowly to keep the line open. An oxytocin infusion, composed of 500 mL of Hartmann's solution containing oxytocin, is commenced via the T-connector. The infusion rate is increased half-hourly until the desired labour pattern is achieved. All birth suites will have individual protocols for management of such infusions.

What is your further management of Lucy?

At 6.30 pm you come to reassess Lucy. Another midwife, Brenda, is now caring for her and reports that contractions are regular and strong. You can see from the CTG trace (Fig. 41.4) that contractions are occurring every 2–3 minutes (4 contractions in 10 minutes) and that the fetal heart shows accelerations with contractions and good

Figure 41.4 Cardiotocograph trace showing normal baseline fetal heart rate (120–160 bpm), continuous variability in fetal heart rate >15 bpm, accelerations with contractions and no decelerations

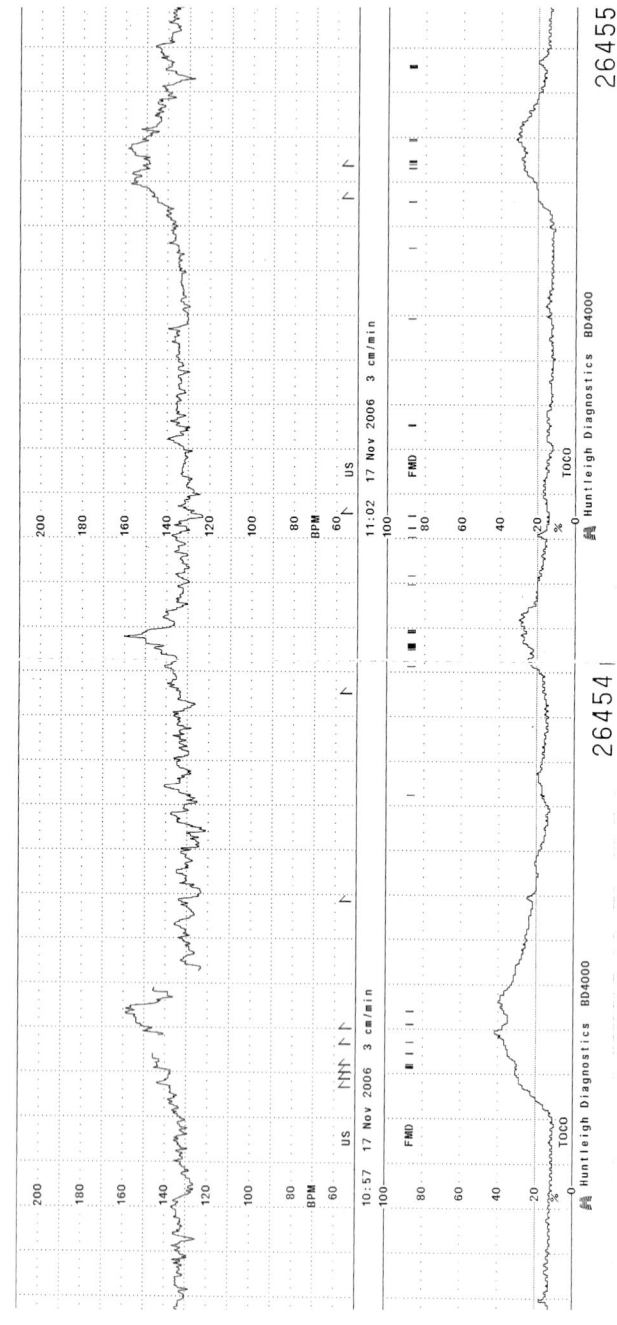

variability between contractions. On abdominal palpation no head can be felt; vaginal examination shows the cervix to be almost fully dilated with just an anterior lip palpable. The head has rotated to the left occipito-anterior position—you are easily able to feel the posterior fontanelle behind and to the left of the pubic symphysis—and has descended to the level of the iliac spines. You reassure Lucy that she has progressed well and that vaginal birth is likely. All maternal observations are satisfactory.

At 7.45 pm, while you are drinking a cup of coffee in the doctors' on-call room, you receive an urgent summons to the birth suite: 'Come immediately, the shoulders are stuck!'

What is your immediate action?

You proceed at full speed to the birth suite and find that Lucy has successfully delivered the baby's head '5 minutes ago,' Brenda says. The head is still in the occipito-anterior position but there has been no external rotation. As you enter the room Lucy is pushing hard but there is no onward progress or rotation of the head. The baby's face rests on the mother's perineum, the chin is not visible and the baby is a deep blue in colour. Brenda has already called for help from other midwives who now arrive. You call for the neonatal paediatric team, then explain to Lucy the urgency of the situation and assist Brenda to acutely flex Lucy's legs in McRoberts manoeuvre. You direct a second midwife to apply suprapubic pressure to help to disimpact the anterior shoulder from the symphysis pubis. The anaesthetist is informed in case you need to take Lucy to the operating theatre. With some difficulty you insert two fingers of your left hand into the vagina to protect the baby's face while you cut an episiotomy on the right side of Lucy's perineum. The purpose of an episiotomy is to allow space for internal manoeuvres if necessary. With the next contraction you carefully grasp the baby's head over the mandibles and malar bones and with maternal effort and suprapubic pressure, the anterior shoulder descends far enough for you to reach into the axilla and deliver the arm. Lifting the baby forward and up succeeds in dislodging the posterior shoulder and the remainder of the delivery takes place uneventfully. By this stage the paediatrician has arrived and takes over resuscitation of the baby, a boy. The Apgar score at 1 minute is 5 but by 5 minutes baby Jordan is crying lustily, the Apgar score is 10 and he can be handed to his parents.

CLINICAL COMMENT

Drill for the management of shoulder dystocia

- Call for help—more midwives, senior obstetrician, paediatrician, anaesthetist.
- Perform McRoberts manoeuvre—abduction and acute flexion of the mother's hips by assistants.
- Consider performing an episiotomy (access may be difficult, the cut may need to be midline).
- Have an assistant apply suprapubic pressure (downward and lateral pressure to push the fetal shoulder under the pubic bone) to aid delivery of the anterior arm.
- Displace the anterior shoulder from the symphysis pubis by pushing against the anterior shoulder from behind. If this fails, rotate the posterior aspect of the posterior shoulder forward (reverse wood screw).
- Deliver the posterior arm after lifting the baby's head anteriorly. In some cases, looping a catheter around the baby's axilla and pulling downwards and laterally can allow safe delivery of the posterior shoulder.
- If the above is not successful, roll the patient onto all fours and encourage pushing while awaiting further help.

It is important at all times to avoid fundal pressure and excessive traction or rotation attempts on the fetal head.

With some relief you deliver the placenta—placing your left hand on the abdomen you feel that separation has occurred and gentle traction on the cord is all that is required (Fig. 41.5).

However, almost immediately there is a gush of bright red blood, which quickly develops into a rapid haemorrhage estimated at 800 mL.

How do you manage this new development?

On palpation of the abdomen you find that the uterus is relaxed although one ampoule of oxytocin/ergometrine has been given intramuscularly (IM) once the baby was born, as is normal practice in your unit. You rub up a contraction through the abdominal wall, check that Lucy's indwelling urinary catheter is draining freely and order 40 units of oxytocin to be placed in a litre of Hartmann's solution, to be run in over 4 hours to help keep the uterus well contracted. Giving an intravenous bolus of 1 gram of tranexamic acid is safe and useful, and you order this. You collect a blood

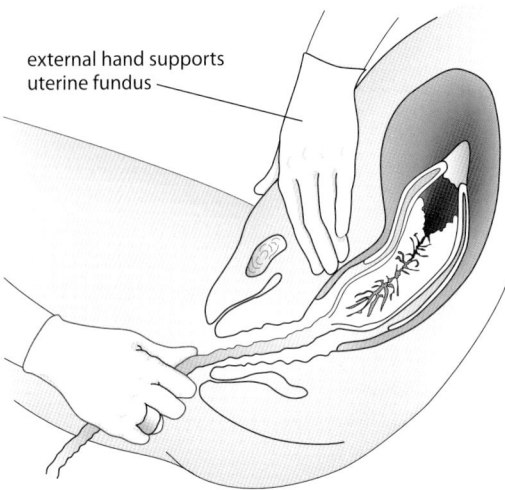

external hand supports
uterine fundus

Figure 41.5 Delivery of the placenta using controlled cord traction following signs of placental separation

sample from Lucy for an urgent haemoglobin level and for cross-match of 2 units of packed red blood cells.

Bleeding diminishes in amount but is still excessive. Analgesia from the epidural still seems adequate but postpartum haemorrhage is unpredictable, so you transfer Lucy to the operating theatre, where you proceed to a rapid inspection of the lower genital tract, looking for other sources of blood loss. The epidural anaesthetic is useful and you are able to explain your findings and actions to Lucy as you go. You find that there is bleeding from several sites in your episiotomy, but that this has not extended into the anorectal region, and that there is also a large anterior laceration around the clitoris and urethral meatus which, although superficial, is contributing significantly to the blood loss. You inspect the upper vagina and cervix, applying sponge forceps to the anterior and posterior cervical lips—there are no other lacerations, blood loss through the cervical os has slowed to an acceptable level and the uterus continues to be well contracted. You explore the uterine cavity to exclude retained placental tissue and, fortunately, find none.

'The empty, contracted, uninjured uterus does not bleed in the presence of a normal coagulation mechanism' is an aphorism that should be remembered by everyone practising obstetrics; this can be further reduced to 'tone, tissue, trauma, thrombin' to remember the causes of PPH.

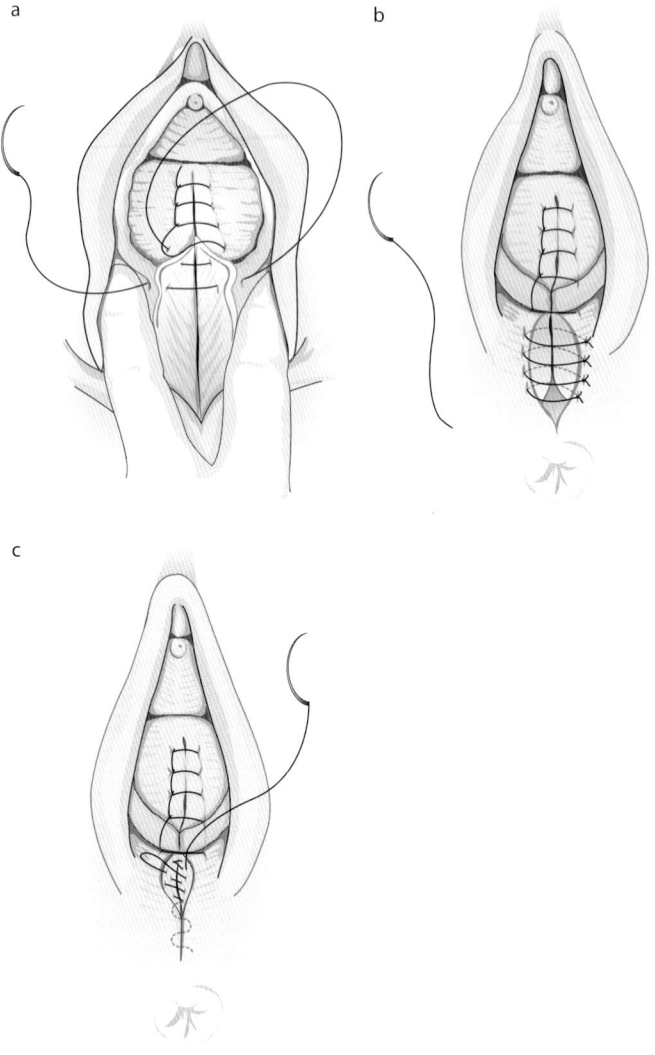

Figure 41.6 Repair of episiotomy or second-degree perineal tear:
(**a**) continuous suture of the vaginal mucosa (**b**) repair of perineal muscles
(**c**) continuous subcuticular suture closing the perineal skin

You repair the lacerations using 2/0 polyglactin and the episiotomy in
anatomical layers (Fig. 41.6), again with 2/0 polyglactin. Then, having
made sure that haemostasis has been achieved, you perform a rectal

examination to confirm that no tear or suture extends into the rectal mucosa. You arrange with the midwifery staff to perform regular checks of the uterine fundus and of blood loss and to call you if there are further concerns, and you order a full blood count for Lucy, to be performed the following morning.

Unanticipated complications in labour are frightening and require detailed debriefing, so you spend time speaking with Lucy and Alice after the birth and offer to see them as often as needed to allow them to understand events and ask questions. A detailed discharge handover to Lucy's family doctor is critical after adverse events like this.

Risks for postpartum haemorrhage

Atonic uterus
- grand multiparity
- multiple pregnancy (overdistended uterus)
- polyhydramnios (overdistended uterus)
- prolonged labour
- prior antepartum haemorrhage (e.g. placenta praevia or abruption)

Retained placenta or membranes (uterus not empty)

Genital tract trauma
- vaginal tear
- cervical tear
- ruptured uterus
- inversion of the uterus

Coagulation defects including disseminated intravascular coagulation

---

 CLINICAL COMMENT

Drill for management of postpartum haemorrhage

- Call for help.
- Rub the uterine fundus to stimulate a contraction.
- Insert a large-bore (14 or 16G) IV cannula and run Hartmann's solution or normal saline stat.

continued

continued

- Take blood for FBC and cross-match of 2 units of packed cells.
- Check the coagulation profile.
- If the placenta is still in situ, it must be removed—manually, if necessary (under anaesthesia).
- Give a further dose of ergometrine 0.25 mg IV and 0.25 mg IM (do not give more than 1 mg ergometrine in total in a 24-hour period). Misoprostol 800 µg may be given orally, sublingually or per rectum.
- Insert a urinary catheter.
- Insert 40 units of oxytocin in 1 L of normal saline and infuse at a 4-hourly rate. Administer 1 gram tranexamic acid.
- If bleeding continues at this point, you will need to conduct examination under anaesthesia. Contact theatre and anaesthetic staff. Warn the patient about the risk of laparotomy and possible hysterectomy.
- Examine the uterus under anaesthesia to exclude retained placenta or membranes. A balloon tamponade (Bakri balloon) may be useful.
- Examine the cervix for bleeding lacerations with two sponge-holding forceps.
- Examine the vagina for lacerations.
- In some cases, the use of prostaglandin medications such as carboprost will be indicated.
- If bleeding is not controlled, the patient requires laparotomy. Cross-match more packed cells, order platelets and fresh frozen plasma and summon specialist help. At laparotomy, repair of lacerations, hysterectomy, iliac artery ligation and B-Lynch suture compression, thereby facilitating contraction of the uterus, are all possible options for controlling haemorrhage but are specialist procedures.

CLINICAL PEARLS

- When a large baby is predicted antenatally, shoulder dystocia should always be kept in mind. Everyone practising obstetrics should know the drill for shoulder dystocia thoroughly.
- A prolonged first stage of labour may herald difficulties with the second stage, requiring intervention. This may then predispose to PPH, from either uterine atony or genital tract trauma.

References and further reading

Evensen A, Anderson JM, Fontaine P. Postpartum hemorrhage: prevention and treatment. *Am Fam Physician*. 2017;95(7):442–9.

Hill MG, Cohen WR. Shoulder dystocia: prediction and management. *Womens Health (Lond)*. 2016;12(2):251–61.

Royal Australian and New Zealand College of Obstetricians and Gynaecologists. Intrapartum fetal surveillance. Clinical guideline—fourth edition 2019. Melbourne: RANZCOG; 2019. www.ranzcog.edu.au

Case 42
Tegan develops an obstetric emergency. . .

On a Sunday morning in the birth suite, you are asked to see a 32-year-old woman, Tegan, who is 36 weeks pregnant with her third child. Tegan has presented because she has had some irregular contractions overnight and is uncertain whether her waters have broken—she had a small gush of fluid vaginally earlier that morning. Her pregnancy to date has been unremarkable and the baby is moving normally, but the midwife in attendance is concerned that the presentation is a breech.

How do you proceed with this consultation?

You review Tegan's antenatal notes and take a short but relevant history. In both previous pregnancies the babies were breech presentations up to 36–37 weeks but turned spontaneously to cephalic presentation. During this pregnancy the baby has been at times recorded as breech and at other times as cephalic. Tegan's blood pressure and other observations, including measurement of uterine fundus height, have been normal throughout the pregnancy. Results of all routine investigations have been normal apart from the fact that an MSU at booking showed a growth of group B streptococcus (GBS). Tegan's blood group is O Rhesus-negative and she was given anti-D 625 units at 28 and 34 weeks of pregnancy.

Tegan reports only slight vaginal loss since coming into the hospital and her contractions have been infrequent (<1 in 10 minutes) and mild.

What examination do you conduct for Tegan?

All standard observations are normal. A short CTG trace was performed by the midwife before your arrival—it was normal and reassuring. After discussing this with Tegan, you proceed to abdominal examination. Inspection suggests a longitudinal lie, which is confirmed by palpation. You are confident that the fetal head can be felt in the upper right quadrant of the abdomen and that the presentation therefore is breech. The fetal buttocks can be palpated just above the pelvic brim. Bedside ultrasound scanning confirms your diagnosis of breech presentation.

Should you perform a vaginal examination?

You must perform a vaginal speculum examination to try to ascertain whether the membranes have ruptured, as this will determine whether your management is expectant or active. You perform the speculum examination under strict aseptic conditions with scrubbing and sterile gloving, and preparation of the perineum with an antiseptic wash. Your examination shows that the cervix appears partly effaced but closed. There is no pool of liquor visible in the posterior fornix after Tegan has been lying for some time on her back and no appearance of liquor via the cervix when you ask her to cough. You collect sterile swabs from the cervix for microscopy and culture.

What is your recommendation to Tegan?

You explain that it does not seem that Tegan has ruptured the membranes nor is she in labour, but you wish to keep her for observation in case labour is, in fact, imminent. You explain to her the risks of breech presentation and give her some written information about this. She is already familiar with much of this from her previous pregnancies. You explain that she will be given penicillin prophylaxis to cover her birth because of the finding of GBS earlier in the pregnancy. You arrange to transfer her to the antenatal ward for observation for some hours. She asks if her partner, Yahya, can go home to arrange care for her other children and you assure them both that nothing is likely to happen in the next couple of hours. Yahya can be contacted if the need arises. Tegan is duly transferred to the ward.

One hour later you are summoned urgently to the antenatal ward. Tegan has called the midwife because she has had a large gush of fluid vaginally and felt 'something coming down'. Immediate inspection by the midwife has shown a pulsating umbilical cord protruding from the vagina.

What do you do?

This is an acute obstetric emergency. Fetal death or severe cerebral injury may result from compression of the cord between the presenting fetal part and the mother's pelvis or cervix. You urgently summon help from other midwifery staff, senior obstetric and anaesthetic personnel, and alert the paediatric team. You insert your gloved hand into the vagina to replace the cord and hold up the presenting part, the breech, as high as possible. You are assisted in this by midwifery staff, who turn Tegan into the knee–chest position. During these manoeuvres you explain to Tegan what is happening, assure her that you can feel the baby's heart beating through the cord pulsations and that the heart rate is normal. You further rapidly explain that as she is not in labour she will need an immediate caesarean section to deliver her baby and that this will need to be under general anaesthesia. With some difficulty you get a consent form signed—there is not time to give an adequate outline of the risks of the procedure.

At this point both your consultant and Tegan's family arrive. The consultant quickly explains the position to Yahya. By now, the anaesthetist has also arrived and asked for Tegan to be moved to the operating theatre. You accompany Tegan to theatre on the trolley with a hand still keeping the breech up away from the cord—this is a stressful, uncomfortable and exhausting thing to do but is very important. You remain in this position until general anaesthesia has been induced and your consultant has performed a rapid abdominal and uterine incision and delivered a live female baby. Antibiotics are given routinely for caesarean section in your hospital in the form of cefazolin 2 g IV, but in view of the high risk of infection in this case you add metronidazole 2 g.

The baby is in good condition and is handed to neonatal paediatric staff. The information is given to the paediatric staff that Tegan's earlier MSU showed GBS and that there was not time to administer penicillin intrapartum. It is decided that swabs will be taken from the baby, who will also be observed in the SCBU. The operation proceeds uneventfully thereafter; however, you note that due to the urgent nature of the proceedings the use of calf compressors, normally routine for caesarean surgery, has been omitted. You include this in your writing up of the case and recommend early mobilisation and adequate fluid intake postpartum.

GBS infection is a significant cause of neonatal mortality and morbidity. Controversy, as yet unresolved by clinical trials, surrounds the issues of whether, when and how to screen and treat the whole pregnant population for the infection. Antepartum maternal colonisation with GBS is a recognised risk factor but antepartum antibiotics do not eliminate this risk. Rapid intrapartum diagnosis of GBS is unreliable; however, intrapartum antibiotics significantly reduce the risk of vertical transmission.

Management of GBS carriers in pregnancy

- All women known to be carriers of GBS or to have had a child affected by early-onset GBS disease should be treated with IV penicillin during labour, until delivery.
- In cases of penicillin allergy, clindamycin or erythromycin may be given.
- Antibiotics should also be offered in labour to women with prolonged rupture of the membranes (greater than 18 hours) or preterm labour at less than 35 weeks, and where the maternal temperature is 38°C or more.

What is your postoperative management of this case?

Later that day you visit Tegan. She is awake but she and her partner are still obviously quite shocked by the suddenness of the day's events. Yahya is concerned that he was not permitted to be present at the birth and that he was not contacted by the hospital when Tegan's membranes ruptured. Baby Plum is in the SCBU. Her blood has been tested and she has been found to be Rhesus positive, so anti-D 625 units have been administered to Tegan.

How do you deal with this couple's concerns?

You take some time to 'debrief' Tegan and Yahya. You explain that cord prolapse is a recognised but unusual event occurring in about 1 in 800 births. There was no evidence of ruptured membranes or fetal distress when Tegan was examined in the birth suite, but with the history she gave and with a breech presentation, observation close to specialist care was appropriate. You go over the events of the morning, explaining why it was necessary to perform an urgent caesarean section under general anaesthesia. Had the cord prolapse occurred at full dilatation with a cephalic presentation, operative vaginal delivery might have been possible, but even in that situation caesarean section under general anaesthesia may have been the safest and quickest option. You further explain that because Plum was born at 36 weeks' gestation she is experiencing some mild respiratory distress but that this is responding to simple measures in the SCBU and that you expect that the baby will be with her mother the following morning. You emphasise the urgency of the events to the couple and the fact that they have a live and healthy baby.

After any unexpected or adverse event it is good practice to spend time 'debriefing' patients and their families. Not only does this provide relevant information to those concerned, it can also be beneficial to the doctor, particularly when there has been a neonatal or maternal death or serious morbidity. Good communication at the time of or soon after an event can help avoid subsequent litigation.

What further follow-up do you expect for Tegan?

Five days later you see Tegan again on your postnatal round. She appears well and happy and baby Plum is now with her. Breastfeeding is established and it is expected that mother and baby will go home the following day. The abdominal wound is healing well and the subcuticular suture has been removed. However, Tegan is slightly febrile with a temperature of 37.8°C. Her temperature prior to this has been normal.

Is this significant?

You should take a short but relevant history and conduct an examination to ensure that there is no serious incipient cause for this temperature rise. There is no headache, cough or chest pain. On auscultation the chest is clear. There is no pain in the breasts, which are soft with no inflamed areas. There are no urinary or bowel symptoms. Tegan reports some abdominal tenderness around the wound site only and palpation shows an involuting uterus, which is only slightly tender, compatible with her recent surgery. There is no tenderness over the renal angles.

You then examine Tegan's legs. She states that there is some slight tenderness in her left calf but she did not think that this was important. On examination you find the calf is swollen and warm, with tenderness on deep palpation.

Postoperative pyrexia must always be taken seriously and a cause searched for. Where a laparotomy has been performed under general anaesthesia there is the possibility of respiratory or intra-abdominal complications, as well as urinary tract infection and thromboembolism, all directly related to the surgery. The possibility of incidental infection should also not be overlooked.

What are your concerns from this examination?

Symptoms and signs suggest the possibility of deep venous thrombosis (DVT) in the calf, possibly extending above the knee. If this is the case there is a risk of pulmonary embolism.

What is your immediate management?

You arrange a compression ultrasound for Tegan, which confirms DVT confined to the left calf.

 CLINICAL COMMENT

> Acute venous thromboembolism (VTE) is a major potential cause of maternal mortality. The treatment of VTE in pregnancy has evolved rapidly over the past 15 years, with the introduction of new antithrombotic agents and growing experience and evidence for their use in pregnancy. This process is ongoing and it is desirable to involve the haematologist in the care of pregnant or recently pregnant women with VTE. In pregnancy, 85% of DVTs are left-sided compared to 55% in the non-pregnant.

What investigations should be performed?

Once the therapeutic anticoagulation treatment has ceased, a full thrombophilia screen should be performed for Tegan—testing for activated protein C resistance (APCR)/factor V (Leiden) gene mutation (FVL), protein C, protein S, antithrombin-3, elevated fasting homocysteine level, elevated factor VIII level, methyltetrahydrofolate reductase (MTHFR), factor II mutation, lupus anticoagulant and increased anticardiolipin antibodies. While most of these tests can be done before Tegan is commenced on anticoagulants, protein S and factor VIII cannot be measured in the acute phase of VTE and later repeat screening (after about 12 weeks) should be arranged, usually in conjunction with the haematologist.

What is your further management?

In consultation with the haematologist, anticoagulation is commenced, using the low-molecular-weight heparin (LMWH), enoxaparin, subcutaneously twice daily. Postpartum, either heparin or warfarin may be used for ongoing anticoagulation, which should continue for 12 weeks.

CLINICAL COMMENT

Anticoagulants during pregnancy

Warfarin is contraindicated during pregnancy as it is teratogenic and may cause fetal haemorrhage, especially in the third trimester. It may be safely used during breastfeeding, although a small amount is secreted in the milk. Heparin, either unfractionated (UFH) or LMWH, does not cross the placenta so can be safely used in pregnancy. In the non-pregnant state, LMWH is equally effective and safer than UFH in the treatment of VTE. These observations have not yet been fully validated in pregnancy. The major factors in favour of LMWH are:

- significantly decreased incidence of heparin-induced thrombocytopenia
- decreased incidence of osteoporosis
- decreased incidence of bleeding
- significantly higher rate of initial effective anticoagulation
- no requirement for routine monitoring.

'How have I developed DVT?' asks Tegan.

You explain to Tegan that the urgency of the caesarean led to the calf compressors not being used, and that this may have contributed to the development of DVT, although you also explain that DVT is a recognised complication of pregnancy and of abdominal surgery. Tegan tells you that she now understands what happened and she is very grateful that Plum is normal and healthy. She also tells you that she and her partner are sure they want no further children and that Yahya is arranging to have a vasectomy. You agree that this is a sensible course of action and means that she does not need to be concerned about thromboprophylaxis in future pregnancies or about whether she has contraindications to the COCP.

CLINICAL PEARLS

Whenever an unexpected event or adverse outcome occurs in practice, it is wise to have as full and frank a discussion as possible with all parties concerned soon after the events. This ensures that communication of all important facts is achieved and lessens the chances of subsequent litigation.

References and further reading

Devis P, Knuttinen MG. Deep venous thrombosis in pregnancy: incidence, pathogenesis and endovascular management. *Cardiovasc Diagn Ther.* 2017;7(Suppl 3):S309–S319.

Sayed Ahmed WA, Hamdy MA. Optimal management of umbilical cord prolapse. *Int J Womens Health.* 2018;10:459–65.

Case 43
Kelly is referred to the emergency department with heavy postpartum bleeding...

Kelly is a 32-year-old woman who has been referred by her GP, Dr Daniels, to the emergency department of your hospital with a history of increasing vaginal (PV) bleeding 10 days after the birth of her first baby. Her general practitioner also states in her referral letter that Kelly has been breastfeeding her baby with no problems but that she was noted to have mild pyrexia.

You see Kelly in the emergency department. What information would you like to have from her?

You take a detailed history and also go through her maternity notes. Her antenatal course was uncomplicated. You note that her labour was induced at 39 weeks' gestation, 24 hours after spontaneous rupture of membranes. A high vaginal swab taken at the time had shown no growth subsequently. Her labour progressed well but she had an outlet forceps delivery for maternal exhaustion in the second stage. She had an episiotomy which was repaired and her third stage was noted to be complete, with the notes showing that the placenta was complete. She was treated with oral antibiotics after an instrumental delivery as is the recommendation.

Kelly was discharged home 2 days later with her baby and had been breastfeeding. She has not commenced any contraceptive yet. She noted that her lochia had become heavier after a week and had also become foul smelling. She then started to feel lower abdominal crampy pain and her bleeding became heavier. She noted a slight temperature and made an urgent appointment to see her GP. Dr Daniels examined her and said that she might have an infection and referred her to the emergency department. You also establish that she has no other symptoms, especially breast, respiratory, urinary or bowel symptoms. She also says that her bleeding has been gradually heavy with the passage of clots today. She has no allergies and is currently not on any medication.

How would you assess her?

You check her vital signs to ensure that she is stable. Her blood pressure is 120/80 mmHg and her pulse rate 96 bpm. She is not short of breath but her temperature is 38.1°C. Examination of her breasts shows them to be soft and non-tender; lactation is well established. Her lungs are clear and she has no evidence of mastitis. Examination of her abdomen shows no distension. Her uterus is palpable at around the 12-week size and is tender. No other mass is palpable and her abdomen is not guarded. Her calves are soft and non-tender, with no oedema suggestive of thrombosis.

With permission, you carry out a vaginal examination. You note that the episiotomy site is well healed and there is no haematoma in the vagina or perineum. A speculum examination is performed and you take a high vaginal swab for microbiology. Small clots are seen in the vagina and the cervix is visualised after removing the clots. The cervical os is noted to be closed but she is still noted to be bleeding from the uterine cavity. You carry out a bimanual examination. The cervix is closed and the uterus is enlarged to around 12 weeks' size and is tender. No adnexal mass is palpable.

You set up an IV line and take blood for FBC, C-reactive protein (CRP), urea and electrolytes, coagulation screen, group and save and blood culture. You send off a midstream urine sample and start maintenance IV fluids. You also arrange for IV antibiotics to be commenced.

As she is still bleeding, you arrange to give her 1 g of oral tranexamic acid IV and 3 misoprostol tablets (600 μg) with a sip of water.

You arrange for admission to the ward with her baby and also an urgent USS. The findings of the ultrasound suggest the possibility of retained products of conception. She is kept fasted and is advised that she is able to continue to breastfeed. The next morning, she undergoes a suction curettage, during which a moderate amount of products of conception is removed and sent for histology.

Kelly makes a satisfactory recovery and is discharged home the following day after she is noted to be afebrile. She is advised to complete her course of antibiotics and to see her general practitioner for follow-up in a week.

CLINICAL COMMENT

- The incidence of secondary PPH in developed countries is between 0.5% and 2%.
- It is defined as abnormal or excessive bleeding from the genital tract between 24 hours and 12 weeks after giving birth.

continued

269

continued

The amount of blood loss is not defined and can vary from inconvenient to fatal.

- It is important to take a good contraceptive history as some women may have had an injectable progestogen (depot medroxyprogesterone acetate) or etonogestrel implant inserted immediately postpartum, leading to irregular or troublesome bleeding.

Causes of PPH

- Subinvolution of the uterus—retained placental tissue and/or endometritis, fibroid uterus
- Lower genital tract lacerations/haematoma
- Surgical injury, dehiscence of a caesarean section scar
- Lower genital tract infections, e.g. endometritis, myometritis, parametritis
- Placental abnormality—placenta accreta, percreta, increta
- Coagulopathies, bleeding disorders and use of anticoagulants
- Neoplasms (rare)—choriocarcinoma, cervical neoplasm

Investigation of PPH (Fig. 43.1)

- USS should be considered if there are concerns about retained placental tissue. It is useful for identifying clots or other debris in the uterine cavity and subinvolution. Overdiagnosis of retained placental tissue may lead to unnecessary surgical intervention and potential complications. However, it has a good negative predictive value and is helpful in excluding a diagnosis of retained placental tissue.
- If a clot or debris greater than 2 cm is demonstrated in the cavity, administration of uterotonics may reduce the rate of surgical intervention.
- Surgical measures should be undertaken if there is excessive or continuous bleeding, irrespective of the ultrasound findings.

Conservative management of PPH

- This approach may be adopted if only endometritis is suspected and all the other causes have been excluded.
- Antibiotics form the mainstay of treatment.

Surgical management of PPH

- As secondary PPH is usually associated with endometritis, it is imperative that any surgical intervention is carried out with adequate antibiotic cover. Unless the woman is bleeding torrentially, it is recommended that antibiotics are commenced at least 6–12 hours before surgery.

- Surgical management may include any of the following:
  - Examination under anaesthesia, dilatation and evacuation of products of conception and gentle suction curettage. Send tissue for histology and avoid vigorous curettage to prevent Asherman syndrome (intrauterine adhesions).

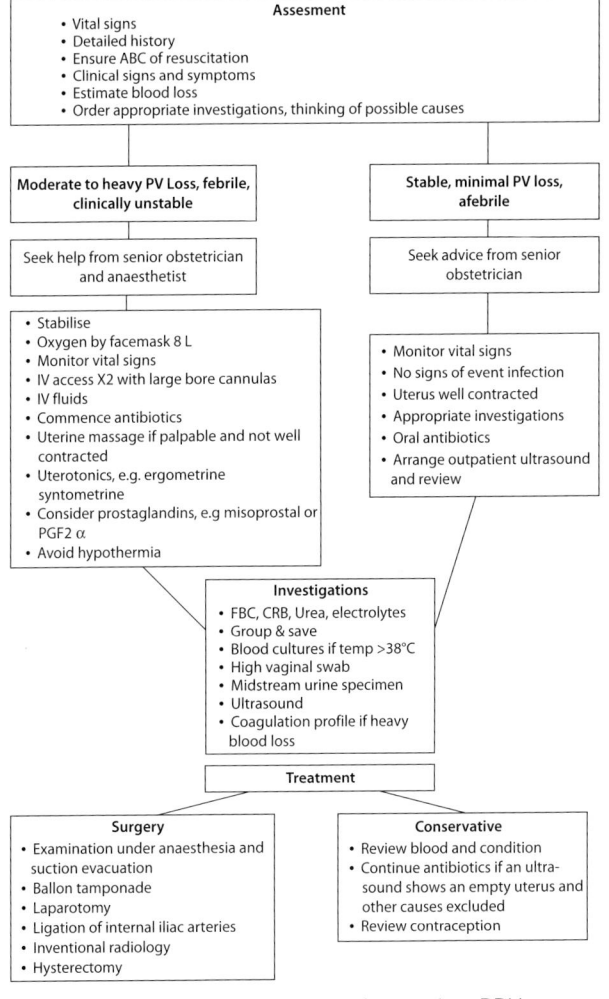

Figure 43.1 Pathway for the management of secondary PPH

continued

continued

- Insertion of an intrauterine tamponade balloon
- Laparotomy and ligation of internal iliac arteries if interventional radiology is not readily available
- Selective arterial embolisation
- Hysterectomy.

Antibiotic therapy

- Secondary PPH is often associated with endometritis. Women with suspected retained products require antibiotic cover before surgical intervention.
- Give IV antibiotics if the woman is febrile and oral antibiotics if afebrile but endometritis is suspected.
- A combination of ampicillin and metronidazole is appropriate if given an IV. Lincomycin or clindamycin may be used if the woman is allergic to penicillin.
- Consider the addition of gentamicin in severe sepsis.
- If an oral antibiotic is to be used, amoxycillin/potassium clavulanate is recommended.

CLINICAL PEARLS

- Secondary PPH can be associated with significant maternal morbidity and needs to be assessed carefully.
- A good history, including contraceptive history, will help to identify the possible cause.
- It is commonly associated with endometritis, so antibiotic treatment is imperative before any surgical intervention.
- Suction curettage should be performed by an experienced operator as there is a potential for complications such as uterine perforation or the development of Asherman syndrome.

References and further reading

Evensen A, Anderson JM, Fontaine P. Postpartum hemorrhage: prevention and treatment. *Am Fam Physician*. 2017;95(7):442–9.

Sebghati M, Chandraharan E. An update on the risk factors for and management of obstetric haemorrhage. *Womens Health* (Lond). 2017;13(2):34–40.

Case 44
Ivana presents for high-risk pregnancy care. . .

Ivana is a 32-year-old woman who has been referred for care in her second pregnancy. Ivana lives in a small town about 100 kilometres from the regional hospital in which you are working. Her GP has referred her for hospital antenatal and intrapartum care as her pre-pregnancy BMI was 42kg/m2, placing her in the WHO category of super-obesity. The GP's letter also notes that two years ago Ivana had an emergency caesarean delivery of her first child, a boy, under general anaesthesia. The caesarean was done following obstruction in the second stage of labour and Ivana was advised postnatally that future births should be by elective caesarean as there was an extended uterine tear sustained during delivery. At the time of that birth her BMI was recorded as 35 kg/m^2, indicating that Ivana has had considerable difficulty in controlling her weight since that birth.

Ivana is now 14 weeks pregnant. She is feeling well, and after some nausea in early pregnancy things now have settled. Ivana states that she has had an early transvaginal ultrasound scan to confirm her dates and she has also had a NIPT that puts her at low risk of a fetal anomaly.

 CLINICAL COMMENT

WHO uses the body mass index (BMI) to define categories of size in adults: underweight, normal, overweight, obese (subdivided into class I and II) and super-obese (class III). Pre-pregnancy BMI and changes occurring during pregnancy both contribute to BMI at delivery.

Women in the super-obese category face increased risks in pregnancy and during delivery, including gestational diabetes mellitus (GDM), pre-eclampsia, venous thromboembolism, prolonged labour, postpartum haemorrhage and maternal death. Should they require neuraxial or general anaesthesia during the course of labour and birth, there is a much greater chance that these techniques will not work or will be associated with complications. Their babies are more likely to

continued

continued

be macrosomic, and there is an increased risk of shoulder dystocia with a vaginal birth. There is a higher incidence of caesarean section—both emergency and elective—in this group of women.

Body mass index (BMI) is defined as a person's weight in kilograms divided by the square of the person's height in metres (kg/m^2).

Table 44.1 Nutritional status associated with BMI

BMI	Nutritional status
<18.5	Underweight
18.5–24.9	Normal weight
25.0–29.9	Pre-obesity (overweight)
30.0–34.9	Obesity class I
35.0–39.9	Obesity class II
>40.0	Obesity class III (super-obesity)

What are the important points of your consultation with Ivana?

- It is important for all staff caring for women of high BMI not to be judgemental in their manner; this has been demonstrated to result in women not attending appointments. This is particularly the case when giving information about diet and exercise, and recommending referral to a dietitian; it is desirable that weight gain during the pregnancy is limited to 5–9 kg. Emphasise to Ivana that such suggestions are intended to benefit her own health in pregnancy and that of her baby.
- There is evidence from systematic reviews that obesity in pregnancy is associated with an increase in the risk of depression in pregnancy and the postpartum period, so screening for perinatal mood disorders should be offered.
- Ivana should have an early glucose tolerance test (GTT) because of the increased risk for her of GDM, even though she did not develop this in her first pregnancy. A normal result with the early GTT does not obviate the need for a subsequent GTT at the beginning of the third trimester. A probable date for elective repeat caesarean section can be given at this visit. This will be a potentially difficult operation due to the combination of Ivana's weight and the complications of the previous caesarean section (CS); it is desirable for her own

wellbeing but also for that of the hospital staff that the procedure be elective and not emergency. An elective CS also means that regional anaesthesia can be offered. Early and positive engagement with the obstetric anaesthetic team is an important aspect of care.

- As Ivana is at significant risk of venous thromboembolism, postpartum thromboprophylaxis should be offered. In certain circumstances where there are additional risk factors, e.g. heavy smoking or decreased mobility, antenatal thromboprophylaxis should be considered.

Ivana's BP is within normal limits. On examination she looks generally well although clearly overweight. Abdominal examination shows a large panniculus of adipose tissue lying over her lower abdomen. On retracting this you find a well healed lower abdominal transverse scar. The uterus is not palpable owing to the thickness of the abdominal wall. The fetal heart rate with the Doppler is 140 bpm.

Ivana agrees to a GTT in the following two weeks, a morphology USS at 18 weeks and accepts a referral to the hospital dietitian. You calculate a date when she will be at 39 weeks' gestation as a potential date for her caesarean section.

You explain to Ivana that, although her home is a considerable distance from the hospital, to achieve the best outcome she will need close monitoring so will need to attend regular hospital clinic visits. Because of the potential for other risks, good and timely communication with her GP is vital, particularly as her GP has a key role in providing ongoing care both in the postnatal period and for her long-term health. Ivana replies that she understands this, and tells you that at around 36 weeks she will move into town to be close to the hospital as the delivery date approaches.

Obesity is now the most common medical problem in pregnancy; around 60% of Australian women are overweight or obese at the commencement of pregnancy. It is now usual for regional health services to have dedicated hospitals for the care of women above certain levels of BMI, particularly the 7% of women who have a BMI over 40. High BMI is a risk factor for operative vaginal delivery and caesarean section. To provide adequate care during CS for women of high BMI, specially designed trolleys, theatre table attachments and surgical instruments are required, as well as mechanisms to lift the panniculus often covering the site of CS incision out of the surgical field. Extra assistants may be required for the surgery; more senior staff—medical, midwifery and nursing—with

continued

continued

experience of this potentially complex surgery should be present, and wherever possible, surgery should be elective. Theatre managers need to allocate increased theatre time to the management of these cases, and other health professional staff, especially physiotherapists, should be readily available for postnatal care.

CLINICAL PEARL

While dietary and physical activity lifestyle interventions may be offered to pregnant women with obesity, there is limited evidence to support their effectiveness in preventing adverse maternal and perinatal outcomes.

References and further reading

Dennis A, Lamb K, Story D, et al. Associations between maternal size and health outcomes for women undergoing caesarean section: a multicentre prospective observational study (the MUM SIZE study). *BMJ Open* 2017;7(6):e15630.

Ma R, Schmidt M, Tam W, et al. Clinical management of pregnancy in the obese mother before conception, during pregnancy and postpartum. *Lancet Diabetes Endocrinol.* 2016;4(12):1037–49.

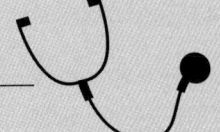

Part 4
Clinical cases
in gynaecology

Case 45
Jenny would like a baby…

Jenny and Arnel are a young couple who have been together for about 2 years. They have been trying to start a family for almost a year without success, and have come to you for advice. Jenny has been your patient for several years, and is a 30-year-old woman who works as a graphic designer. Her periods are regular, making it easy to time intercourse to the midcycle. Her cervical screening test is up to date and normal, and she doesn't have any past gynaecological problems of note. Arnel is a 31-year-old man who is an army officer, a major in the artillery corps. Although he has spent some time stationed overseas, he has been home since their marriage. He is a healthy man whose family are from the Philippines, and all were apparently fertile. There is the possibility that Arnel will be posted overseas before much longer, and both he and Jenny are anxious to try for a family before he has to go away.

How do you approach a problem like this?

You are aware that as many as one couple in six may face a delay in the woman becoming pregnant, and that this can provoke anxiety in the couple, making things worse. You find out that Jenny has been using ovulation detection sticks that detect the midcycle surge of luteinising hormone (LH) that shows her when she is at her most fertile. However, since her cycle is very regular, these have not really provided them with any additional information. She is a non-smoker, and has been taking folic acid (0.5 mg daily) to minimise the risk of neural tube defects such as spina bifida, as well as exercising and avoiding alcohol. There is no history of any conditions that might affect fertility, such as pelvic infection or thyroid disease.

On examination, your find her weight is normal, and her body mass index (BMI) is about 20 kg/m^2, which is in the normal range. Jenny has no signs of endocrine disorders, with no evidence of abnormal facial or body hair (hirsutism), acne or hair thinning. Her thyroid and general examinations are normal and her blood pressure is 110/60 mmHg. Arnel is a very healthy-looking man, as you might expect from an army officer. He has no health problems at all.

Typical fecundity for a healthy woman of Jenny's age is about 20% each month, so a year of trying without a pregnancy is a long delay. Since there is some pressure of time with the possibility of Arnel being posted overseas, you undertake some basic tests. You also discuss reproductive carrier screening and the possibility that while it is likely both carry recessive mutations, the chance of them carrying the same mutations is low. Since Arnel is from the Philippines you suggest screening for thalassaemias, and for Jenny testing for cystic fibrosis, spinal muscular atrophy and fragile X syndrome. If she does not carry these, Arnel does not need screening.

To ensure that Jenny is ready for pregnancy, you check her rubella immunity and vitamin D levels. She has a blood test on day 2 of her regular cycle for her follicle stimulating hormone (FSH) and LH levels and another blood test on day 21 of the cycle to assess her progesterone level (a level of 30 IU/L or more is indicative of ovulation). As a starting point for Arnel, you check his semen analysis.

Some unexpected news for Arnel

You see Jenny and Arnel a couple of weeks later and make an interesting discovery. Jenny is immune to rubella, has normal menstrual phase hormone results and has a progesterone level indicative of ovulation (Table 45.1).

However, Arnel's semen analysis result is abnormal. He has no sperm at all in the ejaculation. Absence of sperm in the ejaculate is called azoospermia.

You explain the findings, and examine Arnel. He is normally masculine, and has a normal Asian body hair distribution. There are no scars in

Table 45.1 Menstrual phase gonadotropin patterns in reproductive-age women

Results	Interpretation
FSH <10 IU/L, LH <5 IU/L	Normal
FSH <2 IU/L, LH <2 IU/L	Hypogonadotropic hypogonadism
	Oral contraceptive use
	Over-exercising, being underweight
	Hypopituitarism
FSH <10 IU/L, LH >5 IU/L	Polycystic ovarian syndrome
FSH >15 IU/L, LH >10 IU/L	Ovarian failure

the groin to suggest previous surgery, such as hernia repair. There is no varicocoele (varicose veins in the upper scrotum) and the testes are both in the normal position in the scrotum and are normal in volume when measured with an orchidometer (Fig. 45.1).

This is obviously a shock for both of them, and you explain that sometimes this sperm result occurs after a fever and that the semen analysis must be repeated. Unfortunately, the repeat test shows the same finding of azoospermia. Table 45.2 describes the characteristics of a normal semen analysis, and the possible causes of azoospermia are listed in Table 45.3.

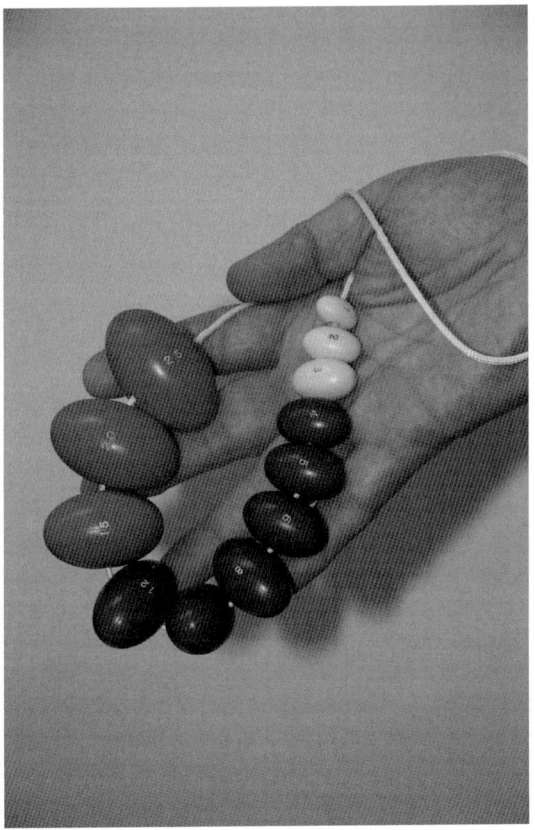

Figure 45.1 Orchidometer

McGraw Hill

Table 45.2 Characteristics of a normal semen analysis

Ejaculate volume	2–5 mL
Sperm concentration	>15 million sperm per mL
Sperm movement	>50% are moving in a roughly forward direction
Sperm morphology	>20% are normal in shape
Clumping of sperm	None

Notes about interpreting a semen analysis:

- Men are generally told to abstain from ejaculation for two or three days before providing the specimen, to optimise the results. Too little abstinence and the sperm may be dilute. Too much abstinence and the ejaculate may have abnormal motility and debris.

- An ejaculate volume of less than 2 mL may indicate obstruction, while a volume more than 5 mL may indicate prostatitis.

- The sample should be kept warm and checked for sperm movement (motility) within 30 minutes, as movement can decrease rapidly if left cold for longer.

- NEVER base any diagnosis on the results of a single sperm specimen. If there are abnormalities in a semen analysis result, always repeat the test after 2–6 weeks.

Table 45.3 Possible causes of azoospermia

1. Sperm are being made normally but not appearing in the ejaculate ('obstructive' azoospermia)
• Vasectomy (the commonest cause in developed countries)
• Bilateral absence of the vas deferens (usually a form of cystic fibrosis)
• Prostatic obstruction, usually after surgery, with retrograde ejaculation
• Accidental damage to the vas deferens during hernia or other groin surgery
2. Sperm are not being made ('non-obstructive' azoospermia)
• Pituitary failure or high prolactin level
• Chromosomal abnormality, such as 47 XXY (Klinefelter syndrome)
• Acquired infection, especially mumps
• Congenital absence of sperm-producing cells (Sertoli-cell-only syndrome)

Investigation and management of azoospermia

Absence of sperm in the ejaculate is an alarming finding and may indicate serious disease. There should always be a careful examination of the man to look for signs of chromosomal problems such as Klinefelter syndrome (47 XXY karyotype) in which the man is tall and relatively hairless and has a wide angle at the elbow, with small testes. It is important also to rule out a pituitary tumour or pituitary failure: look for diminished visual fields, reduced reflexes or other hair changes.

A check of the reproductive hormones—FSH, LH, thyroid stimulating hormone (TSH) and prolactin—is important. If the FSH level is low, it may indicate pituitary failure. If it is high, it may be a sign of primary testicular failure. It is also important to order laboratory tests to rule out cystic fibrosis and a chromosomal abnormality.

In Arnel's case, the hormones were all normal and his karyotype was the normal male 46 XY. However, testing revealed that he is a heterozygous carrier of a ΔF_{508} mutation of cystic fibrosis. This is associated with congenital bilateral absence of the vas deferens (CBAVD). This means that sperm are being manufactured normally in the testes but cannot move from the epididymis and be ejaculated. Fortunately Jenny had undergone the reproductive carrier screening you had discussed and she does not carry a cystic fibrosis mutation; if both Jenny and Arnel carried cystic fibrosis mutations, the baby they conceived would have a 1-in-4 chance of full-blown cystic fibrosis.

The role of IVF in treating fertility problems

In vitro fertilisation (IVF) has been available as a treatment for infertility since the 1980s. IVF is a very common treatment, and as many as 5% of all babies born now result from IVF. During a typical cycle of treatment, a woman will have purified FSH injected each day to stimulate not one follicle, as usually occurs each month, but a number of follicles. A second injection of a GnRH antagonist is given to prevent early ovulation. Once the follicles are mature, a triggering injection (either LH or human chorionic gonadotropin, hCG) is given to initiate the ovulation sequence and free the oocytes (eggs) from the follicle wall. About 36 hours after the trigger injection, the oocytes are collected using a needle passed through the vagina and into the ovaries, under ultrasound guidance. The oocytes are prepared in the IVF laboratory, then microinjected (Fig. 45.2) to allow fertilisation. The resulting embryos are then cultured in a nutrient solution in an incubator. It is possible to take cell samples from the embryos to test for the presence of the cystic fibrosis mutation and only transfer embryos that do not carry cystic fibrosis.

283

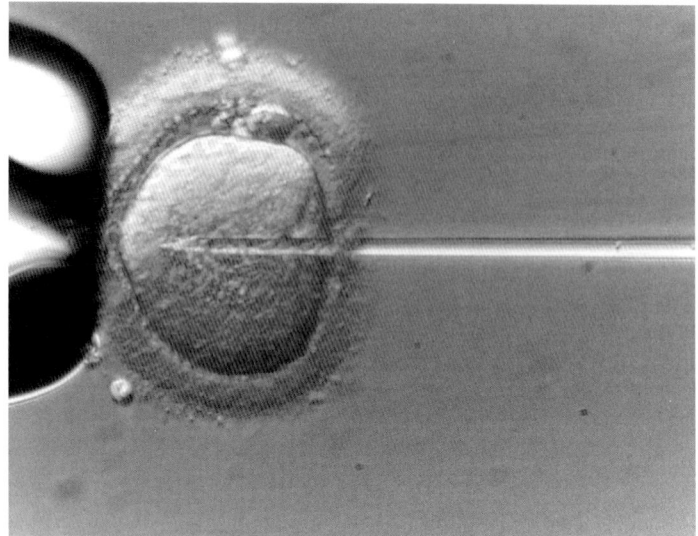

Figure 45.2 IVF
McGraw Hill

In Jenny's case, a single embryo is transferred back through the cervix into the endometrial cavity on the fifth day of embryological development (the blastocyst stage) and the other embryos are frozen for use in the future.

Jenny and Arnel return from the IVF clinic with the happy news that Jenny is pregnant with a single fetus and her hormone levels are all reassuring. You discuss the routine early management of pregnancy with the excited couple and talk to them about nuchal translucency screening.

CP CLINICAL PEARLS

- The chance of a healthy couple's conceiving with midcycle intercourse is very dependent on the woman's age. The chance is more than 20% each month for a woman in her early 20s but falls to about 12% once a woman is aged 35 years.
- Couples trying for pregnancy should have routine pre-pregnancy checks (including a physical examination, tests such as rubella immunity and making sure her cervical screening test is up to date) as well as checks that she is releasing eggs and that the semen

analysis is normal. All couples planning a family should have reproductive carrier screening discussed with them by a suitably qualified health professional.

- Azoospermia is an alarming finding, and should prompt a thorough search for the cause.

References and further reading

Katz DJ, Teloken P, Shoshany O. Male infertility—the other side of the equation. *Aust Fam Physician*. 2017;46(9):641–6.

Wosnitzer M, Goldstein M, Hardy MP. Review of azoospermia. *Spermatogenesis*. 2014;4:e28218.

Case 46
Tarni presents with irregular periods…

Tarni is a 31-year-old woman who presents to a primary care clinic in a remote rural area, with a history of frequent irregular vaginal bleeding over the past year, associated with diffuse lower abdominal pain. Tarni has had seven pregnancies; she has also been noted to have been a poor attender for antenatal care at the clinic during these pregnancies.

What history do you take from Tarni?

You must get a detailed menstrual history and try to determine whether there is intermenstrual or postcoital bleeding, and the relationship of the pain to the bleeding, if any.

Tarni reports that she seems to have periods about every 3 weeks but also has spotting or light bleeding between these periods. Some of this bleeding has been postcoital. The pain she experiences is worse at the time of bleeding and on questioning she also admits to some deep dyspareunia but denies that this is a problem. Her LMP was 1 week previously.

You also take a relevant medical, surgical and obstetric history. Tarni's seven pregnancies resulted in four uncomplicated vaginal births (when she was aged 15, 17, 19 and 21), two miscarriages and an ectopic pregnancy, in that order. The ectopic was 2 years previously and was treated laparoscopically, with a left salpingectomy. From the report of that surgery in her clinic notes, you learn that at laparoscopy extensive pelvic adhesions involving both tubes and ovaries were noted and a diagnosis of chronic pelvic infection was made. She has had no other surgery. Her last cervical screening test (CST) was 3 years previously; the result of this is in your clinic notes and is normal. You also note that Tarni has been treated twice for chlamydia infections in the past 5 years at the clinic but on questioning says that her partner declined chlamydia testing and treatment. Asked about contraception, she replies that she does not want another pregnancy but has not been using any form of contraception. She does not have diabetes or any other medical problems. She also denies any bowel or bladder symptoms.

From her notes you see that Tarni has a history of intimate partner violence and of sexual abuse from her partner, dating back to her teens, but on questioning she states that she does not want any discussion about this at today's consultation or help from other agencies.

Domestic Violence

- Domestic violence is a complex pattern of behaviours that may include, in addition to physical acts of violence, sexual abuse and emotional abuse.
- Women experience domestic violence at far greater rates than men do, and women and children often live in fear as a result of the abuse that is used by men to maintain control over their partners.
- Domestic violence is a major public health problem and is very common in women attending clinical practice.
- Women present most commonly with a range of chronic symptoms to unsuspecting general practitioners, emergency department doctors or medical specialists.
- Women who have experienced partner abuse want to be asked about it and are more likely to disclose if asked in an empathic, non-judgemental way. Doctors can make a difference.

Examples of questions you could ask a woman if you suspect domestic violence

- Are you ever afraid of your partner?
- In the last year, has your partner hit, kicked, punched or otherwise hurt you?
- In the last year, has your partner put you down, humiliated you or tried to control what you can do?
- In the last year, has your partner threatened to hurt you?
- Would you like help with any of this now?

How do you proceed with this consultation?

Tarni has failed to attend previous appointments, so it is desirable that you cover as many aspects as possible of her healthcare in this consultation. She is of healthy weight with a BMI of 24. Her blood pressure is 100/70 mmHg. General physical examination including cardiovascular and respiratory systems, thyroid and breasts is unremarkable, but abdominal examination reveals some mild central lower abdominal tenderness. A urinary ß-hCG is negative, ruling out a complication of early pregnancy as the cause of Tarni's symptoms.

What are the important points of a vaginal examination?

Tarni has already had a diagnosis of chronic pelvic infection made when she was 29, and her obstetric and sexual histories are consistent with this diagnosis. It is also likely that the cause of her irregular vaginal bleeding is chronic pelvic infection (or more accurately, the aftermath of previous episodes of acute pelvic infection, as in most cases an obvious causative organism cannot be isolated). However, other causes must be excluded.

You perform a speculum examination: the cervix appears inflamed but otherwise normal. The vaginal walls also appear normal but there is a greyish vaginal discharge with a 'fishy' odour suggestive of bacterial vaginosis. There is no fresh or old blood present. You take a cervical screening test. Although it has been less than 5 years since her last CST you perform one because of her abnormal bleeding. You also perform an endocervical swab and a vaginal swab.

You then perform a bimanual examination, which reveals a tender uterus slightly larger than normal and mild tenderness in both lateral fornices with a palpable mass in the right fornix.

Pelvic pain due to chronic PID must be distinguished from other causes of chronic lower abdominal pain originating in the bowel or bladder. Chronic pelvic pain of genital tract origin may also be caused by endo-metriosis, adenomyosis, uterine fibroids or adhesions from previous surgery in the region.

CLINICAL COMMENT

- Chronic PID is a loose term used where a woman known or suspected of having one or more episodes of acute PID or subclinical chlamydia or gonococcal infection experiences chronic pelvic pain and/or further episodes of acute pelvic infection. Genital tract infection with sexually transmitted organisms (most commonly *Chlamydia trachomatis*), both symptomatic and asymptomatic, treated and untreated, can be followed by secondary ascending infection from normal flora of the bowel or vagina. Occasionally, PID—both acute and chronic—can follow postnatal or post-abortion sepsis and it can also follow gynaecological surgery.

- Chronic PID can be suspected from the history, clinical examination and ultrasound findings and confirmed by laparoscopy.
- It is not known how often acute PID progresses to chronic PID but it is certainly a common condition in gynaecological practice.
- Chronic PID is known to be associated with infertility, ectopic pregnancy, dyspareunia, menstrual disturbance (as both the ovaries and the endometrium may be involved), chronic pelvic pain and bowel symptoms.
- Acute exacerbations in a woman known to have the condition should be treated vigorously to prevent worsening symptoms subsequently.
- While analgesia should be supplied as appropriate, it is important to avoid drugs of dependence; involvement of a pain management team or clinic, if available, should be considered.
- Partners should be notified and screened and appropriately treated.

What investigations are indicated?

A pelvic ultrasound should be performed to determine the nature of the pelvic mass and you arrange for this to be done when the visiting ultrasonographer attends the clinic in a week's time. You explain to Tarni the importance of attending for the ultrasound and for a further clinic appointment in 2 weeks' time when all her test results will be available. If there are social or transport difficulties limiting her ability to attend that can be solved within the framework of the clinic's resources, assistance should be offered.

The follow-up visit

Tarni returns to the clinic 2 weeks later. The CST result is normal and endocervical swabs are negative for chlamydia and gonorrhoea, but the vaginal swab confirms bacterial vaginosis. The ultrasound shows a 7 cm mass involving the right ovary, which appears adherent to the right side of the uterus.

Bacterial vaginosis (BV)

- This is a common condition, caused by a profound change in the normal vaginal flora. There is a decrease in lactobacilli and an increase in other bacteria including *Gardnerella* and *Mycoplasma* species and anaerobes.
- The condition often recurs following antibiotic treatment.
- The recommended treatment regimens are oral metronidazole or intravaginal metronidazole or intravaginal clindamycin cream.
- There is known to be some association between BV and PID.
- There appears to be an association between BV and preterm birth but the evidence to date does not support screening and treating asymptomatic pregnant women.
- The use of probiotics to treat the condition is currently being studied and may prove effective.

What is your further management for Tarni?

You explain the results to Tarni and recommend that she be referred to the gynaecological outpatients department of your base hospital. You discuss the treatment of BV, recommending a course of metronidazole, but Tarni declines this as she is not experiencing any discomfort from the discharge.

Six weeks later you receive a letter from the consultant gynaecologist at the hospital. Tarni initially underwent hysteroscopy and curettage, which showed no abnormality in the uterine cavity or on histological examination of the endometrium, and laparoscopy, which revealed a right tubo-ovarian mass adherent to the right side of the uterus and adhesions involving the left ovary.

After discussion with Tarni, it was decided to proceed to total hysterectomy: she stated that her family was complete, she wished to be cured of her symptoms and she did not want to travel away from home again. At operation the following week, it was possible to conserve the left ovary and part of the right, an important concern in a young woman. In cases where both ovaries require removal, hormone therapy to at least the expected age of menopause would be indicated. Her immediate postoperative course was uneventful and she was advised to return to your clinic for further follow-up. Tarni has also agreed to be referred to a hospital social worker for possible assistance with her domestic violence issues.

CLINICAL COMMENT

- While chronic pelvic infection and pelvic pain may be treated with analgesics, and acute exacerbations with appropriate antibiotics, definitive treatment must be surgical.
- Where the condition is confined, completely or partially, to the adnexa on one side, the woman may benefit from unilateral salpingo-oophorectomy, which also has the potential to preserve fertility. Where the condition is generalised, removal of all diseased tissue is the only option likely to provide relief of symptoms, although in younger women attempts should always be made to conserve the ovaries.

CLINICAL PEARLS

- The best treatment of chronic PID is prevention. Acute PID should be treated early and vigorously with appropriate antibiotics.
- When consulted by a woman with a history of non-attendance or non-compliance (which may be for any of a number of family, social, geographical or financial reasons), take the opportunity to offer other healthcare as indicated.
- Medicare Australia encourages and facilitates Skype or telemedicine consultations with patients in rural or remote areas.

References and further reading

Australian Sexual Health Alliance. Australian STI management guidelines for use in primary care. Sydney: Australasian Society for HIV, Viral Hepatitis and Sexual Health Medicine (ASHM); 2020. http://sti.guidelines.org.au/

Baird K. Routine enquiry for DFV in healthcare settings. *O&G Magazine*. 2017; 19(4). ogmagazine.org.au/19/4-19/routine-enquiry-dfv-healthcare-settings

British Association for Sexual Health and HIV. BASHH guideline for acute pelvic inflammatory disease. Lichfield, UK: BASSH; 2019. www .bashhguidelines.org/current-guidelines/systemic-presentation-and -complications/pid-2019/

World Health Organization. Responding to intimate partner violence and sexual violence against women. WHO Clinical and Policy Guideline. Geneva: WHO; 2013. www.who.int/reproductivehealth/publications/violence

Case 47
Rebecca presents with acute abdominal pain...

You are working in the emergency department of a country hospital when you are called early one Sunday morning to see Rebecca, a 20-year-old woman who has presented complaining of severe lower abdominal pain. When you arrive you find Rebecca lying on her left side on a bed in a cubicle, her legs drawn up and very distressed by the pain. Vital signs have already been recorded by the nursing staff—blood pressure 100/80 mmHg, pulse 100 beats per minute (bpm), temperature 39.5°C.

What is your immediate management of Rebecca?

You explain to Rebecca that she will be given pain relief very shortly but that you must first get some idea of the cause of her problem. You take a short but relevant history: the pain has been present for 24 hours but has increased greatly since midnight. It has always been in the lower abdomen but is much worse on the right side. She has never had a similar pain. She has not had her appendix removed or any other abdominal surgery. Her periods have been a bit irregular lately, the last one being about 5 weeks ago.

'How long have they been irregular?' you ask. Rebecca then tells you that she had a termination of pregnancy 4 months ago and was also treated for chlamydia; since then her cycles have been irregular and short with episodes of spotting in between. The clinic where she had the termination has given her a prescription for the combined oral contraceptive pill (COCP) but because of the irregular bleeding she has not yet commenced this. She is still with the same partner and they use condoms 'most of the time'. She agrees that she could possibly be pregnant again. There have been no urinary or bowel symptoms.

What examination do you now make?

A quick general physical examination reveals nothing remarkable, although Rebecca is clearly very distressed by the pain. On palpating her abdomen you find marked tenderness in the right lower quadrant with rebound and guarding—Rebecca pushes your hand away. In the left lower quadrant there is also tenderness on palpation but no guarding or rebound tenderness. You ask Rebecca if she could produce a urine specimen—she provides a sample for pregnancy testing and a midstream urine (MSU) sample for microscopy and culture. A rapidly performed commercial kit pregnancy test is negative.

> Commercial pregnancy tests are quantitative, with a sensitivity equivalent to a blood concentration of beta-human chorionic gonadotrophin (β-hCG) of 50 IU/L. Tests will become positive about the time of the first missed period, usually 14 days postconception.

Should you perform a vaginal examination for Rebecca?

Yes. This is essential in making a diagnosis with this presentation. Gently passing a speculum, you examine the cervix, which is inflamed with a yellowish discharge coming from the os. You take swabs from the endocervix for general microscopy and culture, and chlamydia and gonococcal screening.

Bimanual vaginal examination elicits excruciating tenderness in the right fornix with an impression of fullness in the adnexae, although you do not persist with the examination because of the pain it is causing. There is also tenderness in the left fornix and over the body of the uterus itself, which does not feel enlarged, and severe tenderness on gently moving the cervix. You make a clinical diagnosis of acute pelvic inflammatory disease (PID).

Clinical picture of acute pelvic infection

- The most common presentation is in a young, sexually active woman.
- The most common initiating cause is a sexually transmissible infection (STI) (in Australia, chlamydial infection is the most common, followed by gonorrhoea).
- It may follow vaginal delivery or a gynaecological operation (e.g. termination of pregnancy, endometrial sampling, intrauterine contraceptive device (IUCD) insertion).

continued

- It can be associated with severe lower abdominal pain and peritonism, usually bilateral but sometimes more marked on one side.
- Usually the temperature is significantly raised.
- Vaginal examination reveals severe tenderness in one or both lateral fornices and cervical excitation.

What is your ongoing management in this case?

Rebecca is given SC fentanyl for pain, an intravenous line is established, blood is taken for a full blood count (FBC) and rapid plasma reagin (RPR; syphilis screening), and she is commenced on ceftriaxone intravenously (IV) daily, azithromycin 500mg IV daily and metronidazole 500 mg IV 12-hourly (Table 47.1). Arrangements are made to admit her to the ward.

Table 47.1 Treatment regimens for acute pelvic infection

Mild to moderate: Outpatient treatment	Ceftriaxone 500 mg in 2 mL of 1% lignocaine IMI, or 500 mg IV, stat *plus* metronidazole 400 mg po, bd for 14 days *plus* doxycycline 100 mg po, bd for 14 days
Severe: Inpatient treatment	Ceftriaxone 2 g IV, daily *or* cefotaxime 2 g IV, TDS *plus* azithromycin 500 mg IV, daily *plus* metronidazole 500 mg IV, bd

If there is no response in 24–36 hours, reconsider the diagnosis or consider a complication PID (e.g. pelvic abscess).
A full STI screen should be performed on all women presenting with PID.

The following day you see Rebecca on your ward round. She is now sitting up in bed and feeling much better, although she still has some abdominal pain. She no longer requires narcotic analgesia. Her temperature has settled to 37.6°C and her pulse rate to 80 bpm. Palpation of her abdomen produces some tenderness but no rebound or guarding. Rebecca is able to tolerate a normal diet.

What further care does Rebecca need?

You check the results of the tests you ordered the previous day and find that Rebecca's FBC showed a marked leucocytosis with a white cell count of 17×10^9/L with a neutrophilia and a raised C-reactive protein (CRP), but that her haemoglobin and red blood cell measurements were within normal limits. The urinary chlamydia PCR test is positive, and urine microscopy shows small numbers of leucocytes and epithelial cells only. Swabs show a growth of *Streptococcus faecalis*.

These results are consistent with your diagnosis of acute pelvic infection, probably initiated by a new chlamydia infection on a background of mild endometritis following termination of pregnancy. Once tissue damage has occurred as a result of acute pelvic infection, secondary infection can more easily be caused by the ascent of endogenous aerobic and non-aerobic bacteria from the bowel and vagina.

You explain the diagnosis to Rebecca, emphasising the need for adequate antibiotic treatment; rest and abstinence from sexual activity until she is better; if possible, the tracing and treatment of sexual contacts; and the importance of safe sex in the future. You explain that acute infection in the fallopian tubes can lead to infertility or ectopic pregnancy at a later date when she does actually want to become pregnant. Rebecca should commence her oral contraceptive pill at the time of her next period but should also use condoms unless or until she is certain that she and her partner are in a monogamous relationship.

CLINICAL PEARLS

Distinguishing acute PID from appendicitis

- In PID, pain always starts in the lower abdomen and is generally bilateral; in appendicitis, pain starts around the umbilicus or in the upper abdomen, later becoming unilateral.
- Women have a higher temperature in PID.
- Cervical excitation and tenderness in both fornices is characteristic of PID, although pain may predominate on one side.
- Nausea and anorexia are characteristic of appendicitis.
- Remember pregnancy can coexist with PID or appendicitis!
- Do not let a woman of reproductive age in pain languish without a diagnosis—laparoscopy must be performed early if empirical therapy is not successful.
- The earlier appropriate antibiotic treatment is commenced, the less likely it is that the sequelae of PID—infertility, ectopic pregnancy and chronic pelvic pain—will occur.

References and further reading

Australasian Sexual Health Alliance. Australian STI management guidelines for use in primary care. Sydney: Australasian Society for HIV, Viral Hepatitis and Sexual Health Medicine (ASHM); 2020. http://sti.guidelines.org.au/

BASHH (British Association for Sexual Health and HIV). BASHH guideline for acute pelvic inflammatory disease. Available at www.bashhguidelines.org /current-guidelines/systemic-presentation-and-complications/pid-2019/

Curry A, Williams T, Penny M. Pelvic inflammatory disease: diagnosis, management, and prevention. *Am Fam Physician.* 2019;100(6):357–64.

Case 48
Sharon is bleeding in early pregnancy...

Late one Saturday evening you are called to the emergency department to see Sharon, who is a 29-year-old primigravida. Sharon has been trying to conceive for about 6 months. A week ago she performed a home pregnancy test, which was positive. She and her partner, Gary, have been very excited about this. However, this evening she has experienced some crampy lower abdominal pain and spotting and is now very concerned and frightened.

What history do you need to take from Sharon?

You take a history from Sharon. Her LMP was 7 weeks ago, but her cycles are irregular, anything from 4 to 6 weeks in length. She has seen her general practitioner, who also confirmed the pregnancy by urinary β-hCG testing and ordered a pelvic ultrasound for help with dating, although Sharon has not yet had this scan.

Sharon is otherwise in good health with no relevant medical or surgical history and, in particular, no history of STIs. She has never been on the COCP and she stopped smoking completely 9 months ago. She takes no medications apart from folic acid and has no allergies. Her last cervical screening test was 4 years ago and the report was normal.

What physical examination is necessary in Sharon's case?

As well as a brief general examination and measurement of blood pressure, pulse and temperature, Sharon should have both abdominal and vaginal examinations performed.

Sharon's vital signs are all within normal limits. Abdominal inspection is unremarkable and palpation simply shows some mild central lower abdominal tenderness. There is no guarding or rebound tenderness, no tenderness elsewhere in the abdomen and no uterine enlargement or other masses.

Vaginal examination reveals a cervix that is closed on inspection through a speculum, with some dark blood visible at the os. Bimanual palpation shows a bulky, soft, slightly tender uterus.

What is your clinical diagnosis and what investigations are indicated at this point?

Clinically Sharon has a threatened miscarriage—she is known to be pregnant with some bleeding and the cervix is closed. However, there has not been any confirmation so far that her pregnancy is in the uterus and the possibility of an ectopic pregnancy should not be overlooked. An ultrasound scan may be helpful in making a definite diagnosis.

You are able to perform a transvaginal ultrasound scan using the portable machine in the emergency department. This shows a gestational sac within the uterus and a fetal pole of 5 mm crown–rump length, indicating a gestational age of just 6 weeks; however, you are unable to demonstrate a beating fetal heart. You explain to Sharon and Gary that the pregnancy is in the right site, you show them the fetus, explaining how small it is and that it is often not possible to detect a fetal heart until the pregnancy is several more days advanced. Since Sharon's cycles are irregular it is possible that she has a continuing pregnancy and that the fetal heart will become detectable on ultrasound within days. You explain to the couple that unexplained slight bleeding in early pregnancy is not uncommon and may settle spontaneously, the pregnancy continuing normally thereafter. However, there is also the possibility, since there is bleeding from within the uterus, that she may miscarry.

Since Sharon's general physical state is satisfactory you advise her to go home and tell her that while rest has not been shown to have a preventive effect from the point of view of the pregnancy, she may feel better in herself by taking some time off work and resting over a few days until all bleeding ceases. You also advise her to avoid sexual intercourse until bleeding settles. After taking blood for an FBC, quantitative β-hCG levels and blood group and Rhesus status, you arrange for her to be seen in the early pregnancy clinic the following week for ongoing assessment of her pregnancy. You advise her to continue taking folic acid. She appears reassured by your advice.

However, early on Sunday morning you are called back to the emergency department to see Sharon again. For the past hour she has been bleeding more heavily and she now has severe lower abdominal pain and feels 'weak and sweaty'.

On examination Sharon looks pale and is shivering. Her pulse is 90 bpm, blood pressure 90/50 mmHg and temperature 36.8°C. Abdominal examination now shows increased central tenderness above the pubic symphysis. Speculum examination shows an open cervix with placental tissue in the os accompanied by brisk bright red bleeding.

What is your management?

Products of conception in the cervical canal holding the cervix open can cause a degree of shock disproportionate to the amount of blood lost. This is due to cervical shock as a result of excessive parasympathetic stimulation from a dilated cervix. Products of conception should be removed with sponge forceps or digitally using sterile gloves. Removal of all visible products of conception can greatly improve the clinical situation.

With sponge forceps you grasp the placental tissue and remove it. Bleeding, however, continues so you administer ergometrine 0.5 mg IM. You also commence Sharon on intravenous fluids. Her vital signs start to recover.

You explain to Sharon that she has, in fact, miscarried and passed at least part of the pregnancy (Table 48.1). You add that this is disappointing but unfortunately miscarriage is quite common, occurring in about 15–20% of pregnancies in the first trimester. However, most women experiencing miscarriage in a first pregnancy, you tell her, go on to have a normal pregnancy on the second occasion.

'What caused the miscarriage?' Gary asks.

In most miscarriages the reason is unknown, although it is known that a high proportion of spontaneously aborted embryos have chromosomal abnormalities. Examination of the products of conception does not usually help in determining the cause of the miscarriage in the individual case.

Sharon is still bleeding moderately despite the administration of ergometrine. What is your further management?

You recommend to Sharon that she undergo removal of any remaining tissue from within the uterus under a general anaesthetic. This will stop bleeding and reassure her that the miscarriage is complete. She agrees to this and later that morning has suction curettage performed. The results of her blood tests from the previous evening are available—Sharon's haemoglobin level at that time was 131 g/L, and her blood group is A Rhesus positive. Sharon does not require anti-D prophylaxis.

Before discharge home later that day you arrange for Sharon to see her own general practitioner during the week. You tell her that her next period should start within 4–6 weeks following the miscarriage. She asks whether she can then try again to become pregnant and you reassure her about this, advising her that there is no increased risk of miscarriage in her next pregnancy. You advise her to continue with folate supplements as she has been doing.

Table 48.1 Types of miscarriage and their characteristics

Type of miscarriage	Bleeding	Pain	Clinical findings
Threatened	Slight	None	Cervix closed, uterus size commensurate with gestational date
Inevitable	Moderate to heavy	Moderate to severe	Cervix open, no tissue seen
Incomplete	Moderate to heavy	Moderate to severe	Cervix open, tissue seen
Complete	Slight or none	Settling or none	Cervix open or closed, tissue passed
Missed	Slight or none	None	Cervix closed, uterus small for dates
Anembryonic pregnancy/ blighted ovum	Slight or none	None	Cervix closed, uterus small for dates

Note: All types of miscarriage may be complicated by infection.

 CLINICAL PEARLS

- Expectant management is safe for women experiencing miscarriage if bleeding is slight to moderate and pain is tolerable—this will be most women presenting. Surgical evacuation of the uterus is indicated for heavy bleeding, although on occasion it may also be requested by women. 'Medical' evacuation using the drug misoprostol is increasingly being performed; when this synthetic drug is used in gynaecology, it is used 'off-label'.

- A large randomised controlled trial (PRISM) showed that among women with bleeding in early pregnancy, treatment with progesterone during the first trimester *did not result* in a significantly higher incidence of live births than among those who had a placebo (a pessary with no active ingredients). Further analysis, however, showed that a subgroup of women with a history of recurrent miscarriage (three or more miscarriages before this pregnancy), *did* show a significant improvement in outcome for those who had the progesterone treatment.

References and further reading

Coomarasamy A, Devall AJ, Cheed V, et al. Randomized trial of progesterone in women with bleeding in early pregnancy. *N Engl J Med.* 2019;380:1815–24.

Haas DM, Hathaway TJ, Ramsey PS. Progestogen for preventing miscarriage in women with recurrent miscarriage of unclear etiology. *Cochrane Database Syst Rev.* 2019;11:CD003511.

National Institute for Health and Care Excellence. Ectopic pregnancy and miscarriage: diagnosis and initial management. NICE guideline NG126. London: NICE; 2019. www.nice.org.uk/guidance/ng126

Royal College of Obstetricians and Gynaecologists. The investigation and treatment of couples with recurrent first-trimester and second-trimester miscarriage. RCOG Green-top Guideline No. 17, 2011. www.rcog.org.uk/en/guidelines-research-services/guidelines/gtg17

Case 49
Angie presents with an ectopic pregnancy...

You are called urgently to the emergency department to see Angie, a 25-year-old woman who has presented with severe left-side lower abdominal pain and bilateral shoulder tip pain. On arrival you find that Angie's observations have already been taken by nursing staff—pulse 100 bpm, blood pressure 90/60 mmHg, temperature 36.8°C. Angie is lying with her legs drawn up, looking pale and distressed. She is able to tell you that the pain began during sexual intercourse about 1 hour previously. She does remember experiencing some similar but very mild pain the previous day.

What is your overriding concern in your assessment of Angie?

She may have an ectopic pregnancy that has ruptured or is about to rupture, with the risk of life-threatening intra-abdominal haemorrhage.

Quickly you take a short relevant history from Angie. Her LMP was 6 weeks previously. Her cycles are irregular and 6 weeks is not unusual for her. She had some spotting the previous day, which she thought was the start of a period but no more has followed. Although not wishing to be pregnant she has had unprotected sex with two partners during the past month. She has a 6-year-old son born by caesarean section.

What is your next step?

Angie is able to produce a urine specimen with the help of nursing staff and while this is being tested you examine her. She is pale and sweating. Inspection shows some lower abdominal distension. On palpation the abdomen is rigid in the left lower quadrant, which is very tender with rebound tenderness when you remove your hand. The nursing staff now report that Angie's urine pregnancy test is positive. While you were on the way to the emergency department (ED), the ED doctor had performed a focused assessment with sonography for trauma (FAST) scan and demonstrated some free fluid in the pelvis with no evidence of an intrauterine pregnancy.

On the basis of this information you make a tentative diagnosis of ruptured ectopic pregnancy. Angie's clinical condition is such that urgent surgical intervention is needed. You explain to Angie that you believe she has an ectopic pregnancy, probably in her left tube, which has ruptured. You will be urgently calling in a senior colleague to operate, as well as anaesthetic and nursing staff. You proceed at once to insert a wide-bore intravenous cannula for Angie and take blood for an FBC and group and cross-match of 2 units of whole blood. You commence Angie on a litre of Hartmann's solution to run in rapidly. You gain consent from Angie for a laparoscopy and/or laparotomy, explaining that if possible the procedure will be done by laparoscopy but that her condition may make it necessary to proceed to laparotomy. You explain that if a tubal pregnancy is present and bleeding, then part or all of the tube may need to be removed. Your consultant will also inspect the other tube and discuss the findings with Angie postoperatively.

Upon arrival in the operating theatre Angie's blood pressure has dropped to 80/50 mmHg and her lower abdomen is more distended. A senior anaesthetist attends and stabilises her with appropriate fluid management and then initiates rapid-sequence induction of general anaesthesia. The consultant gynaecologist commences with the laparoscopy and finds more than 1 L of fresh blood and clots in the pelvis. There is free bleeding from a distended and ruptured portion of the left fallopian tube and a small amount of placental tissue protruding from the tube. The distal end of the tube is stuck to the ovary and the right tube also shows signs of chronic infection. Both ovaries are noted to be normal. The adhesions around the left fallopian tube are divided and a left salpingectomy is performed; haemostasis is achieved satisfactorily. The excised fallopian tube is sent for histopathology. Peritoneal lavage is carried out. The pneumoperitoneum is reduced and the port sites sutured. Angie's condition improves and stabilises with intravenous fluids, and although blood is available it is not used. Anti-D is not required as she is Rhesus (D) positive.

The following day you see Angie on your ward round. *'What are my chances of future pregnancy?'* she asks.

Angie had definite evidence at laparoscopy of chronic pelvic infection. She has had swabs taken from both tubes at the time of surgery and you have prescribed antibiotics (ceftriaxone, metronidazole and azithromycin) to cover the postoperative period pending microbiological reports. Angie then admits to having been treated twice in the past 2 years for chlamydia infections. You explain that the condition of her tube plus the removal of the left one does mean that she may have difficulty conceiving again and that there is an increased risk of any pregnancy that does occur being an ectopic again. If she does experience difficulty conceiving and wishes to proceed with treatment, then IVF is the procedure most likely to be successful.

She then says that she has a friend who had an ectopic pregnancy who was treated with medication. 'Why couldn't I have been done the same way rather than have an operation?'

What is your response to this question?

Angie's condition had become life-threatening because the ectopic pregnancy had ruptured the fallopian tube, causing severe intraperitoneal haemorrhage necessitating urgent operation. Quite often, laparoscopy is safe even under such conditions provided that she is stabilised by the anaesthetist prior to a general anaesthetic (GA). Rarely, when a patient is very unstable, and there is no ready access to or expertise in laparoscopy, a laparotomy is required.

Medical treatment of ectopic pregnancy involves the administration of methotrexate, a folic acid antagonist. Folate is an essential vitamin needed to help rapidly dividing cells in pregnancy and methotrexate is a powerful drug that works by temporarily interfering with the processing in the body of folate. The drug stops the pregnancy developing any further and the embryo is gradually reabsorbed by the body leaving the fallopian tube intact. Methotrexate is given systemically by intramuscular injections.

Offer systemic methotrexate as a first-line treatment to women who are able to return for follow-up and who have all of the following:

- No significant pain
- An unruptured ectopic pregnancy with an adnexal mass smaller than 35 mm with no visible heart beat
- A serum β-hCG level less than 1500 IU/litre
- No intrauterine pregnancy (as confirmed on an ultrasound scan).

Offer surgery where treatment with methotrexate is not acceptable to the woman.

For women with ectopic pregnancy who have had methotrexate, take 2 serum β-hCG measurements in the first week (days 4 and 7) after treatment and then 1 serum β-hCG measurement per week until a negative result is obtained. If β-hCG levels plateau or rise, reassess the woman's condition for further treatment.

Often ectopic pregnancy is diagnosed when a woman known to be pregnant presents with an ultrasound report showing an empty uterus—there may or may not be ultrasound evidence of the pregnancy developing in one or other tube. Ectopic pregnancy may also present with mild lower abdominal pain in a woman known to be in early pregnancy; the pain is due to slight bleeding irritating the peritoneal surface. There may also be slight vaginal bleeding, as in Angie's case, as fluctuating progesterone levels from developing placental tissue act upon the decidualised endometrium, causing the decidua to shed.

If there is no obvious evidence of a pregnancy within the uterus or fallopian tubes on ultrasound scan, this would be classified as a pregnancy of unknown location (PUL). It is important that this is monitored by β-hCG and ultrasound scan, as it may evolve to be an ectopic pregnancy.

 CLINICAL COMMENT

Bleeding in early pregnancy: distinguishing ectopic pregnancy from miscarriage

Vaginal bleeding associated with ectopic pregnancy tends to be slight and intermittent, and pain is constant and most severe on the side on which the ectopic pregnancy is located. Shoulder tip pain indicates the possibility of haemoperitoneum irritating the diaphragm. Bleeding associated with miscarriage is frequently moderate in amount but may be severe, especially with inevitable or incomplete miscarriage; pain is central and colicky. Quantitative β-hCG levels may be measured in cases where the woman is stable, and when a level of >1000 U is reached; a fetal pole should be visible on transvaginal ultrasound. In a continuing intrauterine pregnancy, β-hCG levels should roughly double every 48 hours.

When the diagnosis of ectopic pregnancy is made early in pregnancy and the fallopian tube has not ruptured, medical treatment with methotrexate may bring about absorption and resolution of the pregnancy without the need for surgical intervention. However, the methotrexate must be given under close medical supervision and surgery should be performed if pain supervenes or serum β-hCG levels do not fall by at least 15% within 4 days. Levels should be followed until they become negative.

CLINICAL PEARLS

- All women of reproductive age should be considered pregnant until proved otherwise! Beware of ruling out pregnancy on the basis of history alone. It's important to note also that ectopic pregnancy should be considered as a possible diagnosis in every woman presenting with abdominal pain.
- Only early ectopic pregnancy with minimal signs and symptoms is suitable for management with methotrexate; patients with features of peritonism or an unstable cardiovascular status require surgical treatment.
- Most cases of ectopic pregnancy requiring surgery can be dealt with by laparoscopy. Patients who have bled significantly intraperitoneally, presenting with shock, should undergo laparotomy.

References and further reading

National Institute for Health and Care Excellence. Ectopic pregnancy and miscarriage: diagnosis and initial management. NICE guideline NG126. London: NICE; 2019. www.nice.org.uk/guidance/ng126

Royal College of Obstetricians and Gynaecologists. Management of tubal pregnancy. RCOG Clinical Green-top Guideline No. 21. London: RCOG; 2016. www.rcog.org.uk/en/guidelines-research-services/guidelines/gtg21

Case 50
Houda has an ovarian cyst…

Houda is a 17-year-old teenager whom you are asked to see urgently at the emergency department, where she has presented with acute abdominal pain, having been sent into hospital by her general practitioner.

When you arrive in the cubicle Houda lies curled on her side and is clearly distressed. Her vital signs have already been taken—blood pressure 110/70 mmHg, pulse rate 100 bpm, temperature 37.0°C.

What are your first steps?

You take a short history from Houda. Her mother, who is present and anxious, does not speak much English but attempts to answer all your questions instead of letting her daughter do so.

> It is important to take the history from the patient herself. She is legally able to give consent for herself and in this case can speak English perfectly.

How do you handle this situation?

You politely but firmly ask the mother to sit next to her daughter and tell her you will ask questions of Houda alone.

Houda tells you she has had some vague lower abdominal pain for a few months. She has seen her general practitioner, who did not find anything wrong on abdominal examination. An abdominal ultrasound has been ordered but has not yet been performed. Today she experienced the sudden severe onset of right iliac fossa pain, somewhat like the vague pains she has been having but much worse. She vomited once and now feels a bit nauseous and not hungry. Her menstrual cycle is regular, last menstrual period (LMP) 2 weeks previously, and she has never been on the COCP, takes no medications and has no allergies. She has no serious medical problems and has never had any surgery. There are no urinary or bowel symptoms.

Do you examine Houda in her mother's presence?

It is advisable to take a sexual history from Houda without her mother present in view of her age. It would be appropriate to ask her mother to sit outside while you examine Houda.

With her mother out of earshot you gently inquire whether Houda is sexually active. She denies this, is quite sure of the date of her LMP and has no other health problems of note.

A short general examination shows no signs of anaemia and confirms Houda's tachycardia. You ask Houda to lie on her back and extend her legs—she has difficulty doing this and finds the pain is less with her legs flexed. Inspection of the abdomen reveals no obvious distension or masses. Palpation reveals acute tenderness in the right lower quadrant with guarding and rebound tenderness. There is minimal tenderness in the left lower quadrant and none in the upper abdomen; the liver and spleen are not palpable and there is no tenderness over the renal angles.

Do you perform a vaginal examination for Houda?

No. Houda has never been sexually active nor used tampons. As already noted, vaginal examination should not be performed in such patients. As well, vaginal examination may be culturally inappropriate. However, it is clear that Houda has an acute problem in the right side of her pelvis. In a young woman with similar symptoms, who had become sexually active, vaginal examination would be helpful in establishing a diagnosis and should be performed.

What investigations should be performed?

A full blood count (FBC), CRP, electrolytes, midstream urine (MSU) and a transabdominal ultrasound scan should be performed. You order intravenous fluids to help fill the bladder prior to the ultrasound scan. You also perform a urine β-hCG test, which is negative.

You prescribe pethidine plus metoclopramide for Houda and keep her fasting.

The FBC shows normal haemoglobin and platelet levels, with a slightly raised white cell count (9×10^9/L). The CRP and UEC are normal.

Differential diagnosis of acute right-sided lower abdominal pain in a young woman

- Appendicitis
- PID
- Ectopic pregnancy
- Complications of ovarian tumours (usually cysts)

The ultrasound scan shows a normal-sized uterus deviated to the left by the presence of a 10 cm cyst in the right adnexa. There is a considerable amount of fluid in the pouch of Douglas. The cyst contains solid material and has the appearance of a dermoid cyst. The left ovary appears normal. You make a provisional diagnosis of a leaking right ovarian cyst and prepare Houda for surgery.

You assist your consultant with laparoscopy, at which your diagnosis is confirmed. There is a quantity of sebaceous material in the pouch of Douglas, and the cyst has undergone torsion. There are a number of fibrinous adhesions around the right tube and ovary. It is decided to proceed to a laparotomy, at which the cyst is untwisted, and ovarian cystectomy, conserving a portion of viable normal ovary, is performed. The cyst is noted to contain hair as well as more sebaceous material. The left ovary is inspected and appears entirely normal.

> Simple cysts in young women can usually be treated laparoscopically but when complications have occurred or there is any possibility of malignancy, laparotomy may be the safer option.

Subsequent histology confirms a benign dermoid cyst. You reassure Houda and her parents that the remaining ovarian tissue is normal and that Houda's ultimate reproductive functioning will not be compromised.

 CLINICAL COMMENT

> Complications of ovarian cysts include torsion, haemorrhage into the cyst, leaking of cyst contents, infection and adhesions to adjacent organs. It is important to consider ovarian or ovarian cyst torsion in any acute lower abdominal presentation in a young woman. USS is not reliable for making this diagnosis; procrastination can lead to complete occlusion of the ovarian blood supply and infraction, with significant reproductive consequences for the woman.

Classification of ovarian cysts

- Physiological—follicular or luteal. These are normally not larger than 6 cm diameter and can be observed by serial ultrasounds. If they are causing symptoms, ovarian function can be suppressed with the COCP.
- Benign epithelial tumours—serous cystadenoma, mucinous (pseudomucinous) cystadenoma, endometrioid cystadenoma, Brenner tumour
- Benign germ cell tumours—dermoid cyst, mature teratoma
- Benign sex cord stromal tumours
- Theca cell tumours—fibroma, Sertoli–Leydig cell tumour
- Borderline
- Malignant

CLINICAL PEARLS

- Appropriate pain relief should be provided while a differential diagnosis is reached and appropriate investigations ordered.
- It is prudent to consider the possibility of pregnancy in every young woman presenting with abdominal symptoms; pregnancy is easily and accurately excluded as a cause of the presentation with urine β-hCG testing. This is true even when pregnancy seems unlikely from the history and social circumstances of the woman. It is essential that pregnancy not be missed in any significant presentation involving the abdomen.

References and further reading

Asfour V, Varma R, Menon P. Clinical risk factors for ovarian torsion. *J Obstet Gynaecol.* 2015;35(7):721–5.

Bottomley C, Bourne T. Diagnosis and management of ovarian cyst accidents. *Best Pract Res Clin Obstet Gynaecol.* 2009;23(5):711–24.

Medeiros LR, Rosa DD, Bozzetti MC, et al. Laparoscopy versus laparotomy for benign ovarian tumour. *Cochrane Database Syst Rev.* 2009;CD004751.

Royal College of Obstetricians and Gynaecologists. Management of suspected ovarian masses in premenopausal women. RCOG Green-top Guideline No. 62. London: RCOG; 2011. www.rcog.org.uk

Case 51
Vivienne presents with abdominal pain...

Vivienne is an 86-year-old woman who is brought for the first time to see you in general practice by her daughter, Susan, who has been a patient of yours for many years. Susan tells you that 'Mum's had this pain for years now. She's got an ovarian cyst but the doctors didn't want to operate, 5 years ago. Now it's getting worse and we wonder if she shouldn't be having something done about it after all.'

What history do you take in this situation?

Vivienne is a spry elderly lady who is able to give a clear history and who has good recall of what was decided by previous doctors. At the age of 80 she developed mild lower abdominal pain and an ultrasound scan was performed. She also had blood tests. She gives you a letter to her previous general practitioner from a specialist gynaecologist, from which you learn that ultrasound had demonstrated a 6 cm cystic mass in Vivienne's right ovary and that CA125 levels were normal. In view of Vivienne's age it was decided not to operate on this mass and apparently further follow-up was arranged (Table 51.1) and (Fig. 51.1).

> 'It's much more uncomfortable lately,' says Vivienne. 'Should I have another ultrasound?'

What is your response to this question?

You need to have a full picture of Vivienne's state of health. While some elderly patients may be too frail for surgery, or have significant intercurrent health problems, it is important to consider each and every patient individually regardless of age. Increasingly, developments in anaesthesia and minimally invasive surgical techniques mean that surgery even in quite elderly subjects can be safely and successfully performed. You must take a full history from Vivienne and conduct a physical examination.

Vivienne is able to tell you that she has had two children, both after normal pregnancies and births. At the age of 43 she underwent an abdominal hysterectomy for fibroids but both ovaries were conserved. She ceased having cervical screening after the hysterectomy but has had regular mammograms. She has never been on hormone therapy. She has hypertension, which is well controlled, and osteoporosis for which she has been prescribed bisphosphonates, having had a wrist fracture at the age of 78. She lives independently in an aged-care facility where she has an apartment; she says she has an active social life in the facility and many friends, and is not far from Susan and her other child, a son. Her husband died from a stroke when Vivienne was 77 and she tells you that she has not been sexually active since his death. There is no other relevant past history.

A systems review reveals no gastrointestinal, bowel or bladder problems although she does get up once or twice at night to urinate. She has become aware of more discomfort in the abdomen over the past 6 months and also often feels bloated (Table 51.2).

What examination do you make for Vivienne?

A general inspection shows a slim and healthy elderly woman who is able to climb by herself onto your examination couch. Examination of the respiratory and cardiovascular systems is unremarkable. Examination of the abdomen reveals a non-tender firm swelling in the right lower quadrant of the abdomen.

 CLINICAL PEARLS

Avoid 'ageism' when taking a history from elderly patients. Whenever possible take the history from the woman herself, although if she has problems with recall, relatives or friends accompanying her may be included in the consultation. In the case of patients with dementia, the history will often need to be taken from carers. Also avoid making assumptions that women are no longer sexually active—first inquire appropriately and sensitively if a woman has a partner and, if so, whether she is having vaginal intercourse.

Should you perform a vaginal examination for Vivienne at this visit?

Elderly women who have not had hormone therapy either systemically or vaginally and who are not sexually active may experience considerable discomfort with vaginal examination due to vaginal atrophy. In some situations, such as the routine performance of CSTs to the age of 70, it may be appropriate to prescribe a course of vaginal oestrogen prior to conducting such an examination and use a small, warmed and lubricated speculum—a paediatric speculum may be suitable.

Vivienne tells you that 6 years ago she experienced significant pain with attempts at vaginal examination and this is one reason she has put off coming back to seek help with her abdominal pain. You have already identified an abdominal mass that requires further investigation. Therefore on this occasion you postpone vaginal examination and order an abdominal ultrasound scan for Vivienne, together with routine blood tests and a CA125.

Two days later you receive a phone call from the medical imaging service to whom you referred Vivienne. Their ultrasound scan has shown a 12 cm mixed solid and cystic mass arising from the right ovary with the suggestion of partial obstruction of the right ureter. They would like to proceed to a computed tomography (CT) scan. You agree with this decision and CT confirms the nature of the mass and the partial ureteric obstruction. On the same day you receive the results of Vivienne's CA125—it is elevated at 123. You arrange to see Vivienne with her daughter and explain these findings to her, and you organise an urgent referral to your usual specialist gynaecologist, Dr Smith.

Two weeks later you receive a letter and operation notes from Dr Smith. Under general anaesthesia and through a midline laparotomy incision, she performed a bilateral salpingo-oophorectomy, omentectomy and lymphadenectomy with no complications. Histology showed a stage 1 serous ovarian cancer (Table 51.3). While there were a number of adhesions from previous surgery and the right ureter was demonstrably being compressed externally, there was no evidence of spread of the disease. Dr Smith states that Vivienne will therefore require no adjuvant therapy. She will, however, be followed up regularly at Dr Smith's clinic and have repeat CA125 levels performed.

Six weeks later Vivienne returns to your practice. She is now fit and well, the abdominal scar is well healed and she no longer has the abdominal pain. She is very happy with her decision to seek a second opinion about her case.

Table 51.1 Histological types of ovarian cancer

Type	Description
Epithelial cancers	These are most common in the age group 45–60 years but can present in the elderly. They constitute over 70% of ovarian tumours and 90% of malignancies.
Germ cell tumours	These are most common at 10–30 years and constitute 20% of ovarian tumours but only 5% of malignancies.
Sex cord stromal tumours	These occur at all ages. The constitute 5% of all tumours, both benign and malignant.
Metastatic disease	For example, from breast cancer.

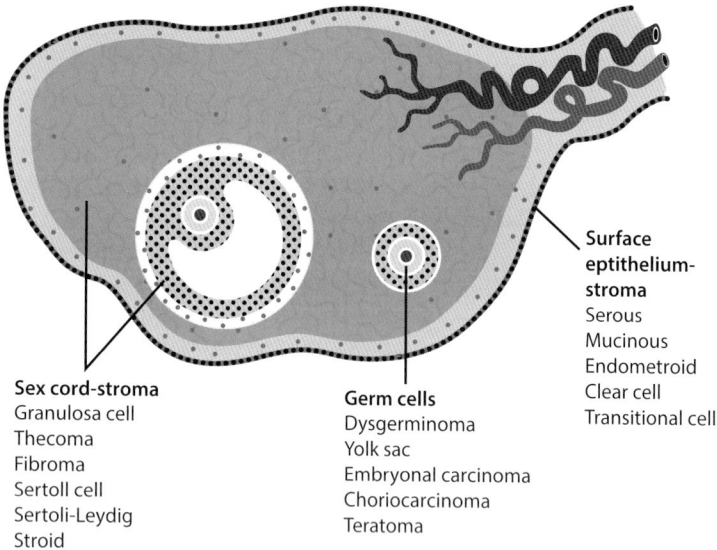

Sex cord-stroma
Granulosa cell
Thecoma
Fibroma
Sertoll cell
Sertoli-Leydig
Stroid

Germ cells
Dysgerminoma
Yolk sac
Embryonal carcinoma
Choriocarcinoma
Teratoma

Surface eptithelium-stroma
Serous
Mucinous
Endometroid
Clear cell
Transitional cell

Figure 51.1 Origins of ovarian tumours

Table 51.2 Common presentations of ovarian cancer

- Pelvic and abdominal pain, which may be vague and intermittent
- Bloating, increasing abdominal girth (often due to ascites)*

- Back pain*
- Leg pain*
- Weight loss, nausea, anorexia*
- Ovarian torsion
- Virilisation or excess oestrogen causing bleeding from the endometrium in the case of hormone-producing tumours

*All these symptoms suggest spread of the disease.

Table 51.3 Surgical staging and 5-year survival in ovarian cancer

Stage	5-year survival rate
Stage 1—confined to ovary	90%
Stage 2—beyond the ovary but within pelvis	68–79%
Stage 3—peritoneal implants or affected lymph nodes	29–49%
Stage 4—distant spread, e.g. pleural effusion, liver metastases	13–17%

Note: Most cases of ovarian cancer present at stages 3 to 4, so overall survival rates are poorer than for other gynaecological cancers.

 CLINICAL PEARLS

- Avoid ageism when consulted by elderly patients. Allow them wherever possible to make their own health decisions, as you would do with younger adults.
- Where vaginal examination in an elderly woman is required but not urgent and there is significant vaginal atrophy, a course of vaginal oestrogen (cream or pessaries) may be appropriate, resulting in a more comfortable examination for the woman and greater opportunity for the doctor to obtain maximum clinical information.
- Where malignancy is suspected and vaginal examination is difficult, it may be appropriate for the general practitioner to organise an abdominal ultrasound and urgent referral to a specialist for further examination and management, without persisting with attempts at vaginal examination.

References and further reading

Royal College of Obstetricians and Gynaecologists. Ovarian cysts in postmenopausal women. Green-top Guideline No. 34. London: RCOG; 2016. www.rocg.org.uk/guidelines

Stewart C, Ralyea C, Lockwood S. Ovarian cancer: an integrated review. *Semin Oncol Nurs.* 2019;35(2):151–6.

Case 52
Marilyn has postmenopausal bleeding…

In the gynaecology outpatient department you see for the first time a 57-year-old woman, Marilyn. She has been referred urgently by her general practitioner, Dr Case, because she presented to her with an episode of vaginal bleeding approximately 18 months after her last apparent menstrual period. Dr Case has performed a cervical screening test and organised a transvaginal pelvic ultrasound, but the results of these investigations are not to hand at the time when you first see Marilyn.

You take a detailed gynaecological and full medical history from Marilyn. She tells you that there has been only one episode of bleeding, which occurred after she had been helping her daughter move a wardrobe in her new house, in preparation for the arrival of Marilyn's first grandchild. Marilyn says she only went to see Dr Case because the bleeding made her realise that she had not had a cervical screening test (CST) for some time—'some time' turned out to be 8 years. Marilyn is sure it was just the heavy lifting that caused the bleeding. She is also sure the referral to hospital is unnecessary and she hopes there won't be any need for any further investigations because her daughter's baby is due any day now.

Marilyn began her periods at age 14; they were always heavy and often irregular, especially in the years before her menopause. She had a dilatation and curettage performed in her late 40s, but this showed nothing abnormal. She has had only one pregnancy, her daughter, conceived after 5 years of marriage; she would have liked more children, but 'it just didn't happen'.

Marilyn has type 2 diabetes, diagnosed 5 years ago. She tries to stick to a good diet but admits she finds it difficult and freely agrees she is overweight at 102 kg. She takes metformin for diabetic control and also states that she has high blood pressure. Dr Case has listed lisinopril among her medications. Marilyn has a family history of heart disease and diabetes on both sides. Her mother died from breast cancer in her 60s and Marilyn says she herself is careful to have regular mammograms—more careful than she is about her cervical screening tests. Marilyn has had a cholecystectomy and appendicectomy in the past and her one child was born by caesarean section and weighed 4530 g.

General physical examination shows a woman of late middle age who is definitely obese; you calculate a BMI of 40. Her blood pressure is 130/90 mmHg. Examination of the cardiovascular system and abdomen is unremarkable, although obesity limits the value of abdominal palpation.

At this point the results of Marilyn's CST and pelvic ultrasound reach you by fax. The CST is reported normal, with no HPV detected. The ultrasound scan shows a uterus of normal size (8 cm in length) with a thickened endometrium; the endometrial stripe measures 13 mm. The ovaries are small and no cysts or other abnormalities are visualised.

Does Marilyn need a further vaginal examination?

There is no need to perform another vaginal examination for Marilyn at this point. You have all the information you need from the general practitioner's letter and the ultrasound report. You note from Dr Case's letter that she observed a degree of atrophic vaginitis at the time of performing the CST but no visible cervical abnormality. Possibly the atrophic vaginitis was, in fact, the source of the vaginal bleeding. However, you must explain the implications of the findings of the thickened endometrium to Marilyn, including the very probable diagnosis of endometrial cancer and what this will entail.

> Atrophic vaginitis is the most common cause of postmenopausal bleeding. However, all women presenting with postmenopausal bleeding, even when atrophic vaginitis is present, must be investigated fully to exclude endometrial cancer, which is the most common gynaecological cancer. Cervical cancer may also be a cause of postmenopausal bleeding.

What information do you now give Marilyn?

The ultrasound scan, you tell her, when she is again dressed and sitting in the consulting room, shows some thickening of the lining of the uterus. The good news is that she has come along early. If endometrial cancer is confirmed, this is a type of cancer with a very good outlook, especially when found early. It is more common in women who have no or few children, women who are overweight and women who have diabetes, so Marilyn fits the bill on all counts.

Marilyn is more philosophical about this than you had expected. 'Of course,' she says, 'I will come for whatever treatment I need. What happens next?' she wants to know.

What further investigations and treatment are likely to be offered to Marilyn?

She will need a hysteroscopy, you explain, to completely visualise the inside of the uterus as well as a biopsy of the endometrium and pathological examination to make an accurate diagnosis. This procedure may be performed under general anaesthesia and increasingly as an outpatient procedure.

Predisposing factors to endometrial cancer

- Age—more common in older women who are either perimenopausal or postmenopausal
- History of early onset of menarche, late menopause
- Obesity
- Type 2 diabetes mellitus
- Endometrial hyperplasia with atypia
- Unopposed exogenous oestrogen therapy
- Polycystic ovarian syndrome
- Tamoxifen therapy
- Western lifestyle possibly contributes.

Note: Women who have used the COCP for at least 2 years have a 40% reduction in the incidence of endometrial cancer.

 CLINICAL COMMENT

Stages of endometrial cancer

Staging is surgical, with hysterectomy and bilateral salpingo-oophorectomy, peritoneal washings for cytology and selective pelvic lymph node sampling (Table 52.1). The operation is commonly performed by laparoscopy but occasionally by laparotomy if clinically indicated. There may be consideration of non-surgical management, such as fertility sparing treatment, in young women who have not yet had children or women with significant co-morbidities. The most common approach in this situation is to treat with high-dose progestogens or insertion of the levonorgestrel-releasing intrauterine device (LNG-IUD). This is usually performed only on advice of the gynaecological oncologist.

319

Table 52.1 Stages of endometrial cancer

Stage	Description
I	Cancer remains in the body of the uterus
IA	Cancer is in the endometrium only
IB	Cancer has invaded less than half of the thickness of the myometrium
IC	Cancer has extended to more than half of the thickness of the myometrium
II	Tumour has extended to the cervix
III	Tumour has spread beyond the uterus but is still in the pelvic area
IV	There is more distant spread of the cancer

Current treatment of endometrial cancer is usually by a combination of surgery and radiotherapy. If the lesion is confined to the inner half of the uterus and is histologically well differentiated, hysterectomy and bilateral salpingo-oophorectomy are sufficient treatment. Higher stages and grades will need pelvic radiotherapy after surgery. Some histological types, including small cell and clear cell adenocarcinoma, are high risk. These cases usually require chemotherapy (Table 52.2).

Table 52.2 Five-year survival rates for endometrial cancer

Stage	5-year survival rate
I	95%
II	70–85%
III	50%
IV	10–30%

CLINICAL PEARLS

- All women presenting with a history of postmenopausal bleeding, however slight, should have endometrial (and cervical) cancer excluded.
- A physical examination, cervical screening test and ultrasound scan measuring the double layer endometrial thickness should always be performed. If the endometrium is clearly visualised and measures less than 4 mm in thickness, further investigation may not be needed and the woman may be monitored, as the risk of endometrial cancer is <1%. If there is a recurrence of PMB or if the endometrial thickness is 4 mm or more, hysteroscopy is advised to assess the endometrial cavity.

References and further reading

Amant F, Mirza MR, Koskas M, Creutzberg CL. Cancer of the corpus uteri: FIGO cancer report 2018. *Int J Gynecol Obstet.* 2018;143(Suppl 2):37–50.

Cancer Council. Optimal care pathway for women with endometrial cancer. Sydney: Cancer Council; 2020. www.cancer.org.au/health-professionals /optimal-cancer-care-pathways

Cancer Council. Understanding cancer of the uterus: a guide for women with cancer, their families and friends. Sydney: Cancer Council; 2019. www .cancer.org.au/assets/pdf/understanding-uterus-cancer-booklet

Royal College of Obstetricians and Gynaecologists. Management of endometrial hyperplasia. RCOG and British Society for Gynaecological Endoscopy joint guideline. Green-top Guideline No. 67. London: RCOG; 2016. www.rcog.org .uk/guidelines

Case 53
Barbara is bothered by 'leaking'...

Barbara is a 54-year-old woman who has noticed worsening urinary incontinence for the last 3 years. She also has noticed a 'lump' protruding through her vagina, which now is beginning to bother her. Initially Barbara noticed the lump while taking a shower, and was frightened she may have found a cancer. Then she remembered that her mother had had a prolapse and realised that this was probably what was happening to her as well. At first it didn't bother her too much, but the bulge from her vagina is present on most days and although not painful, is certainly uncomfortable. Barbara is fond of gardening and the lump is particularly bad after spending a day lifting, carrying and digging in the garden. She has been putting up with both the incontinence and the prolapse, but has now decided enough is enough and has come to the gynaecology outpatients department with a referral from her general practitioner to 'have it all fixed'.

At the beginning of the consultation Barbara explains that she has been reading about 'mesh' and 'all of the problems it causes', saying that her friends have warned her not to have any type of mesh operation to treat her problems.

> 'You have to fix me,' says Barbara, 'but I flatly refuse to have mesh put inside me.'

You take some time explaining that being able to help manage Barbara's problems will involve taking a careful history, examining her carefully and likely arranging further tests.

> First, when does she lose urine?
> 'When I cough and sneeze mainly, and sometimes if I run quickly or run up the steps at home.'

> How long has this been happening?
> *'About 3 or 4 years—it seems to have worsened since I went through the menopause when I was 49.'*

What further questions should be asked?

Barbara should be asked several direct questions:

- 'Do you ever need to pass urine in a hurry, or sometimes not make it to the toilet and have an accident?'—'Yes, this does happen sometimes but not often.'
- 'Do you need to get up at night to empty your bladder?'—'Once or twice a night.'
- 'Do you need to wear any continence protection pads?'—'Yes, I buy them from the supermarket and I need to use them every day.'
- 'Do you have urinary frequency, burning or stinging when you pass urine, blood in the urine or bowel problems?'—Barbara answers 'no' to all these.

CLINICAL COMMENT

- There are four types of incontinence in women—true incontinence (usually due to a urinary fistula, rare in developed countries), overflow incontinence (less common than in men, as it occurs with urinary obstruction), genuine urinary stress incontinence and urinary urge incontinence.
- The latter two are the most important and by far the most common. Stress incontinence is more common than urge incontinence, but women who seek treatment commonly have features of both—mixed incontinence.
- Stress incontinence—the involuntary loss of urine with increased intra-abdominal pressure, such as caused by sneezing, coughing, jumping or exercise—can be embarrassing and distressing. It usually is due to loss of support at the bladder neck resulting in a hypermobile urethra, due to disruption of the pubo-urethral ligaments. This damage is often a result of childbirth and ageing, or more rarely a urinary sphincter mechanism deficiency. Certainly before any surgical treatment the diagnosis must be confirmed on urodynamic study.

continued

continued

- An overactive bladder—commonly leading to the clinical picture of 'urge incontinence'—may be secondary to poor bladder habits, but can also be due to 'detrusor overactivity' where the muscle of the bladder wall (the 'detrusor') contracts and empties at abnormally low volumes of urine and cannot be controlled by conscious effort.

What history do you take from Barbara relevant to her complaints of prolapse?

Barbara tells you that she has noticed this for the past 3 or 4 years and it is quite uncomfortable. There is no history of postmenopausal bleeding or discharge, although the lump does rub on her underwear, causing local irritation. She has four children, all born vaginally, the first baby being a forceps delivery. She is sexually active but the prolapse does make intercourse uncomfortable, and her vagina feels dry unless she uses lubrication. Barbara explains that when her rectum fills she sometimes is unable to empty her bowel, and occasionally needs to use a finger in the vagina to help empty her bowel. She is otherwise healthy and well; in particular, she is not obese, does not have any chronic lung conditions and is on no medication. Her cervical screening test is due and her last screening mammogram was 1 year ago.

What examination do you make for Barbara?

You perform a general examination and then an abdominal examination: the findings are unremarkable. You then carry out a vaginal examination. You note that the genital hiatus—the opening of the vagina—is quite open from her four births. You perform a Sims speculum examination in the left lateral position. You can demonstrate a cystocele coming just out of the vaginal opening when you ask her to 'bear down'. Elevating the cystocele with a pair of sponge-holding forceps, you note that the cervix descends on Valsalva manoeuvre almost to the level of the introitus. You take the cervical screening test. There is a small rectocele and her perineum is somewhat deficient. The vaginal wall is atrophic. With the speculum still in situ, you ask Barbara to cough and you see a small amount of urine leak out of the urethra. You remove the speculum and when Barbara returns to the supine position, you perform a bimanual vaginal examination to check the size of the uterus and to exclude any adnexal masses. The examination findings are normal.

> Barbara then asks, *'So what do you think, doctor? I hope that I don't need an operation. Is there anything else that can be done?'*

You explain to Barbara that from your examination you believe she is experiencing mostly stress incontinence and that she has a pelvic organ prolapse. You further explain that conservative forms of therapy are important to try in the first instance. Although they may not 'cure' the prolapse, her symptoms may be greatly improved.

> Barbara asks about ring pessaries, saying that she had an aunt who used one.

You explain that pessaries are a possible treatment but typically are reserved for elderly or infirm women who wish to avoid, or may be unsuitable for, surgery. The pessary, inserted by a doctor and checked every 4–6 months, when it may be changed, lies transversely in the vagina, resting behind the pubic symphysis and in the posterior fornix, thereby supporting the uterovaginal prolapse. The use of a pessary is probably not a first option for Barbara as she is relatively young, in good health and sexually active. You arrange a referral to a continence adviser at your hospital, as well as an MSU to exclude infection—this is reported as negative.

Conservative approach to prolapse and incontinence

- Topical oestrogen therapy will treat atrophy of the vaginal and urethral epithelium in postmenopausal women, and may result in some improvement of symptoms.
- Pelvic floor exercises as coached by a trained health professional, such as a continence adviser or a physiotherapist, can result in significant improvement in the symptoms of prolapse and stress incontinence. Even if surgery is performed, pelvic floor exercises should be practised regularly to maintain the pelvic floor muscle's strength and tone.
- Bladder retraining (bladder drill) can improve symptoms of urinary urgency and urge incontinence—remember that these are not treated surgically.

> Two months later you see Barbara again. *'How are you getting on?'* you ask her.

'Doctor, I feel as if I have improved but the prolapse is still there, and I still have to wear a pad for the incontinence,' Barbara tells you. 'I think I would like to consider surgery after all.'

Does Barbara need further investigation before surgery is offered?

Yes. Before any continence surgery is offered it is mandatory that urodynamic studies be undertaken to confirm or clarify the diagnosis. If the formal urodynamic study shows that involuntary urine loss occurs with coughing—in the absence of detruser activity—then a diagnosis of genuine stress incontinence is confirmed. Detrusor overactivity is confirmed by the rise of detrusor pressure at abnormally low bladder volumes. The tests are measured, recorded and adjusted by computers.

Barbara has urodynamic studies performed and stress incontinence is confirmed. When you see Barbara to explain the findings, she is apprehensive about the use of a mid-urethral tape to control the stress incontinence. Naturally you spend some time explaining that a large body of evidence supports the safety and efficacy of sling procedures in the management of stress urinary incontinence that has not responded to an adequate trial of conservative treatments. A large amount of material, including video presentations and detailed evidence-based patient information pamphlets, is available to assist in counselling and decision-making.

A vaginal hysterectomy and pelvic floor repair is initially recommended by your consultant, to be followed by a retropubic tape 3 months later, as it is her normal practice not to perform these procedures simultaneously. Barbara agrees to this recommendation.

 CLINICAL COMMENT

Treatment for prolapse and incontinence

- Detrusor overactivity commonly can be treated with anticholinergic medications, such as oxybutinin and solifenacin. Side effects such as a dry mouth or blurred vision are common. It is important to advise patients that these side effects may occur.

- Urinary stress incontinence not responsive to conservative treatments is typically managed with placement of a mid-urethral tape. The retropubic approach is the most effective and safest, and may be placed under local anaesthetic or regional block. The other approach, the use of stitches of the lateral upper vagina to the posterior ligaments of the pubic rami—a Burch procedure—remains an option for some women. In view of the controversy around the use of mesh, it is important that substantial assessment and counselling are undertaken before using a tape procedure.
- Surgery for pelvic organ prolapse also has been a contentious issue. After a re-evaluation of surgical approaches using transvaginal mesh, these largely have been abandoned. The current recommendations are that surgical repairs using a woman's native tissues are the first-line treatment. Management of uterine prolapse commonly involves vaginal hysterectomy. Additional surgical steps are used to provide support to the upper vagina and reduce the risk of prolapse of the vault. These include suspensions to the deep ligaments of the pelvis such as the sacrospinous ligament.

The follow-up visit

Six months later you see Barbara again in the outpatients department. It is now 6 months since the second procedure; all has gone well with her surgery.

'I'm very happy, doctor. My prolapse is gone, and I'm much more comfortable. I'm still using the oestrogen cream you gave me, and I do the pelvic floor exercises every day. I don't need to wear pads anymore, which is fantastic. I feel like I've got my life back!'

You tell Barbara you are very happy things have improved for her and refer her back to her general practitioner, reminding her that although she no longer requires cervical screening she still needs regular mammograms.

CLINICAL PEARLS

- All women should be encouraged to perform pelvic floor exercises regularly. Women should be assessed at postnatal visits for pelvic floor strength and referred to a physiotherapist or continence adviser if instruction in how to perform pelvic floor exercises is required.

continued

continued

- Women who have undergone total hysterectomy (i.e. with removal of the cervix) and who have never had previous cervical abnormalities no longer require cervical screening. However, if there have been prior abnormalities with or without treatment, regular smears of the vaginal vault are recommended.

References and further reading

Aoki Y, Brown HW, Brubaker L, et al. Urinary incontinence in women. *Nat Rev Dis Primers*. 2017;3:17042.

Dietz HP. Pelvic organ prolapse—a review. *Aust Fam Physician*. 2015;44(7): 446–52.

Hu JS, Pierre EF. Urinary incontinence in women: evaluation and management. *Am Fam Physician*. 2019;100(6):339–48.

Multiple-choice questions

1. An 18-year-old nulliparous woman presents asking for effective contraception. She has been advised to take the combined oral contraceptive pill (COCP) but is worried about the side effects. She is a non-smoker. Which of the following statements is likely to be most applicable to her situation?
    A. Third-generation combined oral contraceptive pills are associated with lower risks of thromboembolic disease than the second-generation COCPs.
    B. Although younger women are at slightly increased risk of breast cancer with the use of the COCP, the risk returns to normal 10 years after discontinuation of the pill.
    C. Intramuscular medroxyprogesterone acetate (DMPA) given every 3 months is a more effective alternative and can help to reduce her menstrual loss.
    D. The use of the COCP reduces the risk of cervical cancer, as oestrogen modifies the cervical environment by changing the nature of the transformation zone.
    E. Taking an active pill every day with no break for withdrawal bleeds is not advised as it is important for women to have a withdrawal bleed from time to time.

2. A 27-year-old woman is seen at 6 weeks following a normal vaginal birth. She is well and plans to fully breastfeed her infant for 6 months. She seeks advice about reliable contraception. Which of the following statements is true?
    A. Three-monthly depot medroxyprogesterone acetate (DMPA) injections are unsuitable when she is breastfeeding, as she is likely to develop osteoporosis.
    B. The progestogen-only pill (POP) is unsuitable for her as she is likely to develop atrophic vaginitis and dyspareunia.
    C. The etonorgestrel rod is unsuitable for her as she is likely to have significant vaginal bleeding.
    D. The combined oral contraceptive pill (COCP) is unsuitable for her as it may inhibit lactation.
    E. The levonorgestrel intrauterine contraceptive device is unsuitable for her until at least 6 months.

3. **In regard to cervical screening, the cervical screening test (CST) replaced the Pap test in Australia. Which statement below is applicable to the new screening test?**
   A. The 2-yearly Pap test for people aged 18 to 69 has been replaced by a 5-yearly human papillomavirus (HPV) test for people aged 25 to 74.
   B. The new CST is as accurate as the Pap test in identifying premalignant conditions of the cervix but is a cheaper test and thus more cost-effective.
   C. The time between tests has changed from 2 to 5 years only in women who have had the HPV vaccine.
   D. The age at which screening starts has increased from 18 years to 20 years.
   E. The cervical screening test is accurate as it tests for abnormal cervical cells.

4. **Heavy menstrual bleeding:**
   A. can be diagnosed by history alone of heavy vaginal bleeding.
   B. often responds well to the use of the levonorgestrel intrauterine system.
   C. can be diagnosed by pipelle sampling (endometrial biopsy) alone.
   D. is most effectively treated by endometrial ablation.
   E. should never be treated with the COCP (combined oral contraceptive pill).

5. **A 13-year-old girl presents to her GP with heavy periods, cycle 7/28 days, menarche at age 11. Which of the following statements is true?**
   A. Von Willebrand disease is the most common bleeding diathesis causing menorrhagia at this age.
   B. If clinical examination is unremarkable, she should be commenced on tranexamic acid without further investigations.
   C. If clinical examination is unremarkable, she should be commenced on a non-steroidal anti-inflammatory drug without further investigations.
   D. The combined oral contraceptive pill should not be prescribed for girls of this age as skeletal growth is not completed.
   E. Hypothyroidism is a common cause of menorrhagia at this age.

6. **For the diagnosis of polycystic ovarian syndrome:**
   A. ultrasound appearance alone is sufficient.
   B. acne, hirsutism and/or obesity must be clinically evident.
   C. evidence of either oligo-ovulation or anovulation, or clinical or biochemical hyperandrogenism, must be present.
   D. full glucose tolerance testing should be performed.
   E. the diagnosis can be excluded if normal menstrual cycles are present.

7. **In general practice you see a healthy 12-year-old girl describing severe dysmenorrhoea. Her menarche was at the age of 10 years. She has regular menstrual cycles. She is not sexually active. Which of the following statements is true?**
   A. She most likely has endometriosis and should have magnetic resonance imaging (MRI) done.
   B. It is inappropriate to offer information about sexually transmitted infections and their prevention at this consultation.
   C. She should have a cervical screening test and bimanual vaginal examination before being prescribed the combined oral contraceptive pill (COCP).
   D. Nonsteroidal anti-inflammatory drugs (NSAIDs) used prior to the onset of the periods are effective at preventing formation of prostaglandins in the endometrium, reducing future pain.
   E. She should be told that side effects including nausea, headache and breakthrough bleeding generally settle down within 3 to 6 months of commencing the COCP.

8. **A 60-year-old woman presents with vulval pruritus. Biopsy of the vulvar lesion confirmed lichen sclerosus. Which of the following statements is true?**
   A. She should be told there is a 10% risk of vulvar cancer in women with lichen sclerosus.
   B. She should be told that the condition is chronic and may benefit from intermittent treatment with high-dose topical steroids.
   C. She should be told the condition is related to human papilloma virus infection, stressing the importance of having a yearly HPV screen.
   D. Lichen sclerosus may progress to vulval intraepithelial neoplasia (VIN, low-grade or high-grade lesions) and can be diagnosed on inspection only.
   E. Hormone replacement therapy is protective against lichen sclerosus.

9. **A 30-year-old gravida 5 para 4 woman presenting for a surgical termination of pregnancy is also requesting tubal sterilisation. She had been using condoms for contraception. Which of the following statements is correct with respect to tubal sterilisation?**
   A. There is emerging evidence that bilateral salpingectomy may prevent the occurrence of germ cell tumours of the ovaries in later life.
   B. Her partner should give his consent to the procedure.
   C. She should be quite certain she will not wish to have children in the future.
   D. There will be no change in her menstrual cycles after the procedure.
   E. Performing tubal sterilisation at the time of surgical abortion may be associated with more bleeding due to the richer blood supply in pregnancy.

10. **Rhesus (D) negative non-sensitised women who become pregnant:**
    A. who have already had their routine anti-D prophylaxis at 28 and 34 weeks' gestation do not need further anti-D prophylaxis if they present with antepartum haemorrhage at 36 weeks' gestation.
    B. do not need to be given anti-D following surgical evacuation of incomplete miscarriage (D&C) in the first trimester of pregnancy.
    C. should be offered anti-D after an external cephalic version, even if the procedure is not successful.
    D. need to be given anti-D following early medical abortion.
    E. do not need to be given anti-D if they undergo surgical abortion.

11. **Antenatal care involves routine screening and regular examination of the pregnant woman to help ensure that her pregnancy is progressing normally with regard to maternal and fetal health. Which of the following statements describes appropriate antenatal care in an uncomplicated pregnancy?**
    A. Routine ultrasound scan for fetal growth should be offered in the third trimester.
    B. Higher levels of folate preparations prior to and during pregnancy are required to reduce the risk of neural tube defects.
    C. Routine first-trimester blood tests include screening for maternal anaemia, hepatitis B and syphilis.
    D. Measurement of symphysial fundal height is subjective and not a useful tool to screen for intrauterine growth restriction.
    E. Random blood glucose testing in the first trimester is a good screen for gestational diabetes mellitus.

12. **The incidence of primary cytomegalovirus (CMV) infection in pregnancy in Australia is estimated to be 6 per 1000 pregnancies. Most primary CMV infections are asymptomatic but carry a 50% risk of transmission to the fetus. Which of the following statements is true?**
    A. All pregnant women should be offered vaccination against CMV infection from 20 weeks' gestation.
    B. CMV is shed in the saliva, breastmilk and urine, and can be transmitted vertically from mother to the fetus.
    C. Diagnosis of CMV is best made by taking a nasopharyngeal swab to test for the viral RNA by PCR.
    D. Congenital CMV is difficult to detect during the antenatal period and is best detected in the postnatal period.
    E. Infants with CMV will always be jaundiced at birth.

13. **A 30-year-old woman with type 1 diabetes is in the 37th week of her first pregnancy. Blood sugar levels are well controlled. Which of the following statements is true?**
    A. Caesarean section should be performed at 38 weeks because the infant will have macrosomia.
    B. Delivery should be planned for a mutually acceptable time by 38 weeks.
    C. She can be allowed to continue beyond 40 weeks awaiting the spontaneous onset of labour.
    D. The infant is not at risk of respiratory distress syndrome as it will be born after 37 weeks' gestation.
    E. The infant is not likely to develop neonatal jaundice.

14. **A 24-year-old woman who has been an insulin-dependent diabetic since the age of 12 comes to consult you in general practice. She is currently taking the combined oral contraceptive pill (COCP) but is planning her first pregnancy and seeks your advice. You advise her that:**
    A. She needs to stop the COCP for at least 6 months and use barrier methods of contraception before trying to conceive.
    B. She can expect her insulin dose to remain unchanged during her pregnancy.
    C. Her diabetes poses no risks to the growth and development of her baby.
    D. She should take folic acid before and during the first trimester of pregnancy.
    E. She will be suitable for shared antenatal care with a midwife clinic.

15. **A 39-year-old woman presents to the antenatal clinic for the first time at 12 weeks of pregnancy. This was a spontaneous conception. An ultrasound scan ordered by her general practitioner has revealed a dichorionic diamniotic pregnancy. Which of the following is true?**
    A. Her twins cannot be identical.
    B. Screening for fetal nuchal translucency (FNT) should not be offered to women with multiple pregnancy as there is no reference range of measurements.
    C. Twin-to-twin transfusion syndrome is a serious complication that is likely to occur, and she should be closely monitored for this.
    D. She should take an iron-folate preparation if she is not already doing so.
    E. She should be advised to undergo chorionic villus sampling (CVS) to rule out Down syndrome in the fetuses.

16. A woman aged 40 has difficulty conceiving. She has two children from a past relationship aged 10 and 14. She has a new partner also aged 40 who has one son aged 12. She has a history of hypothyroidism that has been well managed with thyroxine for many years. The couple have been having regular unprotected intercourse for 12 months. Her failure to conceive is most likely to be due to—
    A. reduced frequency of sexual intercourse.
    B. ageing of the endometrium.
    C. erectile dysfunction in the male partner.
    D. the effects of the thyroxine therapy.
    E. decreased quality of the woman's oocytes.

17. A 32-year-old woman is referred to the gynaecological outpatients as she wishes to become pregnant but has not conceived after 12 months of unprotected sexual intercourse. Her partner aged 34 is stated to be in good health. Which of the following is true?
    A. It is highly desirable that her partner present himself for a full history and examination.
    B. Laparoscopy should be arranged at an early date to assess tubal patency.
    C. She should be immediately referred for IVF (in vitro fertilisation) as this is most likely to result in a successful full-term pregnancy.
    D. A history of regular menstrual cycles is positive proof of ovulation.
    E. The results of her partner's seminal analysis should be considered before proceeding to invasive investigations in the woman.

18. A 45-year-old woman presents with a painless abdominal swelling. She had two children by caesarean section and later underwent tubal sterilisation. She has no menstrual symptoms and has had a recent normal cervical screening test. Examination revealed a mass arising from the pelvis up to the level of the umbilicus. Which of the following statements is true?
    A. Magnetic resonance imaging (MRI) is an important first-line investigation as it will help to identify whether the mass is benign or malignant.
    B. An urgent laparoscopy should be arranged to obtain peritoneal washings and biopsy.
    C. Ultrasound scan will confirm if a cystic ovarian lesion is present and identify characteristics of the cyst, which when combined with tumour markers will help to estimate the risk of malignancy.
    D. The tumour marker CA125 is a sensitive but non-specific test for epithelial ovarian malignancy.
    E. Fine-needle biopsy of ovarian masses should be part of the initial investigation.

19. A 22-year-old woman who is 20 weeks' pregnant has a positive PCR result for chlamydia in a first-catch urine specimen. She returns without her partner to the antenatal clinic for advice and treatment. You advise her that:
    A. she cannot be treated with azithromycin because she is pregnant, but her partner can be treated with this drug.
    B. chlamydia may occur in conjunction with other sexually transmitted infections, and both she and her partner should be screened for these.
    C. infection in women is confined to the lower genital tract, and there is no risk to the fetus.
    D. her partner does not need testing because she says he has no symptoms.
    E. she can be treated with doxycycline as she is past the first trimester of pregnancy.

20. Chlamydial infection of the female genital tract:
    A. is often asymptomatic.
    B. may be detected by PCR testing of first-catch urine specimens, which has a sensitivity of around 50%.
    C. is not associated with later infertility in the woman.
    D. can be effectively treated with a single dose of ceftriaxone.
    E. can be effectively treated with a single dose of doxycycline.

21. In regard to postnatal depression:
    A. it cannot be predicted antenatally.
    B. it is common and affects around 13% of women.
    C. about 3% of women progress to postpartum psychosis if not treated.
    D. antidepressants are not advised for lactating women.
    E. extended family members are the best form of support for women with postnatal depression.

22. Women with postnatal depression:
    A. should be encouraged to be admitted to the mother and baby unit for close monitoring and treatment.
    B. can be managed and supported by their GPs in most cases.
    C. must be advised to go out as much as possible with their baby.
    D. should stop breastfeeding.
    E. or symptoms suggestive of postnatal depression should be referred to see a psychiatrist.

23. A 48-year-old woman seeks treatment from her general practitioner for hot flushes. Her last menstrual period was 6 months previously

and she has had no abnormal vaginal bleeding. Which of the following statements is true?

A. She has reached her menopause.

B. It is essential to measure levels of follicle stimulating hormone (FSH) before prescribing hormone replacement therapy (hormone therapy).

C. She should be advised that hormone replacement therapy (hormone therapy) is associated with a significant increase in the incidence of breast and bowel cancer.

D. Part of her management will include lifestyle measures and the recommendation of a daily calcium supplement.

E. Her age of menopause will be the same as her mother's.

24. **In regard to cervical cancer which statement is correct?**

A. Adenocarcinoma is the most common histological type.

B. High-risk serotypes of human papilloma virus (HPV) are responsible for the development of the disease.

C. Cervical tumours only have an exophytic growth pattern.

D. Patients with early stage disease often present with irregular vaginal bleeding.

E. The inguinal lymph nodes are frequently involved in cervical cancer.

25. **A 22-year-old nulliparous woman presents having had unplanned and unprotected sex 12 hours previously. Her cycles are regular, 5/28 days, and her last menstrual period began 11 days earlier. Which of the following is true?**

A. The use of ulipristal acetate as a 'morning-after pill' will be highly effective at preventing pregnancy.

B. Oral levonorgestrel (1500 μg) if taken immediately will be 75–85% effective at preventing pregnancy.

C. If she takes oral levonorgestrel but the pregnancy continues there is a significant risk of fetal abnormality.

D. There is no possibility that she will become pregnant on day 11 when she has regular 28-day cycles.

E. Injection of medroxyprogesterone acetate (DMPA) at this consultation will be highly effective at preventing pregnancy.

26. **A 35-year-old woman is seen for counselling following surgical evacuation of a complete molar pregnancy at 10 weeks' gestation. She has had one other pregnancy in the past which ended in a normal**

vaginal birth, and is keen to try for a second child as soon as possible. Which of the following statements is true?

A. She has a 50% risk of recurrence of molar pregnancy in her next pregnancy.

B. She can be advised that she can try to conceive again following the return of normal menstrual cycles, a negative β-hCG test and completion of 6 months of follow-up.

C. She should be advised to have an intrauterine device inserted at 6 weeks as this is an effective form of non-hormonal contraception.

D. She is not suitable to take the combined oral contraceptive pill (COCP).

E. Monthly ultrasound scans should be performed to rule out the development of persisting molar pregnancy.

27. **Which of the following is not a cause of dyspareunia?**
    A. Psychological cause
    B. Endometriosis
    C. Lactation
    D. Urinary tract infection
    E. Vulvovaginitis

28. **In a young woman presenting with a vaginal discharge, it is important to consider which of the the following in the management?**
    A. She may be on the combined oral contraceptive pill.
    B. She may have a urinary tract infection.
    C. She may have a vaginal prolapse.
    D. The cause may be vaginal varicosities.
    E. She may have a urethral caruncle.

29. **A 14-year-old girl presents to her general practitioner with a history of recurrent lower abdominal pain. She has not had her periods yet and is not yet sexually active. Examination shows normal secondary sexual characteristics and a mass arising out of the pelvis to just above the symphysis pubis. Which of the following statements is true?**
    A. The pain is likely to be psychological in origin.
    B. She should be prescribed tranexamic acid for the pain.
    C. Transabdominal pelvic ultrasound may be an appropriate investigation.
    D. She should be advised to start the combined oral contraceptive pill immediately.
    E. She should be advised to have an etonorgestrel implant.

30. A 23-year-old primigravid woman in labour undergoes two vaginal examinations 4 hours apart. On both occasions the cervix is found to be 6 cm dilated with the fetal head in an occipito-posterior position 2 cm above the ischial spines. The fetal heart tracing (CTG) is variable and reactive with a baseline rate of 140 beats per minute. Which of the following is true?
    A. She should be immediately consented for caesarean section.
    B. It may be appropriate to start an oxytocin infusion.
    C. She should be reassured about her own and her baby's wellbeing and re-examined in another 4 hours.
    D. Fetal scalp blood sampling for lactate level is immediately indicated.
    E. She can be transferred out of the birth suite as she is not yet in established labour.

31. In the medical management of postpartum haemorrhage:
    A. misoprostol is the most effective third-stage prophylactic agent to prevent postpartum haemorrhage.
    B. carboprost should be administered when an oxytocin infusion is set up to manage uterine atony.
    C. bolus doses of intravenous oxytocin are contraindicated in women with pre-eclampsia.
    D. 1000 mg of tranexamic acid should be administered orally.
    E. tranexamic acid has been shown in large trials to reduce maternal mortality.

32. Preeclampsia:
    A. is always associated with growth restriction of the fetus.
    B. is always associated with oedema of the lower limbs.
    C. is always treated with magnesium sulphate.
    D. has headache as the most common presenting symptom.
    E. is more common in women with preexisting hypertension.

33. A 38-year-old woman gravida 4, with three previous full-term deliveries, presents at 36 weeks of pregnancy with headache, blurring of vision and ankle swelling. She has a history of hypertension prior to the pregnancy. Ward testing of urine reveals 3+ protein. Your management is likely to include:
    A. weekly ultrasound scans to assess fetal growth over the next 4 weeks.
    B. prescribing increased doses of her oral hypertensive therapy.
    C. antibiotics for probable urinary tract infection.
    D. admission to hospital and immediate caesarean section.
    E. admission to hospital for observation and consideration of early induction of labour.

34. In the assessment of a woman with a raised blood pressure at 28 weeks' gestation, which of the following is correct?

A. It is important to quantitatively assess the amount of proteinuria by a 24-hour collection of urine or a spot protein:creatinine ratio.

B. If she does not report epigastric pain or headache, she may be treated as an outpatient.

C. Weekly ultrasound scan for fetal growth is important to exclude IUGR once pre-eclampsia is diagnosed.

D. HELLP syndrome is unlikely at this gestation.

E. Magnesium sulphate should be given routinely to prevent progression to pre-eclampsia.

35. In regard to hypertension in pregnancy:

A. antihypertensive treatment in mild to moderate pre-eclampsia is useful for the prevention of cerebrovascular complications.

B. antihypertensive treatment in pre-eclampsia improves placental perfusion.

C. women with chronic (essential) hypertension may be managed on an outpatient basis in the day assessment unit.

D. low-dose aspirin is helpful for control of blood pressure in women with hypertension in pregnancy.

E. once the blood pressure is well controlled in women with essential hypertension, the risk of superimposed pre-eclampsia is significantly reduced.

36. In the management of hypertension in pregnancy:

A. it is important to keep the diastolic blood pressure below 90 mmHg.

B. it is important to commence antihypertensive treatment if the systolic BP is persistently > 150 mmHg.

C. in pre-eclampsia, when the woman is oedematous, treatment of the hypertension should involve the use of diuretics.

D. oedema is an important sign of pre-eclampsia.

E. when hypertension is noted, CTG should be performed as CTG abnormalities are frequently seen when the blood pressure is elevated.

37. Regarding the management of preterm labour:

A. vaginal progesterone is an effective medication to suppress preterm contractions.

B. the purpose of administration of corticosteroids in preterm labour is to suppress maternal steroid production to suppress labour.

C. administration of corticosteroids is known to reduce the risk of neonatal morbidity and mortality from respiratory distress syndrome.
D. the fetal fibronectin test is a useful test to indicate if a woman has experienced spontaneous rupture of membranes.
E. indomethacin is contraindicated in the management of preterm labour as it causes premature closure of the sinus venosus.

38. Postpartum haemorrhage following antepartum haemorrhage:
A. is always due to coagulation defects.
B. should be anticipated before delivery and active prophylaxis instituted.
C. is very uncommon.
D. is more common in women having their first baby than among multiparae.
E. should be immediately treated by the transfusion of whole blood.

39. A gravida 2 para 1 woman presents at 30 weeks' gestation with painless unprovoked vaginal bleeding. She had an uncomplicated pregnancy and normal delivery previously. Her 20-week scan showed a low-lying anterior placenta. Which of the following statements is true?
A. As only 5% of placentas remain low in the third trimester, it is likely that her placenta has 'migrated' and no further ultrasound scan is necessary at this stage.
B. Emergency caesarean section is indicated.
C. Vaginal examination is not contraindicated as it is important to exclude preterm labour.
D. Speculum examination should be performed to exclude other causes of the bleeding .
E. Abruptio placentae is the most likely diagnosis.

40. In regard to diabetes in pregnancy:
A. there is poor correlation between the HbA1c level and the perinatal outcome.
B. pre-eclampsia is a complication of diabetes in pregnancy.
C. IUGR is commonly seen in women with poor glycaemic control.
D. the insulin requirements usually drop towards term.
E. high maternal sugar levels are a response to hyperinsulinaemia in the fetus.

41. In the screening and management of diabetes in pregnancy:
A. the 50 g glucose challenge test carried out at 26 weeks' gestation has a high sensitivity for the diagnosis of gestational diabetes mellitus.
B. metformin is not contraindicated in the management of diabetes in pregnancy.

C. long-acting insulin is best for glycaemic control in pregnancy.

D. only babies born to type 1 diabetics are at risk of hypoglycaemia postnatally.

E. macrosomia is never seen in women with tight control of their diabetes.

42. **A 30-year-old woman with insulin-dependent diabetes is at 37 weeks of pregnancy. Which of the following statements is true?**

A. She has no higher risk of stillbirth than the general population.

B. She should be delivered by elective caesarean section at 38 weeks.

C. She should be managed during delivery using insulin doses calculated according to the results of regular blood glucose measurement.

D. Insulin requirements will decrease slowly over 3–4 days postpartum.

E. Her infant will not develop hypoglycaemia if her antenatal blood sugars are well controlled.

43. **In twin pregnancy:**

A. perinatal mortality is as high as five times that of singleton pregnancies.

B. monochorionic monoamniotic (MCMA) twins can also be non-identical.

C. dichorionic diamniotic (DCDA) twins are always a result of the fertilisation of two eggs (ova).

D. MCDA twins must be delivered by caesarean section.

E. DCDA twins are always non-identical.

44. **In regard to multiple pregnancy:**

A. the condition is more common in younger women.

B. postpartum haemorrhage is more common due to genital tract trauma from vaginal delivery.

C. in the conduct of vaginal delivery of twins, the second twin must be delivered within 10 minutes of the first twin.

D. it is important to carry out ultrasound scans on a fortnightly basis for MCDA twins from 16 weeks' gestation to monitor for twin-to-twin transfusion syndrome.

E. antepartum haemorrhage is a common complication of twins due to abruption.

45. **A 20-year-old woman presents at 36 weeks of pregnancy with recurrent herpes genitalis (HSV-2) infection on the perineum. Which of the following statements is true?**

A. Aciclovir or valaciclovir administration from 36 weeks to delivery will reduce the chance of a further outbreak at the time of delivery.

B. Immediate caesarean section is indicated.

C. Elective caesarean at 38 weeks' gestation is indicated.

D. HSV-2 commonly crosses the placenta close to term and may cause intrauterine encephalitis.

E. HSV-2 poses no risk at all to the baby in a recurrent episode.

46. Placental abruption:
   A. always presents with vaginal bleeding.
   B. is more common in primigravidae than multiparae.
   C. is a potential complication of attempted external cephalic version for breech presentation.
   D. is not more common in twin pregnancy.
   E. is commonly associated with hypertension in pregnancy.

47. Hyperemesis gravidarum:
   A. always requires admission to hospital.
   B. always requires termination of the pregnancy.
   C. occurs in 1:100 pregnancies.
   D. is always psychosomatic in origin.
   E. is not associated with multiple pregnancy.

48. Breech presentation:
   A. occurs in about 10% of full-term pregnancies.
   B. is not associated with fetal abnormality.
   C. is not associated with a higher perinatal mortality rate than cephalic presentation if vaginal birth is attempted.
   D. occurs in about 15% of pregnancies at 30 weeks' gestation.
   E. will not convert spontaneously to cephalic presentation after 37 weeks of pregnancy.

49. A gravida 3 para 2 woman arrives in the birthing unit at 35 weeks' gestation with a history of ruptured membranes and a sensation of something in between her legs. She is having three contractions every 10 minutes. At her last antenatal visit she was diagnosed to have breech presentation and is due to see a specialist next week. Examination shows a loop of cord at the introitus. What would be the correct course of action?
   A. Do a vaginal examination and push the presenting part upwards to avoid compression on the cord but do not handle the cord.
   B. Encourage her to push if she is fully dilated.
   C. Do a vaginal examination and push the cord into the vagina to keep it warm and moist.
   D. Arrange an elective caesarean section after giving steroids to mature the fetal lungs as she is still preterm.
   E. Give a tocolytic as she is contracting.

50. A 67-year-old woman presents to her GP with a history of one day's vaginal bleeding. Her last menstrual period was 15 years previously and she is on no medication. Physical examination is unremarkable apart from a marked degree of atrophic vaginitis. Which of the following immediate management options is most appropriate?
A. Reassurance and advice to return if bleeding continues
B. Topical oestrogen pessaries
C. Combined oral hormone therapy (oestrogen and progestogen)
D. Endometrial biopsy (pipelle) in surgery
E. Transvaginal ultrasound scan to assess the endometrial thickness

51. A 28-year-old woman presents with 8 weeks' amenorrhoea with severe lower abdominal crampy pains and vaginal bleeding. She had an ultrasound scan 2 weeks ago which demonstrated an intrauterine gestation sac. Blood pressure is 70/40, pulse rate 80 bpm, she is pale and afebrile, urinary β-hCG positive. Which statement is correct?
A. Order a CT scan to rule out a ruptured appendix.
B. She may be experiencing cervical shock from products of conception distending her cervix.
C. Order an urgent formal ultrasound scan in the medical imaging department and await the results.
D. Request blood tests for quantitative β-hCG to monitor viability of the pregnancy.
E. The woman should be consented for possible hysterectomy.

52. A 20-year-old woman presents to the emergency department (ED) with a 1-day history of lower abdominal pain. She had stopped the combined pill to try to conceive, and her last normal period was 7 weeks ago. Urine hCG in the ED is positive, and her vital signs show her BP 90/65 mmHg, pulse 100 bpm and her pain is getting worse. You suspect an ectopic pregnancy. Which of the following statements is incorrect?
A. The symptom of shoulder tip pain is indicative of haemoperitoneum irritating the liver and diaphragm.
B. Ultrasound scan may demonstrate an empty uterus.
C. Ectopic pregnancy may be managed medically with methotrexate provided the patient is stable and β-hCG level is less than 1500 IU/L with an unruptured empty sac.
D. Anti-D should be administered if she is Rhesus (D) negative.
E. Vaginal bleeding is common due to decidual shedding.

53. A painless lower abdominal swelling in a girl of 16 with a negative β-HCG test is most likely to be:
    A. pelvic kidney.
    B. hydrosalpinx.
    C. endometrioma.
    D. benign ovarian cyst.
    E. faecal impaction.

54. A 33-year-old woman presents seeking advice. She has had three consecutive first-trimester miscarriages. Which of the following statements is true?
    A. Recurrent miscarriage occurs in about 15–20% of women in the reproductive age group.
    B. Bed rest may help prevent recurrent miscarriage.
    C. The chance of successful full-term pregnancy after three miscarriages is less than 10%.
    D. Recurrent miscarriage may be prevented by taking 600 mg aspirin daily during early pregnancy.
    E. The cause of most cases of recurrent miscarriage is usually not identifiable.

55. A 27-year-old woman presents 6 weeks following her last menstrual period (LMP) with mild left iliac fossa pain and slight postcoital bleeding. Her general condition is good. A urinary β-hCG test is positive. Which of the following is correct?
    A. No vaginal examination should be performed until ultrasound scan has established that the placenta is not low-lying.
    B. Ultrasound is not useful at distinguishing intrauterine from extrauterine pregnancy at this gestation.
    C. Serial β-hCGs at weekly intervals are the most accurate way of making a diagnosis.
    D. Speculum examination should be carried out to check the cervical appearance and dilatation.
    E. Laparoscopy is necessary to reach a diagnosis.

56. A 28-year-old woman presents with 7 weeks of amenorrhoea, severe abdominal pain which is worse in the lower abdomen and slight vaginal bleeding. Her blood pressure is 90/55 mmHg, her pulse rate 110 bpm, and she is pale and afebrile with a positive urinary β-hCG. Which statement is correct?
    A. The most likely diagnosis is ruptured appendix.

B. The most likely diagnosis is ruptured spleen.

C. Urgent laparoscopy and possible laparotomy for possible ruptured ectopic pregnancy is indicated.

D. Ultrasound scan of the abdomen should be performed before making a decision about treatment.

E. The woman should be consented for possible hysterectomy.

57. **Genuine stress incontinence of urine:**

A. does not occur in conjunction with urge incontinence.

B. is not helped by pelvic floor exercises.

C. is not helped by lifestyle measures.

D. must be confirmed by urodynamic studies before surgical treatment is offered.

E. is best treated with anticholinergic medications.

58. **A 40-year-old woman is noted in the course of a well-woman check and cervical screening test to have a moderate degree of cystocoele (anterior vaginal wall prolapse). Which of the following is true?**

A. She should be referred for surgical repair of the cystocoele as this is likely to worsen as she approaches the menopause.

B. She should be given instruction in how to perform pelvic floor exercises if she is not already doing these.

C. Vaginal prolapse is associated with urge incontinence, which worsens as a woman ages.

D. The presence of a cystocoele indicates the need for a midstream urine examination for urinary tract infection.

E. She should be prescribed topical oestrogen cream to prevent irritation of the cystocoele.

59. **A 78-year-old woman consults her general practitioner with symptoms of urinary frequency, urinary burning and lower abdominal pain of recent onset. On examination she is found to have both a cystocoele and a rectocoele, with some irritation of the exposed vaginal epithelium. She underwent hysterectomy for fibroids at the age of 40. Which of the following is true?**

A. She should be fitted with a ring pessary to control her symptoms.

B. She should be referred for specialist management of her prolapse.

C. The most likely cause of symptoms is urinary tract infection.

D. The most likely cause of her symptoms is vaginitis.

E. The most likely cause of her symptoms is pelvic adhesions following her hysterectomy.

60. A nuchal translucency scan:
   A. is best performed in the first trimester as it will give measurements of the nuchal thickening of the fetus.
   B. is better at picking up chromosomal abnormalities when combined with serum alpha-fetoprotein (AFP).
   C. is diagnostic of a chromosomal abnormality when it is significantly increased.
   D. is a screening test that improves in sensitivity when combined with a maternal serum screen of AFP, pregnancy-associated plasma protein-A (PAPP-A) and β-hCG.
   E. is a less accurate screening test than maternal age for aneuploidy.

61. In regard to invasive testing for prenatal diagnosis, which of the following statements is true?
   A. Amniocentesis is generally associated with a 1% risk of miscarriage.
   B. CVS is best performed after 15 weeks' gestation to reduce the risk of miscarriage.
   C. Both amniocentesis and CVS allow for fluorescent in situ hybridisation (FISH) to be carried out in 48 hours in order to obtain a result to exclude the major aneuploidies.
   D. Anti-D injection is not necessary in a Rh-negative woman as long as there is no bleeding after an invasive test, as the risk of isoimmunisation will be low.
   E. Invasive testing is only available in specialised fetal medicine centres.

62. In regard to termination of pregnancy (TOP), which of the following statements is true?
   A. Counselling for women who request TOP is a legal requirement in the United Kingdom and Australia.
   B. TOP can be carried out only for fetal abnormalities and not maternal distress in Australia and the UK.
   C. Misoprostol alone is the most commonly used pharmacological agent for mid-trimester abortion.
   D. Surgical termination in the first trimester carries an increased risk of bleeding and trauma and is only available in specialised centres.
   E. Mifepristone facilitates the process of termination by blocking the progesterone receptors, increasing the sensitivity of the uterus to prostaglandin.

63. In regard to risk factors for secondary postpartum haemorrhage (PPH), which of the following statements is true?
   A. Retained placenta requiring manual removal is a significant risk factor.

B. Urinary tract infection in the postnatal period increases the risk of secondary PPH.

C. Prophylactic antibiotics do not reduce the risk of secondary PPH.

D. Endometritis is not usually associated with increased bleeding.

E. There is good correlation between the amount of blood loss in the immediate postpartum period and secondary PPH.

64. In the management of secondary postpartum haemorrhage (PPH):

A. surgical evacuation should be performed in women who present with heavy per vagina (PV) bleeding at 10 days' postpartum.

B. an ultrasound scan is a very accurate diagnostic tool for the confirmation of retained placenta.

C. fibroids remain the most common cause of secondary PPH.

D. antibiotics should always be started prior to surgical intervention.

E. the use of uterotonic drugs in secondary PPH does not reduce blood loss.

65. With secondary postpartum haemorrhage:

A. it is unusual for the woman to be shocked as the bleeding in secondary PPH is usually very light.

B. if there is concern that there may be a pelvic abscess, it is important to exclude this by laparoscopy, which will also allow the abscess to be drained.

C. intravenous antibiotics should always be administered.

D. the course is always complicated by coagulopathy.

E. broad-spectrum antibiotics may be used if the condition is stable enough for outpatient management of the condition.

66. In regard to influenza in pregnancy, which of the following statements is true?

A. Seasonal influenza is usually a mild disease and is associated with a full recovery, hence pregnant women should not be encouraged to be vaccinated.

B. The influenza vaccine is not contraindicated as it contains antibodies against the different strains of influenza viruses.

C. The A2009/H1N1 virus has now been eradicated by an active vaccination campaign.

D. Pregnant women who contract A2009/H1N1 influenza are at increased risk of being admitted to hospital.

E. The A2009/H1N1 virus has been shown to be associated with congenital limb deformities.

67. **In regard to viral infections in pregnancy, which of the following statements is true?**
   A. Chickenpox affecting the first trimester in pregnancy is associated with a high risk of fetal neurological complications.
   B. If a woman develops chickenpox at 38 weeks' gestation, she should be advised to be delivered by caesarean section as soon as possible to prevent transplacental spread of the virus.
   C. Maternal rubella infection in the first trimester is associated with the congenital rubella syndrome.
   D. Cytomegalovirus (CMV) infection is very common and most women have antibodies against it.
   E. Toxoplasmosis is spread by dog litter.

68. **A woman presents with a generalised, non-urticarial rash in the second trimester of pregnancy. Which of the following is true?**
   A. She should always be suspected to have obstetric cholestasis.
   B. A good history should be obtained, including that of a fever, flu-like symptoms and contact with others with similar symptoms, so that appropriate serological testing for a possible viral infection may be carried out.
   C. Having red cheeks in addition to the rash is indicative of toxoplasmosis.
   D. She should have an ultrasound scan to exclude intrauterine growth restriction.
   E. This presentation is typical of German measles.

69. **Bacterial vaginosis (BV):**
   A. is a rare cause of preterm labour.
   B. is caused by *Trichomonas vaginalis*.
   C. is diagnosed clinically by the presence of a thick white vaginal discharge.
   D. is associated with changes in normal vaginal flora.
   E. is completely cured by the use of probiotics.

70. **In regard to chronic pelvic inflammatory disease (PID), which of the following statements is true?**
   A. The condition always follows an STI of the genital tract.
   B. It is most commonly caused by *Neisseria gonorrhoeae*.
   C. Full courses of appropriate antibiotics can completely relieve symptoms.
   D. It is most often caused by the spread of bowel organisms from diverticulitis.
   E. Complete cure often requires surgical removal of the uterus and/or tubes and ovaries.

MULTIPLE CHOICE QUESTIONS

71. Chronic pelvic pain in a 35-year-old woman who has had three caesarean sections:

A. is most likely to be caused by endometriosis.

B. is most likely to be caused by PID.

C. is most likely to be caused by irritable bowel syndrome.

D. may be related to pelvic adhesions.

E. is likely to be psychological in origin.

72. A 36-year-old woman attends for a well-woman check and renewal of her prescription for the combined oral contraceptive pill (COCP). She smokes 10 cigarettes/day. Which of the following is true?

A. She should be referred for mammography as she has an increased risk of breast cancer.

B. She should be referred for a chest X-ray.

C. She can be reassured that cigarette smoking is not associated with an increased risk of abnormal cervical cytology.

D. She should be advised to discontinue the COCP as she has passed the age of 35.

E. She should be advised that if she wishes to continue the COCP she should discontinue smoking.

73. A 48-year-old woman attends for a well-woman check. She had an IUD inserted 5 years previously and now reports 12 months of amenorrhoea. Which of the following is true?

A. She should be advised that the IUD should be removed at this visit.

B. She should be advised that the IUD should be changed at this visit.

C. Measurement of FSH levels will not be useful in determining whether she is postmenopausal.

D. The IUD can be safely left in place for ongoing contraception until she is 50.

E. It is essential that the strings of the IUD be identified on speculum examination.

74. A 35-year-old woman presents with a history of unprotected sexual intercourse 24 hours previously. She does not wish to be pregnant. Her LMP was 12 days previously. She has regular 28-day cycles. She also requests ongoing contraception and states she smokes 20 cigarettes/day. Which of the following is true?

A. Insertion of a copper IUD at the time of consultation will be highly effective at preventing pregnancy and will provide ongoing contraception.

B. She should not have a copper intrauterine contraceptive device (IUCD) inserted at this visit as she may have contracted an STI.

C. Insertion of a levonorgestrel IUCD at the time of consultation will be highly effective at preventing pregnancy and will provide ongoing contraception.

D. She can be reassured that she will not be pregnant because she could not have ovulated yet in this cycle.

E. She may be commenced on the combined oral contraceptive pill.

75. A 24-year-old woman telephones her doctor one morning seeking advice. She is taking the progestogen-only pill (POP) and she has a 6-month-old baby who is fully breastfed. She missed her pill the previous evening and is now experiencing some vaginal spotting. Which of the following is an appropriate advice?

A. To provide effective contraception she should start taking the POP again as soon as possible and also use barrier methods for the next 48 hours (until she has taken three consecutive daily pills).

B. As she is fully breastfeeding she is unlikely to be ovulating and should simply take the next pill that evening.

C. She should stop the POP altogether for 7 days and restart at the end of that time.

D. She should be advised to stop breastfeeding and change to the combined oral contraceptive pill (COCP) as the baby is now 6 months old.

E. She should take two pills that morning and then continue with one each evening as previously.

76. A 20-year-old nulliparous woman consults her general practitioner seeking effective contraception. She was diagnosed with grand mal epilepsy at the age of 6 and is well controlled on lamotrigine. Which of the following is true?

A. She should not be offered the levonorgestrel intrauterine contraceptive device (IUCD) as she has never been pregnant.

B. She should not be offered a copper IUCD as she has never been pregnant.

C. The use of the combined oral contraceptive pill is not recommended for women taking lamotrigine as plasma concentrations of lamotrigine are reduced by ethinyloestradiol.

D. She should be advised that barrier methods are the most suitable form of contraception for her.

E. She should be referred to a gynaecologist to be fitted with a diaphragm.

77. **An 18-year-old woman attends a family planning clinic requesting an etonogestrel implant, following a surgical termination of pregnancy (TOP) 2 days previously. She has a BMI of 30. Which of the following is true?**
    A. She should be told that if she chooses to have an implant it will have to be replaced earlier than 3 years because of her weight.
    B. She should be advised that she cannot have the implant inserted until all vaginal discharge ceases post-TOP.
    C. She should be advised that she cannot have the implant inserted until normal menstrual cycles resume.
    D. She should be advised that more than 50% of women experience amenorrhoea or oligomenorrhoea with the implant in place.
    E. She should be advised that in a small number of cases the implant may cause an ectopic pregnancy.

78. **In regard to the examination of the abdomen of a woman in the third trimester of pregnancy, which of the following statements is true?**
    A. It is usually conducted on a weekly basis.
    B. It is usually accompanied by an ultrasound scan to confirm fetal growth.
    C. Gestation in weeks corresponds approximately to measurement of symphysiofundal height in centimetres.
    D. Examination should always be conducted in the presence of a chaperone.
    E. It is not useful in determining the presentation of the fetus.

79. **A 35-year-old woman is referred to the gynaecology outpatients department by her general practitioner because she has insulin-dependent diabetes and smokes 10 cigarettes daily. She has two children, aged 12 and 10, and currently takes the combined oral contraceptive pill (COCP). The general practitioner has advised laparoscopic sterilisation. Which of the following statements is relevant to the consultation?**
    A. If the woman is uncertain about her decision for sterilisation, the operation should not proceed, as regret after surgery is likely to be significant and the operation is not easily reversed.
    B. She should be advised to continue with the COCP as the risks to her from the surgery are greater than those associated with the pill.
    C. She should be advised that her partner should have a vasectomy.
    D. She should be strongly advised to have laparoscopic sterilisation at an early date.
    E. She should be advised to discontinue the COCP immediately.

80. **A 16-year-old girl presents to her general practitioner with a history of recurrent lower abdominal pain midcycle. Her cycles are regular, 5/28 days. She is not yet sexually active. Which of the following statements is true?**
    A. The pain is likely to be psychological in origin.
    B. She should be prescribed tranexamic acid for the pain.
    C. Transabdominal pelvic ultrasound may be an appropriate investigation.
    D. She should be advised to start the combined oral contraceptive pill immediately.
    E. She should be advised to have an etonogestrel implant.

81. **With regard to fertility awareness–based methods of contraception, which of the following is true?**
    A. There is level A evidence to show these methods are highly effective when properly used.
    B. These methods provide an option for women whose religious beliefs forbid the use of other methods.
    C. They are suitable for women who are breastfeeding.
    D. They are suitable for women with irregular menstrual cycles, provided a menstrual chart is kept.
    E. In a woman with regular 28-day cycles who wishes to avoid pregnancy, intercourse should be avoided on days 10–14 of the cycle.

82. **When advising patients about the use of male condoms for contraception, which of the following is true?**
    A. If latex condoms are used, oil-based lubricants should be avoided as they increase the risk of condom breakage.
    B. The use of polyurethane condoms may be associated with allergic reactions and occasional anaphylaxis in the male partner.
    C. When used correctly, condoms are 99.9% effective at preventing pregnancy.
    D. Condoms should not be used in conjunction with the combined oral contraceptive pill.
    E. Condoms should not be used in conjunction with an intrauterine contraceptive device.

83. **In regard to the progestogen-only pill (POP) for contraception, which of the following is true?**
    A. Women who are overweight or obese are at greater risk of failure of the POP than women with BMIs in the low–normal range.
    B. The POP can be safely prescribed for women taking long-term medications that induce liver enzymes.
    C. Ninety per cent of women taking POP will have complete amenorrhoea within 3 months of commencing the medication.

D. Following miscarriage, the POP should not be commenced until normal cycles are re-established.

E. Weight gain, headaches and mood changes are common side effects of the POP.

84. In regard to hepatitis C virus (HCV), which of the following is true?
A. Most infected people present with jaundice.
B. About 10% of those initially infected will develop chronic infection.
C. Screening for anti-HCV antibodies is a routine part of antenatal care.
D. Pregnant women with HCV should be advised to deliver by caesarean section.
E. Pregnant women with HCV should be advised to avoid breastfeeding.

85. HSV infection:
A. is routinely screened for in pregnant women in Australia and the United Kingdom.
B. will be transmitted to the fetus in utero in 25% of cases of primary infection in pregnancy.
C. is most likely to be transmitted to the infant during labour when the woman has a recurrent infection.
D. is an indication for termination of pregnancy if diagnosed in the first trimester
E. is most often asymptomatic in women.

86. A 24-year-old primigravid woman presents with a dichorionic diamniotic (DCDA) twin pregnancy following IVF treatment. She wants to know what to expect with twin pregnancy.
A. You explain that she has identical twins.
B. She wishes a homebirth and you agree that this is reasonable as she is fit and well.
C. She is at risk of developing pre-eclampsia.
D. She must be delivered by 36 weeks' gestation as her pregnancy is at risk of increased perinatal mortality.
E. There is an increased risk of twin-to-twin transfusion syndrome.

87. In discussing the mode of birth in twins:
A. women with twin pregnancies should be advised that caesarean section at 37 weeks is the safest option.
B. once the first twin is delivered, the risk for the second twin reduces.
C. epidural anaesthesia is not advised as the mother will lose the sensation to push in the second stage of labour.

D. postpartum haemorrhage is a recognised complication due to uterine atony.

E. continuous electronic fetal heart rate monitoring is indicated as there is an increased risk of cord entanglement in labour.

88. **A 28-year-old para 2 woman with type 1 diabetes is seen for pre-pregnancy counselling. She is on an insulin pump and says that her glucose control has been good. What would be the correct course of action?**

A. She is advised that she should take high doses of vitamin A as this helps to improve the outcome of her pregnancy.

B. You advise that she should stop her insulin pump and convert to short-acting insulin during the day and a long-acting insulin at night.

C. You arrange a glucose tolerance test (GTT) to ensure that the diagnosis is correct.

D. You ensure that she takes high-dose folic acid and that her preprandial and postprandial sugar levels are within the target range and check that her HbA1C is also acceptable.

E. You advise her to avoid pregnancy for 2 years from her last childbirth because of the increased risk of worsening diabetes.

89. **A 26-year-old woman presents at 8 weeks of pregnancy to her local health centre in a remote rural area. Her first child was born by emergency caesarean section 1 year previously and weighed 4.8 kg. On examination she is found to have a BMI of 39. Which of the following statements is true?**

A. She should be advised to terminate the pregnancy because the risks to her health of continuing it are too high for herself.

B. She should be advised to undergo bariatric surgery once she reaches the end of the first trimester.

C. She should be referred to the nearest tertiary obstetric centre and remain there throughout the pregnancy.

D. There are no contraindications to attempting VBAC if that is her wish.

E. Telemedicine between the health centre and a tertiary centre may be appropriate for some of her antenatal care.

90. **A 40-year-old woman presents to her GP at 9 weeks in her sixth pregnancy; she has had five spontaneous uncomplicated vaginal births, with babies of increasing size, the last weighing 4.4 kg. Her BMI is**

calculated during this visit and found to be 41. Which of the following statements is true?

A. Risks of any pregnancy complication are the same as for her fifth pregnancy.

B. She cannot have invasive screening for fetal anomaly because of her obesity.

C. Referral to a dietician has been shown to be effective in weight reduction in pregnant women of high BMI.

D. She should have a glucose tolerance test in the first trimester of pregnancy.

E. She is likely to need caesarean section in this pregnancy as the baby will be bigger.

91. Which of the following statements regarding the novel coronavirus disease 2019 (COVID-19), an infectious disease caused by the severe acute respiratory syndrome coronavirus 2 (SARS-CoV-2), in pregnancy is correct?

A. Due to the changes in the immune system, pregnant women are more at risk of contracting the disease than are non-pregnant women.

B. The use of nitrous oxide for pain relief in labour is contraindicated in a woman who is positive for COVID-19 as it is aerosol-generating.

C. Breastfeeding in a woman who is COVID-19-positive is not contraindicated as long as the appropriate hygiene measures are in place.

D. Large studies from the UK show that most women with COVID-19 in pregnancy who manifest symptoms are more severely affected in the first trimester.

E. Vaccines against COVID-19 are contraindicated in pregnancy as they are live attenuated viral vaccines.

92. The management of pre-eclampsia at term may include:

A. induction of labour.

B. use of anti-hypertensive medications.

C. use of magnesium sulphate to reduce the risk of seizures.

D. ultrasound surveillance for fetal wellbeing.

E. all of these options.

93. A 24-year-old primigravid woman at 32 weeks' gestation presents to a small country hospital 80 km from a specialist obstetric unit, with regular contractions 2–3/10 minutes. A CTG is normal. Speculum examination shows a slightly open, fully effaced cervix. Which of the following statements is correct?

A. Steroids should not be given because the pregnancy has already reached 32 weeks.

B. There is no point in giving tocolytics because labour is already established.

C. She should be given nifedipine and transferred by road ambulance to a specialist obstetric unit.

D. She should be observed over 4 hours to determine if labour is becoming established.

E. She should have the membranes ruptured to ascertain whether meconium liquor is present.

94. A 26-year-old woman underwent a caesarean section for placenta praevia in her first pregnancy. She is now 16 weeks advanced in her second pregnancy and seeks advice about delivery on this occasion. Which of the following statements is true?

A. A previous elective caesarean for placenta praevia should always be followed by a further elective caesarean section in the next pregnancy.

B. Her chances of placenta praevia in this pregnancy are exactly the same as in her first pregnancy.

C. There is a 50% risk of placenta accreta in this pregnancy.

D. She should be told to have a vaginal birth this time.

E. The potential risks and benefits of both attempted vaginal birth and planned caesarean section should be explained.

95. A 31-year-old West African woman who is a recent immigrant presents at about 7 months of pregnancy to the emergency department, having had no antenatal care to date. She has had five previous full-term pregnancies. She has had an episode of painless vaginal bleeding. Immediate management should be:

A. arrangement for urgent caesarean section.

B. monitoring of vital signs and the presence of a fetal heart beat.

C. speculum examination to determine the cause of the bleeding.

D. bimanual examination to determine the cause of bleeding.

E. transfusion of un-cross-matched O-negative blood.

96. A 33-year-old woman presents 8 weeks into her third pregnancy. Her last pregnancy was complicated by diet-controlled GDM. Which of the following is true?

A. A glucose tolerance test should be performed early in pregnancy.

B. She should be commenced on oral hypoglycaemics.

C. She is not at increased risk of GDM in this pregnancy.

D. Glucose tolerance testing should be performed no earlier than 28 weeks of pregnancy.

E. Treatment should be based on symptom control.

97. **You are arranging admission and operation for a 30-year-old woman having a planned repeat caesarean section. She has had three previous caesarean sections. Which of the following is true?**

A. It is not necessary to describe the risks of the surgery to her because she has had the operation before and knows all about it.

B. General anaesthesia is essential.

C. The risk of hysterectomy is very high.

D. The risk of damage to bowel and/or bladder is no greater than with her previous caesarean sections.

E. It is appropriate to discuss with her the possibility of tubal sterilisation being performed in conjunction with the caesarean.

98. **A 30-year-old woman in her fourth pregnancy has a history of severe shoulder dystocia in the last delivery, causing a third-degree tear. She seeks advice about the current pregnancy and mode of delivery. Which of the following statements is true?**

A. She should plan a vaginal birth but elective episiotomy should be performed.

B. Another third-degree tear properly repaired does not increase her subsequent risk of pelvic floor dysfunction.

C. Glucose tolerance testing may be performed but will not influence the mode of delivery.

D. Elective caesarean section should be discussed with her.

E. Vaginal birth should be attempted with the possibility of emergency caesarean section if progress is slow.

99. **A 20-year-old woman presents for antenatal care at 16 weeks of pregnancy. Her history reveals extensive recreational drug use. Which of the following statements is true?**

A. Screening for hepatitis C (HCV) should be performed because caesarean section is indicated if she returns a positive result.

B. Heroin use may cause opiate dependence in the neonate but otherwise poses no risk to the fetus.

C. Care provided in conjunction with a multidisciplinary team is likely to improve outcomes for both mother and baby.

D. She should be told that there is good scientific evidence that cannabis use results in small-for-dates infants.

E. Counselling is not indicated as she is unlikely to attend appointments.

100. At **30 weeks of pregnancy, a 29-year-old woman is found to have a fundal height of 26 cm. She reports that fetal movements are present and unchanged, and the fetal heart is heard with a Doppler. Which of the following is true?**
    A. Ultrasound is indicated to test for fetal growth restriction.
    B. The most appropriate management is repeat clinical examination in two weeks.
    C. An urgent CTG should be performed and, if normal, the patient can be discharged safely.
    D. She should be reassured that fundal height measurements are of no value in antenatal care.
    E. She should be offered a prenatal DNA screening test as soon as possible.

101. **A 69-year-old woman presents with a 2-week history of light vaginal bleeding. She is on no medications. Which of the following is true?**
    A. The most likely cause is cancer of the endometrium.
    B. The most likely cause is cancer of the cervix.
    C. The most likely cause is a cyst of the ovary.
    D. Uterine fibroids are a likely cause.
    E. Malignancy should be excluded before commencing treatment.

102. **A 55-year-old woman presents to her general practitioner with a 5-day history of vaginal bleeding. Her last menstrual period was 5 years previously and she is on no medications. Physical examination is unremarkable apart from a marked degree of atrophic vaginitis with a visible bleeding point. Which of the following immediate management options is most appropriate?**
    A. Reassurance and advice to return if bleeding continues.
    B. Topical oestrogen pessaries.
    C. Combined oral hormone therapy (oestrogen and progestogen).
    D. Endometrial biopsy (pipelle sampling) in the surgery.
    E. Transvaginal ultrasound scan.

103. **In the management of secondary postpartum haemorrhage (PPH):**
    A. tranexamic acid has no role.
    B. ultrasound has no role in the diagnosis of retained placental tissue.
    C. fibroids are a common cause of bleeding.
    D. antibiotics should always be started prior to surgical intervention.
    E. the use of uterotonic drugs does not reduce blood loss.

104. **With secondary postpartum haemorrhage:**
    A. it is unusual for the woman to be shocked as the bleeding in secondary PPH is usually very light.
    B. if the woman is breastfeeding, any surgical procedure is contraindicated.
    C. intravenous antibiotics should never be administered.
    D. the clinical course is almost always complicated by coagulopathy.
    E. iron infusion may be a useful part of care.

105. **You are discussing fertility treatment with a couple. Investigation has revealed normal semen parameters in the male. The female partner is 25 years old, has a normal level of FSH and LH, and is immune to rubella but a hysterosalpingogram (HSG) has suggested bilateral tubal occlusion. The most appropriate treatment is:**
    A. ovulation induction with clomiphene citrate.
    B. intrauterine insemination with washed, concentrated sperm in a natural cycle.
    C. therapy with metformin.
    D. laparoscopy to determine whether there is a treatable form of tubal obstruction.
    E. the use of donated eggs.

106. **For women with a urodynamic study strongly suggestive of urge incontinence/detrusor instability, all of the following are appropriate managements except:**
    A. avoidance of caffeinated drinks.
    B. bladder retraining with a continence physiotherapist.
    C. the use of anticholinergic medications, such as oxybutynin.
    D. placement of a polypropylene mid-urethral tape.
    E. close attention to weight control and general fitness.

107. **Management of vasa praevia—where placental vessels cross over or near the internal cervical os in pregnancy—may include all of the following except:**
    A. admission to hospital in later pregnancy.
    B. elective caesarean delivery as early as 34 weeks.
    C. transvaginal ultrasound to provide precise information about the anatomy of fetal vessels.
    D. use of the Apt test for fetal haemoglobin in the presence of any vaginal bleeding.
    E. amniotomy and induction of labour at 36 weeks.

108. **In the screening and management of GDM, which of the following is true?**
    A. The 50 g glucose challenge test carried out at 26 weeks' gestation has a high sensitivity for the diagnosis of GDM.
    B. Metformin may be useful in the management of diabetes in pregnancy.
    C. Long-acting insulins are best for glycaemic control in pregnancy.
    D. Only babies born to women with type 1 diabetes are at risk of hypoglycaemia postnatally.
    E. Macrosomia is never seen in women with tight control of their diabetes.

109. **In general practice you are consulted by a 30-year-old transgender male who has been on regular testosterone injections for 2 years. He is complaining of slight irregular vaginal bleeding. Which of the following statements is true?**
    A. He does not need cervical screening tests as testosterone will bring about cervical atrophy.
    B. The most likely cause is endometrial hyperplasia.
    C. The most likely cause is low testosterone levels.
    D. He should be referred for immediate pelvic ultrasound scanning.
    E. He should be referred for hysteroscopy.

110. **In general practice you are consulted by an 18-year-old transgender man who is requesting screening for sexually transmitted infections. Which of the following would *not* be part of your routine check?**
    A. Syphilis serology
    B. MSU for group B streptococcus
    C. Hepatitis A and B serology
    D. HIV serology
    E. NAAT/PCR swabs for *Chlamydia trachomatis*

Answers

1. B	29. C	57. D	85. E
2. D	30. B	58. B	86. C
3. A	31. E	59. C	87. D
4. B	32. E	60. D	88. D
5. A	33. E	61. C	89. E
6. C	34. A	62. E	90. D
7. D	35. C	63. A	91. C
8. B	36. B	64. D	92. E
9. C	37. C	65. E	93. C
10. C	38. B	66. D	94. E
11. C	39. D	67. C	95. B
12. B	40. B	68. B	96. A
13. B	41. B	69. D	97. E
14. D	42. C	70. C	98. D
15. D	43. A	71. D	99. C
16. E	44. D	72. E	100. A
17. A	45. A	73. D	101. E
18. C	46. C	74. A	102. E
19. B	47. C	75. A	103. D
20. A	48. D	76. C	104. E
21. B	49. A	77. D	105. D
22. B	50. E	78. C	106. D
23. D	51. B	79. A	107. E
24. B	52. A	80. C	108. B
25. A	53. D	81. B	109. C
26. B	54. E	82. A	110. B
27. D	55. D	83. E	
28. A	56. C	84. C	

Index

Note: Page numbers followed by *f* and *t* represent figures and tables, respectively.

risk of malignancy index (RMI), 137
rubella, in pregnancy, 27, 81–82

SARS-CoV-2, 86–88
screening test characteristics, 21–22
seizure management, 204
selective serotonin reuptake inhibitor, 104, 105
semen analysis, 56, 280–285
    characteristics of normal, 282*t*
Sertoli-Leydig cell tumour, 310, 314*f*
sex cord stromal tumours, 314*t*
sex hormone binding globulin, 57
sexual activity, 19, 32, 111–116, 117–122
    safe, 13, 32, 111–116, 121, 186, 295
    unprotected, 112, 113, 117–119, 123, 157, 302
sexual health clinic, 235
sexual history, 4
sexually transmitted infections, *also* sexually transmissible infections, 4, 17, 54, 55, 113, 114–115*t*, 157, 288, 293
shared care, in pregnancy, 64, 67, 70, 101, 244,
    card, 5, 173, 178, 197, 237, 244, 245*f, 246*
shoulder dystocia, 92, 176, 254, 258, 274
slapped cheek syndrome, 85–86
social history, 4
special care baby unit (SCBU), 193
speculum examination, 7, 22, 23, 217
Staphylococcus aureus, 243
sterilisation
    counselling for, 126–127
    laparoscopic, 124–127, 125*f*
    surgical, risks of, 127
    tubal ligation, 225
stress incontinence, 323, 327
suction curettage, 128, 132, 269, 271, 299
syphilis, 114*t*

tachycardia
    fetal, 228
teenagers
    consultation without parents, 50–51
    heavy menstrual bleeding, 32–35
termination of pregnancy *see also* abortion
    legal requirements, 170–171
    therapeutic, 169–171
threatened preterm labour (TPL), 217
thromboembolic disease, 14–16, 149, 177
thyroid function tests, 102, 157
tocolysis, 218–219
tocophobia, 179
TORCH (toxoplasmosis, rubella, cytomegalovirus, herpes) infections, 79–85
Torres Strait Islander background, 70, 206
toxoplasmosis, 79–81
transgender people, care of, 4, 155–160

cervical screening test 156
contraception 157–158
vaginal examination 156
trial of labour, 173, 176–177, 241 *see also* vaginal birth after caesarean section
trichomoniasis, 61, 115*t*, 120
trisomy 13, 167
trisomy 18, 167
trisomy 21, 167
TTTS (twin-to-twin transfusion syndrome), 98, 190
tubal ligation, 225
tubal patency, 57–58, 59
tumour marker, 137
Turner syndrome, 51*t*
twin pregnancy, 95–96, 96*f*, 188–191 *see also* multiple pregnancy
    amnionicity, 98
    chorionicity, 67, 97–98, 190
twins
    dizygotic, 95, 96
    monozygotic, 95
twin-to-twin transfusion syndrome (TTTS), 98, 190

ultrasound, in pregnancy, 9–10, 65–67
    of breast, 137
    fetal morphology, 70, 167
    pelvic, 51, 137, 153
    screening, 91
    surgical removal of implant, 109
    transvaginal, 137, 147
unplanned pregnancy, 123–129
urinary incontinence, 322–328
urinary tract abnormalities, 52
urinary tract infection, 211, 233–234, 243, 164
uterine agenesis, 51–52
uterine artery embolisation, 40
uterine rupture, 174, 176, 177
uterus
    anteverted and retroverted, 38*f*
    atonic, 257
    large-for-dates, 95
    measurement, 9
    suction curettage, 132

vaccinations
    chickenpox, 77
    HPV, 30
    influenza, in pregnancy, 75–76
    MMR, 82
    in pregnancy, 74–89
vacuum extraction, 230, 230*f,* 231
vaginal atrophy, 108, 155, 313, 315
vaginal birth
    caesarean section *versus,* 180–181*t*
    instrumental, 105